Breath Sounds

Kostas N. Priftis
Leontios J. Hadjileontiadis • Mark L. Everard
Editors

Breath Sounds

From Basic Science to Clinical Practice

Springer

Editors
Kostas N. Priftis
Children's Respiratory and Allergy Unit
Third Department of Paediatrics
"Attikon" Hospital
National and Kapodistrian University of Athens
Athens
Greece

Leontios J. Hadjileontiadis
Department of Electrical & Computer Engineering
Aristotle University of Thessaloniki
Thessaloniki
Greece

Mark L. Everard
Division of Child Health
University of Western Australia
Perth Children's Hospital
Perth
Australia

ISBN 978-3-030-10119-0 ISBN 978-3-319-71824-8 (eBook)
https://doi.org/10.1007/978-3-319-71824-8

Softcover re-print of the Hardcover 1st edition 2018

Printed on acid-free paper

This Springer imprint is published by the registered company Springer International Publishing AG part of Springer Nature
The registered company address is: Gewerbestrasse 11, 6330 Cham, Switzerland

Preface

It is now just over 200 years since René-Théophile-Hyacinthe Laennec invented the stethoscope and 2018 will be the bicentennial of the publication of his masterpiece, *A treatise on the diseases of the chest and on mediate auscultation.* The intervening centuries have seen the stethoscope becoming a ubiquitous tool that is synonymous, in the minds of the general public, with the medical profession. Despite repeated reports of its imminent demise, the stethoscope continues to evolve and contribute to clinical care throughout the world.

In light of the imminent anniversary of Laennec's textbook, it seems appropriate to revisit the role of this inexpensive tool in the assessment of respiratory health and disease and consider its future in a world in which the conventional stethoscope is, in a number of settings, being replaced by increasingly sophisticated electronic devices. This publication is not intended to be a classical 'textbook', but rather a 'state-of-the-art' review on specific clinical and research topics on the subject of respiratory sounds. The starting point was the training of the clinician: from the student to the chest physician. At the same time, the goal was to allow the clinician to talk to the scientist and get an idea of the cutting edge of relevant technology and research.

The book is divided in four parts. The first part covers a wide spectrum of general issues regarding the history of stethoscope, the clinical usefulness, epidemiology and nomenclature of breath sounds. The second part of the book is mainly devoted to the science, i.e. sound recording, analysis and perception. The third part deals with clinical issues regarding adventitious respiratory sounds, laryngeal origin sounds, sleep and cough sounds. Finally, the fourth part chapters emphasise a view of the future.

In order to provide the most comprehensive picture of the past, present and future evolution of the stethoscope, from the original roll of parchment to its highly sophisticated electronic descendants that connect to the Internet and provide computerised analysis, experts from a range of backgrounds were invited to share their knowledge. We are grateful to all the authors for their effort, time and efficiency in this common endeavour.

We are indebted to the publisher, Springer International Publishing AG, for adopting and supporting this project. Special thanks and gratitude go to Donatella Rizza for her expert advice and editorial organisation. We are also grateful to Barbara Pittaluga and Rekha Udaiyar for their patience and help.

Athens, Greece — Kostas N. Priftis
Thessaloniki, Greece — Leontios J. Hadjileontiadis
Perth, Australia — Mark L. Everard

Contents

Part III Respiratory Sounds

Part IV Where Are We Going?

Introduction

1

Andrew Bush

A long time ago in a galaxy far, far away, I started in the University College Hospital London medical school and purchased my first stethoscope, which consisted of a bell and a diaphragm joined by a rubber tube to two earpieces. At that time, telephone calls were made on Bakelite telephones with a circular dial, and one inserted a finger into the appropriate hole and rotated it; urgent communications were by telegram at a given cost per word; and lecturers used glass-mounted slides or drew on the blackboard to illustrate their talks. After nearly 40 years as a doctor, and more than a quarter of a century of consultant practice, smartphones are replete with unbelievable quantities of APPs, computing and storage power; the telegram is as dead as the dinosaurs, and instead social media such as Facebook, Instagram, Snapchat and Twitter rule; and PowerPoint reigns supreme in the conference and lecture room. And lo! My stethoscope still consists of a bell and a diaphragm joined by a rubber tube to two earpieces. It is difficult to believe that this medical stagnation in the face of so much technological transformation elsewhere reflects much credit on anyone. So where are we, and where are we going: and the main purpose of this book is to review exactly this. This introduction is intended to set the scene by being a provocative look at past, present and future chest auscultation, in order to stimulate thought (and possibly rage!) in the interested reader.

AB is an NIHR Senior Investigator and additionally was supported by the NIHR Respiratory Disease Biomedical Research Unit at the Royal Brompton and Harefield NHS Foundation Trust and Imperial College London.

A. Bush, MD, FRCP, FRCPCH, FERS, FAPSR
National Heart and Lung Institute, London, UK

Imperial College, London, UK

Department of Paediatric Respiratory Medicine, Royal Brompton Hospital, London, UK

Royal Brompton Harefield NHS Foundation Trust, London, UK
e-mail: A.Bush@rbht.nhs.uk; a.bush@imperial.ac.uk

K. N. Priftis et al. (eds.), *Breath Sounds*, https://doi.org/10.1007/978-3-319-71824-8_1

1.1 The Thoracic Cage as Checkpoint Charlie: The Good, the Bad and the Totally Unintelligent

An important evolutionary task is to protect the organism from external assaults such as heat, cold and a well-directed spear by encasing it in protection either natural (e.g. bones, a thick hide, scales or a shell) or artificially manufactured armour. The thoracic cage gives good protection to the heart and lungs, but this natural protective layer has the undesirable effect of muffling or eliminating many signals of disease from within the organism, the discernment of which may allow a beneficial intervention. This was of small concern when there were no such interventions, and all the physician had to offer amounted to little more than tea and sympathy. In the twenty-first century, the field has changed:

- We have ever more powerful diagnostic tests which completely bypass the protective layers, such as HRCT, MRI and other imaging modalities, to say nothing of sophisticated biological tests including genetics, ciliary function and increasingly likely -omics technology.
- There are increasingly precise therapeutics, such as the designer molecules for gene class-specific mutations in cystic fibrosis [1, 2] and an increasingly formidable array of monoclonals for asthma [3, 4].
- We are moving further away from asking 'are you feeling better' to the use of specific biomarkers and molecular tests for diagnosis [5] and to monitor disease progression [6].
- Non-invasive testing in preschool infants and even babies is increasingly moving out of the research field and into the routine clinical arena [7]. So, for example, sputum induction for the diagnosis of tuberculosis is being performed in primary health-care centres in South African townships [8], and multiple breath washouts are feasible in clinical settings [9, 10].

So has the time come for the clinician to be pensioned off in favour of a more cheerful version of Douglas Adams's Marvin the severely depressed and bored robot with a brain the size of a planet (*The Hitchhikers Guide to the Galaxy*)? Paradoxically, the greater technological advances mean that clinical skills become more, not less, important. So not every child with a runny nose can or should have nasal nitric oxide, assessment of ciliary beat frequency and pattern, ciliary electron microscopy and electron microscopic tomography, whole exome sequencing, ciliary immunofluorescence and finally ciliary culture lest a diagnosis of primary ciliary dyskinesia is missed [11, 12]. The clinical skill that is absolutely essential is to pick out the handful of such children in whom this diagnosis should be pursued at all hazard [13–16]. To do this, old-fashioned skills of history and physical examination must be deployed but with two important caveats: firstly, we must not be complacent but accept that these can and should be honed, and secondly, we need to recognise when the patient's journey has reached the point when clinical skills are no longer useful.

So the basic skills of the thoracic physician are history and physical examination, with the latter split into the time-honoured inspection, palpation, percussion and auscultation. The purpose of this introduction is to place auscultation, the subject of this book, in the context both of clinical skills and the exciting new diagnostic and therapeutic technologies. My thesis will be that the stagnation of the stethoscope, far from suggesting that Laennec's great invention [17] has reached its apogee, in fact reflects badly on the complacency and lack of drive of the respiratory community (this author included). However, I will propose that the stethoscope is not dead, merely sleeping, and modern physics and mathematical signal processing may transform a sleeping pygmy into a wide awake giant.

1.2 Consensus Documents: A Step Forward or the Blind Leading the Deaf?

Attempts to agree nomenclature have been made for decades [18, 19], culminating in a recently published ERS Task Force [20]. Linguistic differences, as well as those in the performance of the eighth cranial nerves, have complicated the field. From early on, analysis of breath sounds, by analogy with electrocardiography, was proposed [18]. The recent Task Force includes an online library of lung sounds, a major educational asset. However, experts sitting around a table cannot be considered the last word in evidence, no matter how eminent they may appear in at least their own eyes.

1.3 Even a Mole May Instruct a Philosopher in the Art of Digging (Earnest Bramah, *The Wallet of Kai Lung*)

It is well known that the thorax contains two organs of interest: the right lung and the left lung. There is a third minor organ, the oesophagus, and finally the heart. Yet perhaps we can learn a lesson from cardiologists about auscultation, which we may apply to the lungs.

In the days before sophisticated imaging and cardiac catheterisation, the stethoscope was the primary diagnostic tool for heart disease and was in the best ears exceedingly accurate. The great Sir Thomas Lewis recognised the findings in mitral stenosis as he did 'the bark of his favourite dog' [21]. But nowadays, the next step would be a non-invasive test, transthoracic echocardiography, to confirm the diagnosis and further assess severity. On that basis, the need or otherwise of more sophisticated or invasive testing is determined. Increasingly, cardiac auscultation is used as a screening test for any abnormality, rather than to make a specific diagnosis, although the experienced cardiologist will still be proved right by further testing on many occasions.

Applying this to respiratory medicine, should the stethoscope be relegated to merely dichotomising patients into normal and abnormal? I think such would be an error, because we do not have the equivalent of echocardiography in our armamentarium as the next step. For sure, the chest radiograph is simple and involves minimal radiation, but its lack of sensitivity compared to, for example, thoracic computed tomography, is well known. Although access to the lungs via the airway allows detailed functional assessments through spirometry, multiple breath washouts, impulse oscillometry, plethysmography and many others, not merely at rest but when stressing the system with maximal exercise, physiology can make only two diagnoses: exercise-induced bronchoconstriction and hyperventilation. For sure, restrictive and obstructive physiological patterns may point to *groups* of diseases, such as the airway and the interstitium, but not actual specific diagnoses, unlike echocardiography. By contrast, echocardiography is non-invasive and does not require radiation exposure but gives superb information on cross-sectional anatomy and hence specific diagnoses. Paradoxically, the barrier to lung ultrasound is not the sturdy chest wall but air, although there is some diagnostic utility in pneumonia and pleural effusion. So we need firstly to understand how good we are with current auscultation and, next, whether technological advances could be deployed to improve our performance.

1.4 Thoracic Auscultation: The Way We Were

The history of the nomenclature of lung sounds makes Babeldom seem a model of clarity and precision. 'Wheeze', 'Rhonchi', 'Râles', 'crepitations', 'crackles' and many more were used to describe what was heard. 'When I use a word', Humpty Dumpty said, in rather a scornful tone, 'it means just what I choose it to mean—neither more nor less'. 'The question is', said Alice, 'whether you can make words mean so many different things' (Lewis Carroll, *Through the Looking Glass*). Humpty Dumpty ruled, and Alice's assumption that there were so many things to describe when auscultating the chest was never challenged. Richard Asher has taught us that the first essential is to describe what we actually see (or in this case, hear), in simple modern words, and not to speculate about their origin, because such speculations will almost certainly be proved wrong [22]. Do we describe a newborn as a 'vesicular baby'? That would be ridiculous, so why call normal breath sounds 'vesicular'. And how often do we see the words 'wheeze' and 'bronchospasm' used synonymously? This fallacious thinking means that the speaker has jumped from a noise heard (or thought to have been heard!) and a pathophysiological mechanism (airway smooth muscle constriction) and the likely erroneous prescription of a short-acting β-2 agonist and even worse, a diagnosis of 'asthma'. Instead, the argument should go that there is narrowing of the airway, which may be from causes within the airway lumen (e.g. airway mucus), within the wall (e.g. airway smooth muscle constriction, developmental narrowing or acquired airway remodelling), or extramural (loss of alveolar tethering). The greater the uncertainty, the more Asher's rule holds. As Socrates said (*The Plato Collection*), 'he who first gave names and gave them according to his conception of the things which they signified; if his conception was erroneous, shall we not be deceived by him?' And the answer is a resounding affirmative. An

Table 1.1 Simplified nomenclature of lung sounds [23–25]

Sound	Timing	Nature
Crackles	Inspiration, expiration or both	Fine or coarse
Wheeze	Inspiration, expiration or both	Monophonic or polyphonic
Pleural rub	Inspiration, expiration or both	Coarse, continuous noise

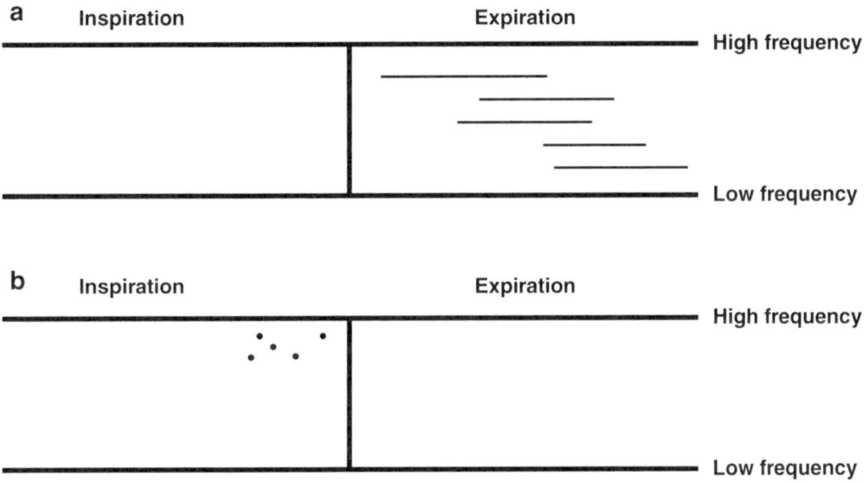

Fig. 1.1 Visual representation of lung sounds [23–25]. (**a**) Expiratory polyphonic wheeze. (**b**) Fine end-inspiratory crackles

example from chest auscultation is the phrase 'reduced air entry', which is so often used. The fatal assumption that is palmed off with all the skill of the London three-card-trick conman is going from what is *heard* (softer than expected breath sounds) to an assumption of what this *means* (e.g. reduced localised or generalised ventilation, whereas exactly the same findings could be produced by normal ventilation but a chest wall thickened by tumour). This is not of course to say that modelling and other studies to determine mechanisms are not without their use; but as time goes by, any model is likely to be superseded, and there should be clear blue water between the naming of sounds and the speculation about mechanisms. Asher would certainly have approved of the great Paul Forgacs who simplified nomenclature (Table 1.1) and proposed a pictorial way of describing auscultatory findings (Fig. 1.1) [23–25]. Perhaps this is a bit too simple, missing as it does the end-inspiratory squawk [26, 27]. Despite Forgacs and Asher, the Humpty Dumpties ruled, and those that darkened council by words without knowledge (*Book of Job*) were allowed full play in the Chest Clinic. Only one thing was needed to complete the chaos, and that was putting stethoscopes in the ears of everyone; the stethoscope was still the physician's prerogative, at least for a short time. But to paraphrase Oscar Wilde 'seems we Doctors have everything in common with other doctors except the language' (Oscar Wilde, *The Canterville Ghost*).

1.5 Thoracic Auscultation: The Way We Are

Modern audio technology now allows documentation of the sounds that cross the thoracic wall (and note I distinguish this from sounds actually heard!) so that physician opinion could actually be cross-checked with reality. In a second development, it was realised that ill-informed talk was not the prerogative of the physician, but allied health professionals, nurses and parents could also acquire ignorance and a stethoscope and join the circus. The utility and perceived meaning of the word 'wheeze' has long been studied. To the physician, wheeze means, in Paul Forgacs' nomenclature [23–25], a musical, polyphonic expiratory noise. To even intelligent lay people, wheeze is an umbrella term for a wide variety of upper and lower airway noises [28–30]. In a clinical setting (a walk-in, paediatric ambulatory urgent care facility), objective transthoracic recording of the presence and severity of wheeze was compared with parental, nurse and paediatrician opinion [31]. Physicians and parents agreed one third of the time, physicians and nurses only half the time (nothing new there, then) and physicians and objective recordings 77% of the time. This means that on 23% of occasions, physicians got this commonplace sign wrong. As well as implications for clinical care, these findings call into question the use of 'Dr-diagnosed wheeze' in epidemiological and genetic studies, a point to which I return below. Nonetheless, noises made by airways may have value prognostically; the Aberdeen group used a pragmatic classification of 'whistle', 'rattle' and 'purr' to help parents identify the noise their child was making at age 2 years. In total, 210 out of 1371 (15.3%) had 'current wheeze' of whom only 24 had 'whistle' (1.8% of the total population or 11% of 'wheezers'. The reproducibility of parental identification of noises was far from perfect, but nonetheless, the 'whistlers' were around twice as likely to have persistent symptoms age 5 years [32].

An important recent experimental study asked 12 doctors (half paediatricians) to listen to 20 audio recordings and determine which of 10 noises were heard [33]. Perhaps unsurprising, although most combinations of the ears and recordings determined there was an abnormality present, agreement between observers was poor; reproducibility was much better if the two simple categories of 'crackles' and 'wheezes' were used. The authors rightly point out that there is still a utility of auscultation, for example, crackles being predictive of pneumonia [34]. Limitations to the study of course include that auscultation is never carried out in isolation, and the ability to detect change in a patient was not studied; nonetheless, similar findings have been reported by others using less sophisticated methods [35–37]. There are also important lessons to be learned. Firstly, simplicity is best; an elaborate and non-reproducible classification is more worthless than a politician's promises. Secondly, the unfortunate medical student or examination candidate who has not 'heard' the signs correctly should not be unduly penalised; he/she may be doing no better or worse than the professor who is the examiner. Similar poor agreement between observers has also been reported in studies using less sophisticated methodology.

So in summary, at the present time, it is indisputable to say that we cannot:

- Agree on the best nomenclature of lung sounds.
- Agree on what we are actually hearing.
- Reliably report what is recorded transthoracically by a machine.

So should the stethoscope join other great medical artefacts like Maxwell's box and Morland's needle (used to treat tuberculosis with an artificial pneumothorax) in honoured places in a medical museum? For those of us, including the authors and editors of the present volume who believe the answer to be no, the above findings are a rude wake-up call. It is clear that the present use of the stethoscope in chest medicine is intellectually untenable; so where do we go from here?

1.6 Thoracic Auscultation: Where Do We Want to Get to, and What Is the Roadmap?

There are a number of ways in which we need to think modern, including new technology and the positioning of auscultation in clinical practice in a new era of medicine.

1. Clearly we need to remove as much of the element of subjectivity from thoracic auscultation and also try to maximise the information we obtain, given the lack of a 'pulmonary echocardiogram' (above). A corollary of this is to avoid elaborate and unreproducible classifications. The obvious way to maximise information is digital recording of lung sounds and the use of signal processing. Crackles and wheezes can be described numerically, for example, in terms of frequency, duration and timing within the inspiratory and expiratory cycle; but with modern mathematical techniques, more sophisticated analyses are surely possible. Smartphones have more than enough number crunching ability to handle the data generated. So there is work to do; we need to obtain digital recordings of cohorts of well-characterised patients and move from 'Velcro crackles' (how twentieth century is that phrase!) to numerical description of the physical signs.
2. The phrase 'Dr-heard wheeze' needs to disappear from the research vocabulary. It is depressing to see immensely sophisticated genetic studies, with huge cohorts, in which the sophistication of the science is matched only by the crudity of clinical classification. Smartphone technology should be used to determine exactly what noises are emanating from the thorax, and this should be the entry criterion if we are going to rely only on clinical examination, replacing what a variably trained and attentive pair of ears and brain think might be what noises are present. This is not just developed world fantasy—smartphones are ubiquitous in low and middle income settings. Is it impossible to imagine that sound recordings (from which respiratory rate and also heart rate can also be derived) should not be recorded in a primary care outpost miles from a hospital, analysed mathematically and bluetoothed centrally and as a result, a diagnosis being made? Or even cutting out the central reading and taking action on the smartphone analyses using robust clinical algorithms?

3. Auscultation needs to be repositioned in a clinical context. The oldest catch in the book is the silent chest or upper airway, which betokens no improvement in the child with asthma or croup but impending catastrophe. So woe betide the physician who assesses auscultatory signs without also considering the state of the child. One of the greatest bedside teachers of them all, Max Klein, published a simple scheme combining auscultation with other clinical findings to localise the site of disease in the child with airway (in the broadest sense of the word) disease (Fig. 1.2) [38]. Few if any signs or findings can be considered stand-alone—and clinical context is everything. So parents frequently palpate their child's chest if they hear a wet cough and actually feel rattling underneath their hands—where all too often the physician may be misled by the absence of

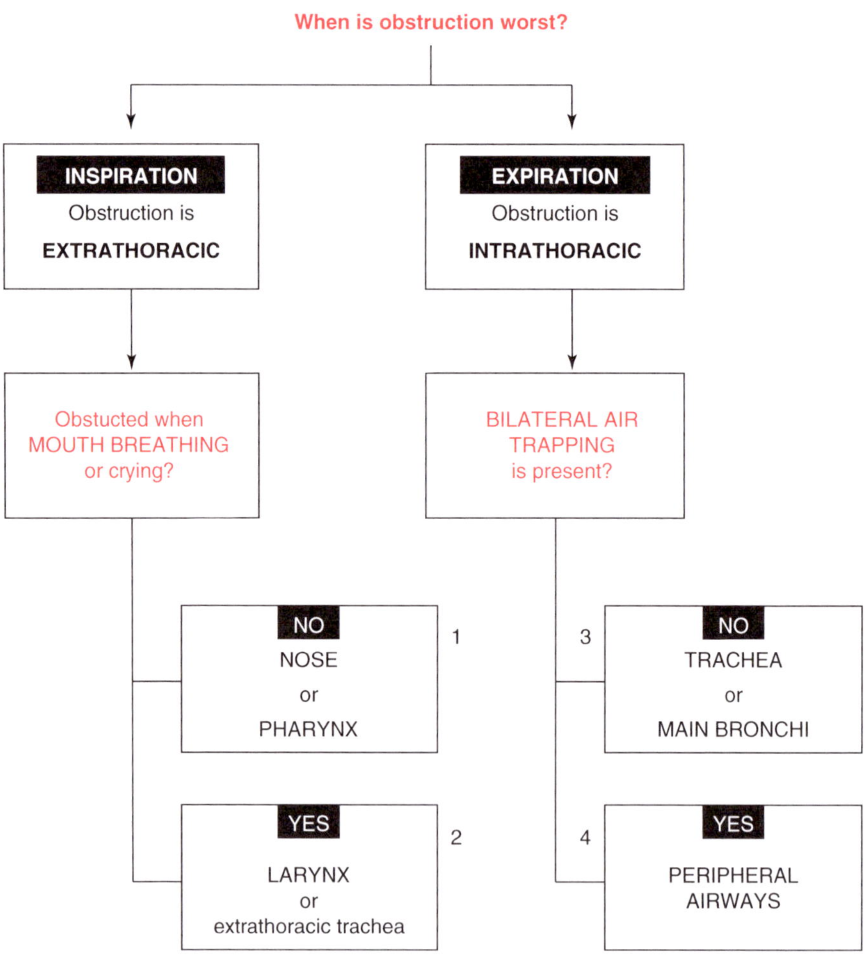

Fig. 1.2 Integrating auscultatory findings into the clinical picture to determine the site of obstruction [38]

auscultatory signs, another example of the 'silent chest' which is not a sign of well-being but rather masks disaster.

4. Finally, we always need to start by determining what question do I need to answer and thus what tools are needed to answer that question. So, for example, is this 10-year-old with cystic fibrosis suffering from a pulmonary exacerbation? The ideal tool to answer that question in the future is likely a molecular biomarker [39, 40], but it is also likely that some sort of screening will be needed to determine who should have this test carried out. So the question then becomes, should this 10-year-old undergo specific diagnostic tests for a pulmonary exacerbation? Whereas the finding of new crackles on auscultation will certainly be good evidence that an exacerbation is likely and may of itself lead to treatment, the history is likely as least as important, and the absence of new auscultatory findings will not exclude a pulmonary exacerbation. In the era of precision medicine, history and examination are likely to be increasingly used to select patients for further testing; we will need our clinical skills for the foreseeable future.

So to sum up, hopefully our professional children, starting out on their careers, will move from the bell and diaphragm, the earpieces and the rubber tube to a high-fidelity microphone attached to a smartphone; they will understand the strengths and weaknesses of auscultation as a clinical tool and how to frame the right questions in a given clinical situation and determine whether or not auscultation is the way to answer those questions or, better, how auscultation will contribute to finding the answer to the question. For this to happen, clinicians and physicists and other scientists need to collaborate to develop the tools they will need. In this volume, this collaboration is evident, with discussions of history and the current clinical situation mixed with sophisticated science leading to a clear vision of the future.

References

1. Ramsey BW, Davies J, McElvaney NG, Tullis E, Bell SC, Dřevínek P, Griese M, McKone EF, Wainwright CE, Konstan MW, Moss R, Ratjen F, Sermet-Gaudelus I, Rowe SM, Dong Q, Rodriguez S, Yen K, Ordoñez C, Elborn JS, VX08-770-102 Study Group (2011) A CFTR potentiator in patients with cystic fibrosis and the G551D mutation. N Engl J Med 365:1663–1672
2. Wainwright CE, Elborn JS, Ramsey BW, Marigowda G, Huang X, Cipolli M, Colombo C, Davies JC, De Boeck K, Flume PA, Konstan MW, McColley SA, McCoy K, McKone EF, Munck A, Ratjen F, Rowe SM, Waltz D, Boyle MP, TRAFFIC Study Group; TRANSPORT Study Group (2015) Lumacaftor-ivacaftor in patients with cystic fibrosis homozygous for Phe508del CFTR. N Engl J Med 373:220–231
3. Pavord ID, Korn S, Howarth P, Bleecker ER, Buhl R, Keene ON, Ortega H, Chanez P (2012) Mepolizumab for severe eosinophilic asthma (DREAM): a multicentre, double-blind, placebo-controlled trial. Lancet 380:651–659
4. Bleecker ER, FitzGerald JM, Chanez P, Papi A, Weinstein SF, Barker P, Sproule S, Gilmartin G, Aurivillius M, Werkström V, Goldman M, SIROCCO study investigators (2016) Efficacy and safety of benralizumab for patients with severe asthma uncontrolled with high-dosage inhaled corticosteroids and long-acting β_2-agonists (SIROCCO): a randomised, multicentre, placebo-controlled phase 3 trial. Lancet 388:2115–2127

5. Zar HJ, Workman L, Isaacs W, Dheda K, Zemanay W, Nicol MP (2013) Rapid diagnosis of pulmonary tuberculosis in African children in a primary care setting by use of Xpert MTB/RIF on respiratory specimens: a prospective study. Lancet Glob Health 1:e97–104
6. Horsley AR, Davies JC, Gray RD, Macleod KA, Donovan J, Aziz ZA, Bell NJ, Rainer M, Mt-Isa S, Voase N, Dewar MH, Saunders C, Gibson JS, Parra-Leiton J, Larsen MD, Jeswiet S, Soussi S, Bakar Y, Meister MG, Tyler P, Doherty A, Hansell DM, Ashby D, Hyde SC, Gill DR, Greening AP, Porteous DJ, Innes JA, Boyd AC, Griesenbach U, Cunningham S, Alton EW (2013) Changes in physiological, functional and structural markers of cystic fibrosis lung disease with treatment of a pulmonary exacerbation. Thorax 68:532–539
7. Jochmann A, Artusio L, Robson K, Nagakumar P, Collins N, Fleming L, Bush A, Saglani S (2016) Infection and inflammation in induced sputum from preschool children with chronic airways diseases. Pediatr Pulmonol 51:778–786
8. Moore HA, Apolles P, de Villiers PJ, Zar HJ (2011) Sputum induction for microbiological diagnosis of childhood pulmonary tuberculosis in a community setting. Int J Tuberc Lung Dis 15:1185–1190
9. Ahmad F, Irving S, Alton E, Davies JC, Macleod K, Rosenthal M, Saunders C, Bush A, Saglani S, Fleming L (2015) Multiple breath washouts in children can be shortened without compromising quality. Eur Respir J 46:1814–1816
10. Downing B, Irving S, Bingham Y, Fleming L, Bush A, Saglani S (2016) Feasibility of lung clearance index in a clinical setting in pre-school children. Eur Respir J 48:1074–1080
11. Shapiro AJ, Zariwala MA, Ferkol T, Davis SD, Sagel SD, Dell SD, Rosenfeld M, Olivier KN, Milla C, Daniel SJ, Kimple AJ, Manion M, Knowles MR, Leigh MW, Genetic Disorders of Mucociliary Clearance Consortium (2016) Diagnosis, monitoring, and treatment of primary ciliary dyskinesia: PCD foundation consensus recommendations based on state of the art review. Pediatr Pulmonol 51:115–132
12. Lucas J, Barbato A, Collins SA, Goutaki M, Behan L, Caudri D, Dell S, Eber E, Escudier E, Hirst RA, Hogg C, Jorissen M, Latzin P, Legendre M, Leigh MW, Midulla F, Nielsen KG, Omran H, Papon JF, Pohunek P, Redfern B, Rigau D, Rindlisbacher B, Santamaria F, Shoemark A, Snijders D, Tonia T, Titieni A, Walker WT, Werner C, Bush A, Kuehni CE (2017) ERS Task Force guideline for the diagnosis of primary ciliary dyskinesia. Eur Respir J. https://doi.org/10.1183/13993003.01090-2016
13. Bush A, O'Callaghan C (2002) Primary ciliary dyskinesia. Arch Dis Child 87:363–365
14. Goutaki M, Meier AB, Halbeisen FS, Lucas JS, Dell SD, Maurer E, Casaulta C, Jurca M, Spycher BD, Kuehni CE (2016) Clinical manifestations in primary ciliary dyskinesia: systematic review and meta-analysis. Eur Respir J 48:1081–1095
15. Behan L, Dimitrov BD, Kuehni CE, Hogg C, Carroll M, Evans HJ, Goutaki M, Harris A, Packham S, Walker WT, Lucas JS (2016) PICADAR: a diagnostic predictive tool for primary ciliary dyskinesia. Eur Respir J 47:1103–1112
16. Leigh MW, Ferkol TW, Davis SD, Lee HS, Rosenfeld M, Dell SD, Sagel SD, Milla C, Olivier KN, Sullivan KM, Zariwala MA, Pittman JE, Shapiro AJ, Carson JL, Krischer J, Hazucha MJ, Knowles MR (2016) Clinical features and associated likelihood of primary ciliary dyskinesia in children and adolescents. Ann Am Thorac Soc 13:1305–1313
17. Tomos I, Karakatsani A, Manali ED, Papiris SA (2016) Celebrating two centuries since the invention of the stethoscope. Rene Theophile Hyacinthe Laennec (1781–1826). Ann ATS 13:1667–1670
18. Mikami R, Murao M, Cugell DW, Chretien J, Cole P, Meier-Sydow J, Murphy RL, Loudon RG (1987) International symposium on lung sounds. Synopsis of proceedings. Chest 92:342–345
19. Bohadana A, Izbicki G, Kraman S (2014) Fundamentals of lung auscultation. N Engl J Med 370:744–751
20. Pasterkamp H, Brand PL, Everard M, Garcia-Marcos L, Melbye H, Priftis KN (2016) Towards the standardisation of lung sound nomenclature. Eur Respir J 47:724–732
21. Hollman A (1985) Thomas Lewis: physiologist, cardiologist and clinical scientist. Clin Cardiol 8:555–559
22. Asher R (1972) Talking sense. Pitman Medical, Kent, UK

23. Forgacs P (1969) Lung sounds. Br J Dis Chest 63:1–12
24. Forgacs P (1978) The functional basis of pulmonary sounds. Chest 73:399–405
25. Forgacs P (1978) Lung sounds. Harcourt Publishers, UK
26. Earle JE, Marsh K, Pearson MG et al (1982) The inspiratory "squawk" in extrinsic allergic alveolitis and other pulmonary fibroses. Thorax 37:923–926
27. Paciel R, Vyshedskiy A, Bana D et al (2004) Squawks in pneumonia. Thorax 59:177–178
28. Cane RS, Ranganathan SC, McKenzie SA (2000) What do parents of wheezy children understand by "wheeze"? Arch Dis Child 82:327–332
29. Elphick HE, Ritson S, Rodgers H, Everard ML (2000) When a "wheeze" is not a wheeze: acoustic analysis of breath sounds in infants. Eur Respir J 16:593–597
30. Saglani S, McKenzie SA, Bush A, Payne DN (2005) A video questionnaire identifies upper airway abnormalities in pre-school children with reported wheeze. Arch Dis Child 90:961–964
31. Levy ML, Godfrey S, Irving CS, Sheikh A, Hanekom W, Bush A et al (2004) Wheeze detection: recordings vs assessment of physician and parent. J Asthma 41:845–853
32. Turner SW, Craig LCA, Harbour PJ, Forbes SH, McNeill G, Seaton A, Devereux G, Russell G, Helms P (2008) Early rattles, purrs and whistles as predictors of later wheeze. Arch Dis Child 93:701–704
33. Melbye H, Garcia-Marcos L, Brand P, Everard M, Proftos K, Pasterkamp H (2016) The ERS task force for lung sounds. Wheezes, crackles and rhonchi: simplifying description of lung sounds increases the agreement on their classification: a study of 12 physicians' classification of lung sounds from video recordings. BMJ Open Respir Res 3:e000136
34. Williams G, Macaskill P, Kerr M et al (2013) Variability and accuracy in interpreting consolidation on chest radiography in children under 5 years of age. Pediatr Pulmonol 48:1195–1200
35. Elphick HE, Lancaster GA, Solis A et al (2004) Validity and reliability of acoustic analysis of respiratory sounds in infants. Arch Dis Child 89:1059–1063
36. Prodham P, Dela Rosa RS, Shubina M et al (2008) Wheeze detection in the pediatric intensive care unit: comparison among physician, nurses, respiratory therapists, and a computerized respiratory sound monitor. Respir Care 53:1304–1309
37. Puder LC, Fischer HS, Wilitzki S et al (2014) Validation of computerized wheeze detection in young infants during the first months of life. BMC Pediatr 14:257
38. Klein M (2014) Fundamentals of lung auscultation. N Engl J Med 370:2052
39. Nick JA, Sanders LA, Ickes B, Briones NJ, Caceres SM, Malcolm KC, Brayshaw SJ, Chacon CS, Barboa CM, Jones MC, St Clair C, Taylor-Cousar JL, Nichols DP, Sagel SD, Strand M, Saavedra MT (2013) Blood mRNA biomarkers for detection of treatment response in acute pulmonary exacerbations of cystic fibrosis. Thorax 68:929–937
40. Quon BS, Dai DL, Hollander Z, Ng RT, Tebbutt SJ, Man SF, Wilcox PG, Sin DD (2016) Discovery of novel plasma protein biomarkers to predict imminent cystic fibrosis pulmonary exacerbations using multiple reaction monitoring mass spectrometry. Thorax 71:216–222

Part I

General Consideration

2 The Stethoscope: Historical Considerations

Robert Lethbridge and Mark L. Everard

It is now more than 200 hundred years since René Laennec invented the stethoscope [1–6], a device that became the unofficial badge of office for doctors for the best part of two centuries. Hailed as one of the great additions to the physician's non-invasive diagnostic armamentarium, there is no doubt that it has had a huge impact on clinical practice for much of this time. Laennec's classic textbook, *A Treatise on Mediate Auscultation and Diseases of the Lungs and Heart* first published 1819 [1], provided entirely novel and profound insights into both pulmonary and cardiac disease. In this he describes the events that lead to the invention of the stethoscope just 3 years earlier and his insights into the significance of the clinical findings he was able to elicit both with 'mediate auscultation' via the stethoscope and using the recently described technique of percussion, which he helped popularise. He was also able to use his skills in the field of morbid anatomy to inform his interpretation of the clinical signs he elicited when examining his many patients. Thus he helped play a central role in developing a rational scientific foundation for examination of the chest that continues to underpin routine clinical practice to this day.

2.1 The Significance of Laennec and the Stethoscope

The stethoscope can be regarded as the first of a long line of instruments that have given us an ever greater ability to examine the internal structure and function of the human body in health and disease. Laennec noted that at the time, the

R. Lethbridge
School of Paediatrics and Child Health, Princess Margaret Hospital for Children, University of Western Australia, Subiaco, WA, Australia
e-mail: Robert.Lethbridge@health.wa.gov.au

M. L. Everard (✉)
Division of Child Health, University of Western Australia, Perth Children's Hospital, Perth, Australia
e-mail: mark.everard@uwa.edu.au

K. N. Priftis et al. (eds.), *Breath Sounds*, https://doi.org/10.1007/978-3-319-71824-8_2

only tools available to explore the inner workings of the body were the probes used by surgeons. The latest devices such as PET scanners are just a step along the evolutionary progress that has its roots in the work of Laennec and his contemporaries.

Even prior to the invention of the stethoscope and publication of his textbook, Laennec was recognised as one of the great clinical empiricists and teachers. The first translation of his textbook into English by Dr. Forbes was published in 1821 [7], and the first review of his original publication appeared in an American journal the same year. As a member of the Paris school of physicians in the early nineteenth century, he was part of the movement that was revolutionising medical thinking. In the eighteenth century, medicine was still wedded to a 'philosophic' approach to the management of disease that was based on balancing the four 'humours' through practices such as blood-letting and dietary changes that dated back to the ancient Greeks. In a matter of a few decades however, around the turn of the century, Medicine had transitioned to a more questioning profession in which scientific insights from the rapidly developing disciplines of anatomy, pathology and physiology were transforming our understanding of health and disease.

This time of change was reflected in comments by Forbes in the preface to his first translation of Laennec's work, which suggested that the introduction of the stethoscope would not be welcome by physicians who would prefer to continue with their 'philosophical' approach rather than improving their diagnostic skill using a new device and the new ideas associated with it. Fortunately, most physicians and their patients welcomed the move towards the improved diagnostic accuracy and prognostication. Laennec's work can be seen as one of the most significant contributions to the rapid transition of medical practice from centuries of dogma to a scientific discipline.

2.2 Immediate and Mediate Auscultation

The value of assessing breath sounds audible at a distance from the subject, or heard through 'immediate' auscultation achieved by applying one's ear to the chest wall, was known to Hippocrates and the ancient Greeks and is referred to in a number of publications from various sources through the ensuing centuries, though this approach does not appear to have been widely adopted at any stage. The idea of augmenting sounds from the chest had already been explored in the previous century by Hooke, but his initial experiments were not pursued [8].

In his introduction, Laennec mentions that he and his fellow students were aware of listening directly to the chest as a possible adjunct to the examination (Fig. 2.1) but that few practiced this in large part because it was felt that it rarely added any information other than in some cardiac cases. He noted that other reasons for its '*limited application*' included '*it is always inconvenient both to the physician and patient: in the case of females it is not only indelicate but often impractical; and in the class of persons found in hospitals it is disgusting.*' Despite these issues, and in contrast to most of his colleagues, he noted that '*Nevertheless, I had been in the habit of using this method for a long time and it was the employment of it which led me to the discovery of a much better one*'. He then goes on to describe the

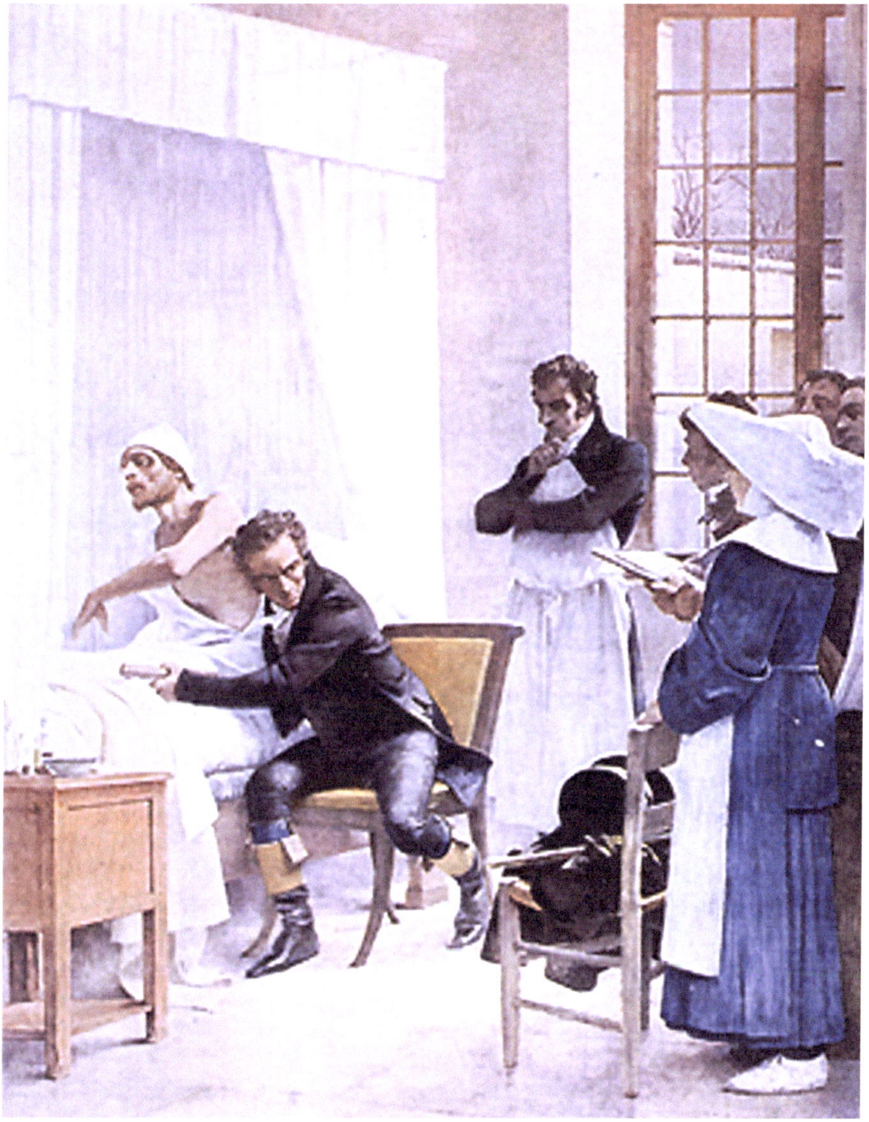

Fig. 2.1 Laennec listens to the chest of patient with tuberculosis prior to the invention of the stethoscope *A L'Hopital Necker, Ausculte Un Phtisique*Théobald Chartran (1849–1907)

well-known story of wishing to examine a young lady with a cardiac problem whose '*great degree of fatness*' had negated obtaining any useful clinical information from palpation and percussion and in whom immediate auscultation was '*inadmissible because of the age and sex of the patient.*'

To circumvent these difficulties, Laennec rolled up a 'quire' of paper (24 sheets) and '*was not a little surprised and pleased to perceive the action of the heart in a manner much more clear and distinct than I had ever been able to do by the immediate application of the ear.*' In 3 years between this episode, which took place towards

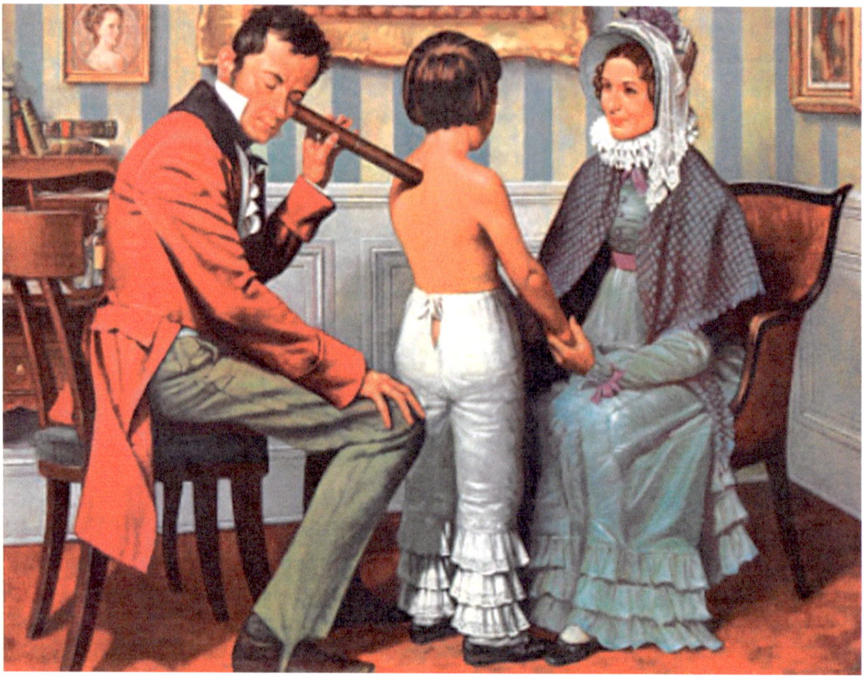

Fig. 2.2 Painting of Laennec using his stethoscope on a boyThis picture was taken from a painting by Robert Thom, copyrighted in 1960

the end of 1816, and the publication of his textbook in 1819, he refined his stethoscope (Figs 2.2 and 2.3). Having experimented with a variety of designs and materials, he then correlated his auscultatory findings with observations from the numerous post mortems he undertook. This led him to note '*The consequence is, that I have been enabled to discover a set of new signs of diseases of the chest, for the most part certain, simple, and prominent, and calculated, perhaps, to render the diagnosis of the diseases—of the lungs, heart and pleura, as decided and circumstantial, as the indications furnished to the surgeon by the introduction of the finger or sound (probe), in the complaints wherein these are used.*'

This 3-year period also marked an explosion of activity, which included writing a very substantial textbook. This is all the more remarkable as it took place at a time when the effects of pulmonary tuberculosis were increasingly starting to impinge on his wellbeing. This disease would eventually take his life at the age of 45 years. He notes in his first edition that his work was not complete. Both his deteriorating health and the frequent misinterpretation of his discoveries, as they were otherwise spread by word of mouth, prompted him to rush publication. Following this, however, his health did improve for a time, and he was able to expand and develop some of his ideas in the second edition published in 1826, the year of his death.

Laennec recognised that the limited responses of the lungs due to a variety of diseases made it difficult to distinguish them on the basis of history alone—an

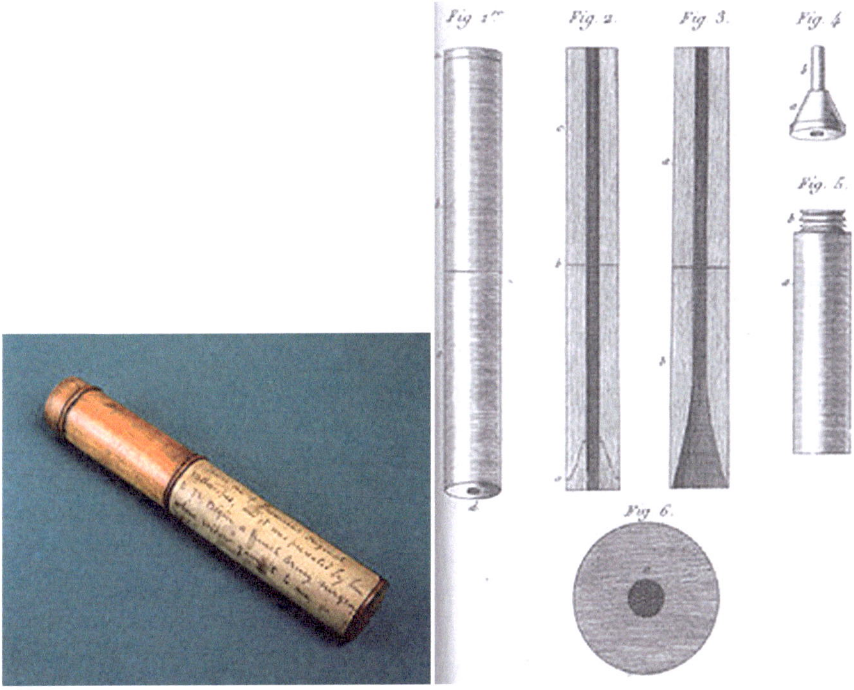

Fig. 2.3 A Laennec stethoscope from 1820

observation that is just as relevant today. This paucity of descriptive symptomatology drove him to try and improve the usefulness of the physical examination. "*…the diseases of the thoracic viscera are very numerous and diversified, and yet have almost all the same class of symptoms. Of these the most common and prominent are cough, dyspnoea, and, in some, expectoration. These, of course, vary in different diseases; but their variations are by no means of that determinate kind which can enable us to consider them as certain indications of known variations in the diseases. The consequence is, that the most skilful physician who trusts to the pulse and general symptoms, is often deceived in regard to the most common and best known complaints of this cavity.*"

To further expand the investigative potential of the physical exam, Laennec augmented his use of the stethoscope with the art of percussion. Auenbugger's original book detailing this technique was published in 1761 [9], and following the availability of a French translation by Corvisart in 1808 [10], Laennec was keen to promote its use. By utilising the findings of each of these methods, he was able to accurately diagnose a wide range of pulmonary conditions, including those first described by him such as bronchiectasis.

Laennec focused on the use of the stethoscope for augmenting the diagnostic process in relation to pulmonary and cardiac disease. In the years immediately after the publication of his book, others found a range of diagnostic applications for the new devices such as listening for crepitus in suspected fractures (less painful and more specific than the traditional prod still used by some in the emergency departments), examining the abdomen and listening to foetal heart beats. Until the use of X-rays for diagnostic purposes were developed in the early twentieth century, the stethoscope reigned supreme as the physician's most useful piece of equipment to enhance diagnostic accuracy.

It is of note that Laennec does not appear to discuss the significance of sounds heard at a distance such as wheeze and stridor. He does comment that sounds such as snores generated in the upper airway are poorly transmitted to the chest, and hence the stethoscope is of little use. Other sounds from the lower airways such as the 'death rattle' due to copious secretions in the large airways, the sonorous rale (again due to secretions in large airway) and the sibilant rale could all be heard on occasions while simply observing the patient. Similarly, he did not make much of trying to attribute inspiratory noises to upper airways pathology and expiratory noises to lower airways pathology even though he recognised this tendency. This is probably because much of the pathology he saw in the hospitalised patients was attributable to excessive secretions associated with chronic diseases such as pulmonary TB or chronic bronchitis, and this gives rise to both harsh inspiratory and expiratory noises generated in the central airways.

2.3 Acceptance of the New Device and Its Evolutionary Decedents

While Laennec's ideas spread rapidly, there was resistance from some quarters, particularly in France [11, 12]. No doubt the inevitable professional jealousies and resistance to new ideas that accompany any leap forward in knowledge were behind some of the initial negative responses noted. In France, many apparently dismissed his book as merely an overlong source of amusement. Forbes, in his introduction to his first translation [7], noted that "*I have no doubt whatever, from my own experience of its value, that it will be acknowledged to be one of the greatest discoveries in medicine,*" but he was far from convinced that it would become part of routine practice. "*That it will ever come into general use, notwithstanding its value, I am extremely doubtful; because its beneficial application requires much time, and gives a good deal of trouble both to the patient and the practitioner; and because its whole hue and character is foreign, and opposed to all our habits and associations. It must be confessed that there is something even ludicrous in a grave physician formally listening through a long tube applied to the patient's thorax, as if the disease within were a living being that could communicate its condition to the sense without. Besides, there is in this method a sort of bold claim and pretension to certainty and precision of diagnosis, which cannot, at first sight, but be somewhat startling to a mind deeply versed in the knowledge and uncertainty of our art, and to the calm and cautious habits of philosophising to which the English physicians accustomed.*"

The idea that it would not be adopted because the doctors' actions might appear 'ludicrous' or that the idea a doctor might make a diagnosis with some precision would break the '*habitual cautious habits of philosophising*' that dominated the English physician's art reflect an approach to medicine that may not have completely disappeared. Even though there was rapid and widespread acceptance that mediate auscultation is of considerable clinical value, it is reported that many, particularly in France, adopted 'immediate' auscultation as the preferred method of listening to the chest for a number of decades because, contrary to all the evidence, they believed the stethoscope 'distorted' the sounds emanating from the lungs or heart. Many adopted a similar view when the flexible rubber binaural stethoscope was developed declaring that hearing in stereo adversely affected their ability to hear with clarity.

2.4 Evolution of Stethoscope Design

There are a number of reviews of the evolution of the stethoscope [11, 13–19]. Laennec's original design outlined in his first edition consisted of a length of wood approximately 1.5 in./4 cm in diameter and roughly 1 foot/30 cm in length with a hollow core. At the distal end, the central core was widened into a funnel shape to be applied to the chest. A plug to fill the funnelled end was used when listening for 'pectoriloquism' while the patient spoke, as well as for listening to the heart. When his first book was published, the purchaser was also able to buy one of Laennec's stethoscopes from the same retailer, as was the case when the English translation was published in London a couple of years later. This device was designed with a join in the middle so that it could be taken apart for convenience when not in use.

Within a very short period of time, a number of manufacturers were producing similar devices. Variations soon appeared with the diameter of the tubing being reduced 'to the thickness of a finger' by 1828, and the following year, the first binaural device was produced (but not adopted). The advent of durable rubber in the middle of the nineteenth century led to the development of a useable binaural device (Fig. 2.4), although a wide variety of material including wood, metal and even glass continued to be used. Experiments with diaphragms fitted to the bell apparently occurred through the second part of the nineteenth century with the first commercial devices, based on a design by Bowles in 1894, being available around the turn of the century. While most devices had a bell or diaphragm, some were manufactured with the option of physically changing from one to the other until the combined 'Bowle-Sprague' device was developed in 1926 allowing movement from one to the other with a switch. The double rubber tubing used for almost 100 years largely disappeared with the development of a single tube with a Y-shaped split to each ear piece designed by Dr. Littmann, an academic cardiologist at Harvard, in 1961.

The concept of attaching a number of listening ports for the purposes of teaching is of course not a new idea, with the earliest devices being described in the mid-nineteenth century while 'electronic stethoscopes' start to appear in the literature in the first half of the twentieth century. Microphones with computerised analysis

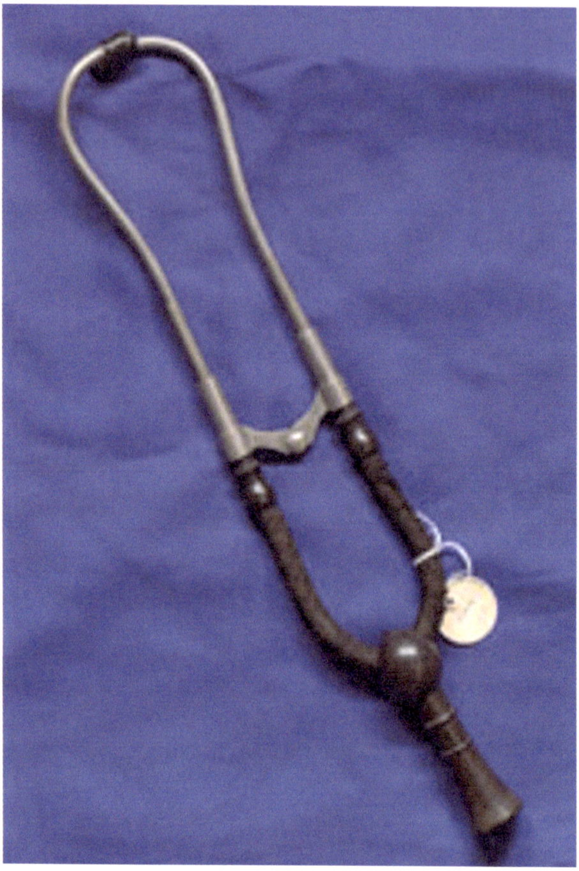

Fig. 2.4 Cammann stethoscope, 1852. Binaural stethoscope made by George Tiemann. Donated by Dr. Harold Nathan Segall. In the 1850s, flexible tubes began to be used, and in 1851 the Irish physician Arthur Leared created the first binaural stethoscope fitting in both ears. This invention was commercialised the following year by George Cammann. Reproduced by permission of the Osler Library of the History of Medicine, McGill University

designed to help the clinician interpret the sounds emanating from the chest have been in development for decades but have yet to enter routine clinical practice [20–23]. The use of a microphone applied to chest or neck and attached to a mobile phone has also, so far, made little impact. In addition to the cost of these developments, most of the devices have either not been conveniently mobile or lack the necessary precision to be a useful diagnostic tool. As will be discussed later in this book, there is still a considerable amount of work being undertaken in this area, though many clinicians find a video of the child when symptomatic taken on a smartphone more useful than attempts by parents or clinicians to describe clinical signs and adventitial sounds.

2.5 Impact of Disease on Sounds of Respiration, Voice and Cough as Heard Through the Stethoscope

Laennec described the normal sounds of respiration, speech and coughing and how they might alter in disease. To him these were at least as important and telling as identification of any adventitial sounds. '*The signs afforded by mediate auscultation in the diseases of the lungs and pleura, are derived from the changes presented by the sound of respiration, by that of the voice and coughing, within the chest, and also by the rale, as well as certain other sounds which occasionally are heard in the same situation,*' Indeed, he devoted significantly more pages to the impact of disease on the auscultation of speech heard through the stethoscope than either 'pulmonary sounds' or 'adventitious sounds'. This was in large part because of the impact of consolidation, accumulation of secretions filling airways and the impact of cavities associated with these changes. It should be remembered that more than a third of his patients had advanced pulmonary TB and that to be admitted to the hospital Nectar in Paris, patients were often very ill. The significant mortality amongst these patients from a variety of conditions provided Laennec the opportunity to correlate his auscultatory findings with the underlying pathology. Few if any of those who followed and 'interpreted' his work and nomenclature had such insights.

To Laennec, the term pulmonary respiration was used to describe the normal breath sounds heard over the lungs. The term vesicular was coined by his fellow countryman Andral and advanced by Forbes as a preferable term. Laennec believed that the sound '*answered to the entrance of air into and out of air-cells of the lungs*' (termed vesicles by others). In this section he argues that one can auscultate through clothes provided there is no friction between the instrument and clothing such as silk. He recognised that the sounds were very individual, for example, being more pronounced and often more prominent in exhalation in children, difficult to hear in fit healthy men breathing quietly and 'puerile' (childlike) in those with more diffuse lung disease. Bronchial breathing was the term he gave to the somewhat harsher sound resembling those heard over the upper trachea. He identified this as *one of the earliest signs of "hepatisation" occurring in pneumonia and 'accumulation of tubercles in the upper lobes.*'

2.6 The 'Humpty Dumpty' Problem[1]

One of Laennec's many insights was his recognition that it may prove difficult to convey the meaning of the terms used. In particular, he anticipated that it would be difficult to convey in words the characteristics of the five classes of adventitial sounds or 'rales' (French for rattle) he recognised. He felt, however, that they were so distinct that once heard it would become obvious what he was describing.

> *For want of a better or more generic term I use the word rale to express all the sounds, beside those of health, which the act of respiration gives rise to, from the passage of the air through fluids in the bronchia or lungs, or by its transmission through any of the air passages partially contracted. They are extremely various: and although they possess, in gen-*

[1] 'When *I* use a word', Humpty Dumpty said, in rather a scornful tone, 'it means just what I choose it to mean—neither more nor less'.'The question is', said Alice, 'whether you *can* make words mean so many different things'.'The question is', said Humpty Dumpty, 'which is to be master—that's all'.

Lewis Carroll's *Through the Looking-Glass* (1872)

> *eral, very striking characters, it becomes difficult so to describe them as to convey anything like a correct notion to those who have never heard them. Sensations, we know, can only be communicated to others by comparisons: and although those which I shall employ may seem to myself sufficiently exact, they may not be so to others. I expect, however, that my description will enable any observation, of ordinary application to recognise them when he meets with them, as they are much more easily distinguished than described.*

Sadly, his optimism was misplaced, and what is clear from the literature generated during the following centuries is that we seem destined not to build on Laennec's insights but to undermine them. The confusion appears to have commenced with the first translation of his work [24], Forbes having decided he was going to reorganise the content, improve the language and reduce its length by half. In particular Forbes disliked the term *rale* and replaced it with *rattle* or *rhonchus*. In the introduction to his second edition, Laennec noted that he too used the term rhonchus interchangeably with rale because in the minds of his patients, the term rale was often assumed to equate to the 'death rattle'. To lessen this connection, he would use the term rhonchus (an alternative term for rattle) when discussing his findings in front of patients. 'Rattle' did not prove popular with Forbes' British colleagues, and the term rhonchus became a general term for an adventitial sound which required further characterisation by an additional term. Over time the term rhonchus came to be used by some to describe one particular type of adventitial sound and thus has been a source of confusion ever since.

There have been repeated attempts to 'standardise' or 'rationalise' breath sound nomenclature [25–37], but unfortunately none have significantly impacted on the confusion that characterises this area as emphasised by the steady stream of publications repeatedly highlighting the inability of clinicians to agree on both the description and significance of auscultator findings [38–55] (though this is perhaps no worse than the ability to agree on many other clinical findings).

"***Auscultation of certain sounds adventitious to the respiration***."

Laennec identified four adventitious sounds in his first edition, adding a fifth in the second edition (see Table 2.1). As noted above he used the terms rale and rhonchus interchangeably as terms that denoted an adventitial sound, and the precise type of sound required a further qualifying term.

Eighty years later in a heartfelt plea to stop confusing medical students and doctors alike, Dr. West [26] echoed Laennec's concern that language may be a source of confusion. '*Auscultation is not really a difficult subject. It requires some little preliminary instruction and after that its mastery is only a question of attention and practice; yet there is no doubt that it often appears confusing to students' and 'The difficulties however are chiefly of our own making, and lie not in things but in words; for the facts of auscultation, their significance and their relation to pathological lesions, are well known and understood, while the confusion lied in the technical terms used to express the phenomena observed*'. He considered the two principle offenders the 'technical terms' of 'bronchial breathing' and 'rales' largely because they had acquired more than one meaning. His problem with bronchial breathing centred on the use of the term for sounds that lay somewhere between 'vesicular' breathing and what he considered to be 'true bronchial breathing'. In trying to

Table 2.1 Lannec's classification of adventitious breath sounds with early translations to English

Laennec	Forbes/Herbert rhonchus = rale
Rale humid **Crepitation**[a]	Crepitant rhonchus/rale **Crepitation**
Rale muqueux **Gargouillement**[b]	Mucus rhonchus/rale **Gurgling**
Rale sec sonore **Ronflement**[c]	Dry sonorous Rhonchus/rale **Snoring**
Rale sibilant **Sifflement**[d]	Dry sibilant Rhonchus/rale **Whistling**
Rale crepitant sec grosses bulles **Craquement**[e]	Dry crepitus with large bubbles rhonchus/rale **Crackling**

On line French English translation
[a]Crepitation, crackling; crepitation, making of a crackling sound
[b]Gargouillement, rumble
[c]Ronflement, roar, snore, snoring
[d]Sifflement, whistling, whistle; whiz, hiss
[e]Craquement, crack, snap

clarify this issue, he provided diagrammatic representations to try and obviate the limitations of language.

More importantly he noted that Laennec's 'sonorous' and 'sibilant' rales were by then commonly referred to as a 'rhonchus' and 'sibilus' (hissing). The term rale had acquired two meanings and could be applied to Laennec's five 'adventitious' sounds or, more specifically, to the remaining three sounds which had become labelled as 'crepitations'—both dry and moist. As such he argued that the term rale should be abandoned. It was to be another 80 years before the term was largely abandoned, at least in the UK, where Thorax editors took the step of refusing to include the term in published case reports—an example of the stick being much more effective than the carrot of a brighter future with lesser confusion. West's paper also highlighted the fact that rhonchus had by then also achieved the same feat of being used commonly to describe a single type of adventitial sound, while others continued to use it in the broader sense of referring to any adventitial sound.

West also noted that the term stridor had become widespread to describe 'noisy laryngeal and tracheal breathing' on inspiration due to a stenosis or narrowing. Laennec did not distinguish between inspiratory and expiratory phases, at least not in the translated version of Forbes, and it is therefore unclear whether stridor was a form of Laennec's 'sonorous rale'. Both Laennec and West noted that these sounds were highly variable and at times musical, but at other times, the term 'musical' would be somewhat stretched to incorporate the harsh sonorous sound attributable to secretions in the airway and which frequently clear with coughing. It was noted by Andral and others from soon after the publication of Laennec's book that '*he has not specified the precise moment, during the act of respiration, at which these (rales) are heard.*' While there are those that advance the notion that inspiratory sounds are generated in the extra thoracic airways (upper extrathoracic trachea and above) and expiratory sounds are generated in the lower airways—as a result of maximal collapse occurring in this phase of the respiratory cycle—this is not true of those sound which Laennec speculated were due to air passing through or over mucus and secretions. The 'sonorous' rale or 'mucous' rale, for example, are described in conditions generating excessive secretions or fluid in the airways and which can occur in both inhalation and exhalation.

In 1932, Kinghorn [27] produced a detailed review of the variation in terminology then in use, choosing to adhere closely to Laennec's classification. He noted, as others had done, that the sonorous rale (otherwise known by many as the 'rhonchus') was highly variable and could often be cleared by coughing, while the sibilant rale (hissing) was generally unaffected by coughing. Echoing Laennec, he attributed the former to secretions in the large airways and the latter due to narrowing, from whatever cause, of the smaller airways.

By 1984, a review of terms used in English language case reports of respiratory conditions [40] noted that American journals *'most often use the terms 'rale', 'wheezes' and 'rhonchi'* though the use of 'crackles' was increasing. In British journals, fashion had led to a decrease in the use of the terms 'rales' and 'crepitations', while the use of 'wheezes' and 'crackles' had increased. In fact 'crackles' was mandated by the editorial board of Thorax, who apparently altered all references to 'crepitations' and 'rales'.

The American practice was presumably influenced by the publication in 1975 of the musings of the ACCP-ATS Joint Committee on Pulmonary Nomenclature [29] which noted that *'There is considerable confusion in the use of the terms rale and rhonchus to describe adventitious sounds heard over the chest'. Some continue to use rhonchus and rale as general terms for all abnormal lung sounds. However, rhonchus is used by others to describe only a continuous sound (wheeze) and rale to describe only short interrupted explosive sounds (crackles) heard usually during inspiration. The simplest way to resolve the confusion is to select the two most commonly used words, rhonchus and rale, and arbitrarily define the term rale to indicate only crackling or bubbling (discontinuous) sounds or vibrations and rhonchus to define only musical (continuous) sounds or vibrations, usually of longer duration. Alternative acceptable terminology substitutes crackles for rales and wheezes for rhonchi.'* A rhonchus is now synonymous with wheeze (a hissing sound) and musical in nature despite embracing Laennec's sibilant and sonorous rales which have very different characteristics, origins and implications for diagnosis.

Leap ahead another quarter of a century and an ERS Task Force [34] recommends abandoning the term bronchial breathing as being 'confusing', keeping the rhonchus as a low pitched wheeze, and defines a wheeze as a 'continuous' 'musical' sound with a duration of >100 ms and a dominant frequency of >100 Hz together with coarse and fine crackles. This Task Force believed they could '*standardise*' terminology as part of a process which would result in the production of a '*mass-produced multipurpose computerised stethoscope which may replace the current acoustic stethoscope as a basic tool for future doctors*'—that is removing the human from having to interpret what he/she hears. In this iteration the word wheeze which for generations had been used to describe a sound audible without mediate or immediate auscultation of the chest is now to be used to describe the 'higher-pitched' musical sound attributable to fluttering of the central airways secondary to flow limitation and to the 'low-pitched' 'sonorous' sounds that appear to be attributed to secretions in the airways, thus becoming descriptive of at least three different types of sounds with at least two different underlying mechanisms. It is perhaps not surprising that universal clarity has not been achieved.

Unfortunately, many doctors faced with the dilemma of labelling something as a crackle or wheeze will label the harsh 'sonorous rale' of Laennec or 'rhonchus' of the ERS Task Force a wheeze as it does not have the discontinuous properties of a typical fine crackle and then compound the mistake by forgetting the maxim that 'all that wheezes is not asthma.'

Laennec, having an enquiring and methodical mind, would, if he returned, be fascinated by the technological advances of the past two centuries such as CT scanning, MRI and echocardiography but would no doubt be profoundly saddened by the confusion evident in the literature regarding the use of his simple but very important aide to interpretation of clinical findings. As he appears to have been both immensely practical and logical, he is likely to question, given the digital world we live in, why there is no 'gold standard' resource for physicians to refer to rather than continuously trying to propose new nomenclature and assuming that the reader will know precisely what the author has in mind. A number of online resources exist, but again there is no standardisation of terminology. A recent ERS Task Force was established in large part to produce such a resource, but this aim was not achieved [56]. As Renetti observed in 1979 when considering the respiratory physicians' uncanny similarity to Humpty Dumpty, 'Laennec, if aware of this chaotic state, must be restless in his grave' [38].

2.7 Reports of the Stethoscope's Demise Have Been Somewhat Premature

Predictions of the demise of the physical examination and its replacement by radiology appear soon after the introduction of chest X-rays. By 1946, while it was recognised that the technical quality of imaging was still relatively primitive and that abnormalities on chest X-rays were often not specific, many were arguing that the stethoscope and physical examination in general had been relegated to third spot behind history and radiology in its value in the diagnosis of pulmonary disease [57]. One of the key charges laid against the use of the stethoscope by doctors was the tendency for doctors to confabulate the finding of a 'clear' chest with absence of pulmonary pathology—again a situation that has not changed 70 years later. Dr. Maxwell noted '*Most doctors are apt to assume and, even worse, to announce to their patients that the failure to detect physical signs implies a healthy respiratory tract. Nothing could be further from the truth.*' This observation can be borne out when re-examining a young child's chest after a CXR has shown evidence of a lobar pneumonia, listening to the 'clear' chest of an asthmatic patient in the afternoon when the patient is complaining of having been awake with shortness of breath and wheeze in the early hours of the morning or listening to the chest of a patient with cystic fibrosis in whom a 'clear chest' can be accompanied by considerable airways secretion that can be revealed with a good cough or huff.

A number of 'authorities' have, over a number of years, argued that auscultation is an anachronism in the age of detailed imaging both of the heart and lungs, particularly given the low level of expertise in describing and interpreting the findings observed in many studies. As such its use is often dismissed as a desire to hold onto a fashion item or status symbol. In contrast its use is often stoutly defended by enthusiasts who feel it provides an invaluable screening tool that is cheap and portable: properties that are likely to contribute to its continued use for some time [58–62]. The largest challenge for the young medical student trying to understand the role of what is often thought of as the defining symbol of the profession they are entering is to convert the contradictory statements contained in textbooks, journal articles and the Chinese-whispered lessons of bedside teaching into a useful model on which to make accurate inferences.

It is of interest to note that in the *American Academy of Pediatrics* textbook on Pediatric Pulmonology, the topic of auscultation as part of the assessment of a child with a respiratory problem warrants barely a page of the 1182-page tome and refers to only 3 sounds—discontinuous crackles which can be course or fine, rhonchi and wheeze. There is no discussion of the mechanisms by which they are generated and little comment regarding the implication of the sounds. This suggests the authors consider mediate auscultation to be of little value to the 'pulmonologists', yet there is no sign that the stethoscope will disappear in the immediate future. We will no doubt continue to see the publication of articles expressing surprise at the inability of clinicians to agree on the terminology that describes a sound they hear and observe further suggestions for addressing this embarrassing reality.

King and Crewe noted in their book '*The Blunders of our Governments* [63] *that if cars continually crash at a junction, eventually it becomes pointless to blame the driver, and a new solution to the design of the junction is required.*' In the case of the stethoscope, the ongoing failure of clinicians to communicate their findings coherently could be addressed by automated sound analysis. This would mitigate the language difficulties but removes the extraordinary abilities of the human brain to interpret sound, the latter being one of the main reasons that this approach has not entered routine clinical practice. An alternative solution, as noted above, is to generate a gold standard teaching programme (as with the platinum/iridium standard metre in Paris) to which everyone in practice and training can refer.

Once pre-eminent amongst the tools we had available to assist the diagnostic process, the stethoscope became the symbol of the medical profession. More recently it has, in many ways, been overtaken by other technological advances. However, despite all the problems associated with its use, it is likely to be around for some time to come. The stethoscope remains a potentially valuable, powerful, portable tool that, if used appropriately, may provide valuable clinical information at low cost and minimal inconvenience. Its role has changed from being the single piece of equipment that could enhance our ability to reach a diagnosis when examining a patient with pulmonary disease to being a screening tool that is frequently used in the initial assessment of potential disease by helping to inform the choice of further, more detailed, investigations. As with any tool, however, it is the skill of its user that defines its true value, and Laennec might well turn in his grave given the problems the profession has contrived to introduce since he produced such a clear guide for the future use of his simple but potent invention.

References

1. Laënnec RTH (1819) De l'ausculatation médiate, un Traité du diagnostic des maladies des poumons et du coeur, fonde, principalement sur ce naveau moyen d'exploration. (A treatise on the diseases of the chest and on mediate auscultation) Paris, Brosson et Chande
2. Williams CT (1907) A Lecture on Lannec and the evolution of the stethescope: Delivered before the Medical Department of the University of Oxford. Br Med J 6(2):6–8
3. Sakula A (1981) R T H Laënnec 1781-1826 his life and work: a bicentenary appreciation. Thorax 36:81–90
4. Kligfield P (1981) Laennec and the discovery of mediate auscultation. Am J Med 70:275–278
5. Reiser SJ (1979) The medical influence of the stethoscope. Sci Am 240:148–150. 153-6
6. Roguin A (2006) Rene Theophile Hyacinthe Laënnec (1781-1826): the man behind the stethoscope. Clin Med Res 4:230–235
7. Laënnec RTH (1821) A treatise on the diseases of the chest, in which they are described according to their anatomical characters, and their diagnosis established on a new principle by means of acoustic instruments (trans: Forbes J). London: Underwood.
8. Owen RG (1939) The microphone, stethoscope, telephone and artificial aids to hearing; their historical relationship. Cal West Med 51:169–171
9. Auenbrugger L (1761) Inventum novum ex percussione thoracis humani ut signo abstrusos interni pectoris morbos dete-gendi. Trattner, Vienna
10. Corvisart JN (1808) (trans): Nouvelle m&hode pour reconnaftre les maladies internes de la poitrine par la percussion de cette cavite, par Avenbrugger. Paris: Migneret
11. Williams CT (1907) A lecture on Laennec and the evolution of the stethoscope: delivered before the medical Department of the University of Oxford. Br Med J 2(2427):6–8
12. Bishop PJ (1981) Reception of the stethoscope and Laënnec's book. Thorax 36:487–492
13. Williams CJ (1874) On the acoustic principles and construction of stethoscopes and ear trumpets. Med Chir Trans 57:21–30
14. (1935) An electronic stethoscope. Can Med Assoc J:304–305
15. Sheldon P (1949 Jan) B & Doe J. The development of the stethoscope: and Br Heart J 11(1):48–54
16. Phillips AF (1949) A loud-speaker stethoscope for clinical teaching. Br Heart J 11:48–54
17. Hampton CS, Chaloner A (1967) Which stethoscope? Br Med J 4(5576):388–390
18. Hollman A (2002) Book review: an ear to the chest: an illustrated history of the evolution of the stethoscope. J Roy Soc Med 95:625–626
19. Bishop PJ (1980) Evolution of the stethoscope. J R Soc Med 73:448–456
20. Hunt FL, Myres MJ (1921) Experiments on the recording and reproduction of cardiac and respiratory sounds. Science 54(1398):359
21. Fenton RT, Pasterkamp H, Tal A, Chernik V (1985) Automated spectral characterization of wheezing in asthmatic children. IEEE Trans Biomed Eng 32:50–55
22. Sovijärvi A, Vanderschoot J, Earis JE (2000) Standardisation of computerised breath sounds analysis. Eur Respir Rev 10(77):585
23. Anderson K, Qiu Y, Whittaker AR, Lucas M (2001) Breath sounds, asthma, and the mobile phone. Lancet 358(9290):1343–1344
24. Robertson AJ (1957) Rales, rhonchi, and Laennec. After an evening with Robert Coope. Lancet 2:417–423

25. Thompson T (1853) Hints on auscultation, with a view to the simplification of terms and arrangement. Assoc Med J 1:364–366
26. West S (1897) Bronchial breathing and râles: a clinical demonstration on some of the difficulties of auscultation given at St. Bartholomew's Hospital. Br Med J 2(1906):65–68
27. Kinghorn HM (1932 Apr) The classification of rales. Can Med Assoc J 26(4):438–445
28. Forgacs P (1967) Crackles and wheezes. Lancet 2:203–205
29. (1977) Report of the ATS-ACCP ad hoc committee on pulmonary nomenclature. Am Thor Soc News 3:5–6
30. Cugell D (1978) Sounds of the lungs (editorial). Chest 73:311–312
31. Kraman SS (1986) Lung sounds for the clinician. Arch Intern Med 146(7):1411–1412
32. Murphy RL (1981) Auscultation of the lung: past lessons, future possibilities. Thorax 36(2):99–107
33. Pasterkamp H, Kraman SS, Wodicka GR (1997) Respiratory sounds. Advances beyond the stethoscope. Am J Respir Crit Care Med 156(3 Pt 1):974–987
34. Sovijärvi A, Dalmasso F, Vanderschoot J, Malmberg LP, Righini G, Stoneman SA (2000) Definitions of term for applications of respiratory sounds. Eur Respir Rev 77:597–610
35. Bohadana A, Izbicki G, Kraman SS (2014) Fundamentals of lung auscultation. N Engl J Med 370(8):744–751
36. Klein M (2014) Fundamentals of lung auscultation. N Engl J Med 370:205
37. Pasterkamp H, Brand PL, Everard M, Garcia-Marcos L, Melbye H, Priftis KN (2016) Towards the standardisation of lung sound nomenclature. Eur Respir J 47(3):724–732
38. Renzetti AD Jr (1979) Lung sound terminology. Chest 76(6):615–616
39. Bunin NJ, Loudon RG (1979) Lung sound terminology in case reports. Chest 76(6):690–692
40. Wilkins RL, Dexter JR, Smith JR (1984) Survey of adventitious lung sound terminology in case reports. Chest 85(4):523–525
41. Pasterkamp H, Montgomery M, Wiebicke W (1987) Nomenclature used by health care professionals to describe breath sounds in asthma. Chest 92(2):346–352
42. Pasterkamp H, Wiebicke W, Fenton R (1987) Subjective assessment vs computer analysis of wheezing in asthma. Chest 91(3):376–381
43. Wilkins RL, Dexter JR, Murphy RL Jr, DelBono EA (1990) Lung sound nomenclature survey. Chest 98(4):886–889
44. Wilkins RL, Dexter JR (1990) Comparing RCPs to physicians for the description of lung sounds: are we accurate and can we communicate? Respir Care 35(10):969–976
45. Brooks D, Thomas J (1995) Interrater reliability of auscultation of breath sounds among physical therapists. Phys Ther 75(12):1082–1088
46. Postiaux G, Lens E (1999) Pulmonary stethacoustic nomenclature: Why not a worldwide consensus? Rev Mal Respir 16(6):1075–1090
47. Mangione S, Nieman LZ (1999) Pulmonary auscultatory skills during training in internal medicine and family practice. Am J Respir Crit Care Med 159(4 Pt 1):1119–1124
48. Elphick HE, Ritson S, Rogers H, Everard ML (2000) When a 'wheeze' is not a wheeze - analysis of breath sounds in infancy. Eur Respir J 16:593–597
49. Elphick HE, Lancaster GA, Solis A, Majumdar A, Gupta R, Smyth RL (2004) Validity and reliability of acoustic analysis of respiratory sounds in infants. Arch Dis Child 89(11):1059–1063
50. Elphick H, Everard ML (2002) Noisy breathing in children. In: David T (ed) Recent Advances in Paediatrics. The Royal Society of Medicine, London
51. Staszko KF, Lincho C, Engelke Vda C, Fiori NS, Silva KC, Nunes EI, Zhang L (2006) Pulmonary auscultation terminology employed in Brazilian medical journals between January of 1980 and December of 2003. J Bras Pneumol 32(5):400–404
52. Mangione S, Torre DM (2003) Teaching of pulmonary auscultation in pediatrics: a nationwide survey of all U.S. accredited residencies. Pediatr Pulmonol 35(6):472–476
53. Mellis C (2009) Respiratory noises: how useful are they clinically? Pediatr Clin N Am 56:1–17
54. Benbassat J, Baumal R (2010) Narrative review: should teaching of the respiratory physical examination be restricted only to signs with proven reliability and validity? J Gen Intern Med 25:865–872

55. Francis NA, Melbye H, Kelly MJ, Cals JW, Hopstaken RM, Coenen S, Butler CC (2013) Variation in family physicians' recording of auscultation abnormalities in patients with acute cough is not explained by case mix. A study from 12 European networks. Eur J Gen Pract 19(2):77–84
56. Melbye H, Garcia-Marcos L, Brand P, Everard ML, Priftis K, Hans Pasterkamp H (2016) The ERS task force for lung sounds. Wheezes, crackles and rhonchi: simplifying description of lung sounds increases the agreement on their classification. BMJ Open Respir Res 3(1):e000136
57. Maxwell J, Kerley P, Blair LG (1946) Discussion on the stethoscope versus x-rays. Proc R Soc Med 39:355–357
58. Markel H (2006) The stethoscope and the art of listening. N Engl J Med 354(6):551–553
59. Murphy RL (2008) In defense of the stethoscope. Respir Care 53(3):355–369
60. Bank I, Vliegen HW, Bruschke AV (2016) The 200th anniversary of the stethoscope: can this low-tech device survive in the high-tech 21st century? Eur Heart J 37(47):3536–3543
61. Tomos I, Karakatsani A, Manali ED, Papiris SA (2016) Celebrating two centuries since the invention of the stethoscope. René Théophile Hyacinthe Laënnec (1781-1826). Ann Am Thorac Soc 13(10):1667–1670
62. Fakoya FA, du Plessis M, Gbenimacho IB (2016) Ultrasound and stethoscope as tools in medical education and practice: considerations for the archives. Adv Med Educ Pract 7:381–387
63. King A, Crewe I (2014) The blunders of our Governments. Oneworld, London

Check for updates

3 Clinical Usefulness of Breath Sounds

Sotirios Fouzas, Michael B. Anthracopoulos, and Abraham Bohadana

3.1 Introduction

Respiratory medicine relies both on clinical information and on complementary, laboratory tests results. However, despite today's technological wonders, a proper history and a sound physical examination have no substitute as the initial step in making a correct diagnosis and, by consequence, providing the appropriate treatment. This chapter focuses on lung sounds as they are reported by patients (or by their guardians in the case of young children) and as a sign noted on chest auscultation performed with the stethoscope. Respiratory complaints are frequently the cause that brings a patient to the doctor, and the respiratory system is the most commonly affected organ system in clinical practice. Consequently, respiratory sounds, either heard at a distance or auscultated over the chest, are integral to the evaluation of patients and may provide valuable clues. It may be worthwhile to remember that the various respiratory diseases present to the physician with a disappointingly limited "vocabulary." Thus, it may be worth keeping in mind the respect owed to clinicians who, in a variety of situations and in different languages, with only few and incomplete objective markers, find their way to patient diagnosis and to communicating their findings, in order to teach respiratory medicine.

The stethoscope has practical and symbolic value for the general physician and the pulmonologist alike. Auscultation provides valuable information about physical examination [1–3]. The binaural stethoscope is favored by most physicians and can adequately serve the specialist. When pressed firmly on the skin, the diaphragm of the headpiece filters out the lower frequencies and allows for better perception of

S. Fouzas, M.D., Ph.D. · M. B. Anthracopoulos, M.D., Ph.D. (✉)
Department of Pediatrics, University Hospital of Patras, Patras, Greece
e-mail: sfouzas@gmail.com; manthra@med.upatras.com; manthra@otenet.gr

A. Bohadana, M.D.
Pulmonary Institute, Shaare Zedek Medical Center, Jerusalem, Israel
e-mail: abohadana@szmc.org.il

K. N. Priftis et al. (eds.), *Breath Sounds*, https://doi.org/10.1007/978-3-319-71824-8_3

high-pitched sounds. Conversely, the bell should be applied lightly—to avoid stretching the skin—in order to select for lower frequencies. Appropriately sized chest pieces should be selected, according to the chest dimension. To have noncooperating patients, particularly infants, assume a straight position and young children cooperate for proper auscultation is an art; still, it may not always be possible to listen adequately over all lung segments. The upper lobes are best auscultated over the upper anterior chest, lower lobe sounds are best heard over the posterior lower chest, and the middle lobe and lingula are best represented on the respective sides of the lower third of the sternum. Over the lateral chest in the axillae, all lobes can be auscultated [1–3].

Air movement in the chest generates respiratory sounds, whether normal or adventitious. Respiratory sounds can be heard at several points including the mouth, the trachea, and, of course, the chest cage. Other sounds such as grunting, snoring, snuffling, and voice-transmitted sounds, although not strictly respiratory in origin, may accompany adventitious sounds and are also discussed. Cough is usually not considered as a breath sound; it is addressed in a separate chapter in this volume. Distinguishing between respiratory sounds is often difficult. Their characteristics and the pathogenesis of adventitious sounds will be briefly addressed as deemed necessary [4–10], while detailed discussions on their specific acoustic properties, nomenclature, and current research prospects are discussed in other chapters of this volume.

3.2 Normal Breath Sounds

Normal breath sounds are characterized by a broad frequency spectrum that ranges according to the location of auscultation. Muscle sounds are very-low-intensity sounds related to the contraction of thoracic skeletal muscles, which mesh into the normal breath sound spectrum. Their frequency is too low for them to be perceived by the human ear. *Tracheal sound* is heard over the extrathoracic trachea and constitutes a broad-spectrum noise (usually up to 1000 Hz) with short inspiratory and longer expiratory duration. *Vesicular breath sound* (a misnomer as it does not originate in the vesicles, i.e., the alveoli) is a quiet, low-frequency (usually up to 400 Hz), non-musical sound auscultated over the chest during inspiration and hardly audible during normal expiration (Fig. 3.1). Finally, the *bronchial sound* is of intermediate frequency, auscultated over the upper anterior chest wall, of higher frequency and intensity than vesicular sound, and of approximately equal duration in inspiration and expiration [3–6].

3.3 Adventitious Breath Sounds

These are superimposed upon normal breath sounds and are usually associated with pulmonary disorders. They are primarily divided into musical, continuous sounds and non-musical, discontinuous sounds. A third category includes mixed sounds [9, 10].

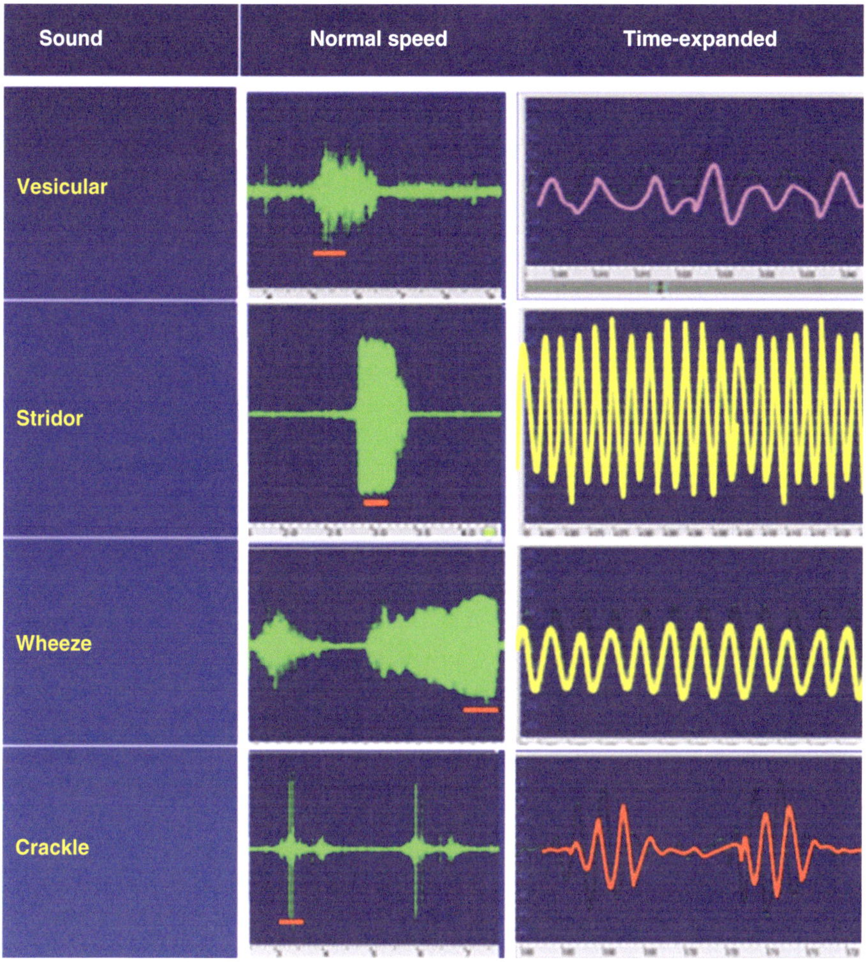

Fig. 3.1 Waveform of selected breath sounds. Amplitude (measured in arbitrary units)-time (measured in seconds) plots of basic breath sounds in unexpanded (i.e., recorded at normal speed) and time-expanded modes (i.e., recorded at high speed). The unexpanded plot contains screenshots of the entire sound with the horizontal line showing where the time-expanded section was obtained. All tracings start by inspiration. Vesicular sound has strong inspiratory component relative to the expiratory component; the time-expanded waveform shows random fluctuations of sound amplitude typical of non-musical sounds. The unexpanded waveform of the stridor has strong inspiratory component, while that of wheeze has strong expiratory component. On expanded mode, the two sounds show sinusoidal oscillations typical of musical sounds, with the lower frequency of the wheeze being evident by the lower number of oscillations per unit of time. The unexpanded plots of fine crackles appear as two vertical spikes in the middle of the inspiratory phase corresponding to rapidly dampened wave deflections seen only in the unexpanded waveform

3.3.1 Musical Sounds

3.3.1.1 Stridor

Stridor is a continuous (musical), monophonic, high-pitched sound, which can be usually heard without a stethoscope, especially during inspiration (Fig. 3.1). It is caused by oscillations of narrowed large, extrathoracic airways, and its presence suggests significant obstruction of airflow within the larynx and/or the extrathoracic portion of the trachea [2, 4, 6, 11, 12].

The generation of stridor can be explained by the dynamics of high-flow inspiration/expiration and the Bernoulli principle which, simply put, states that the pressure exerted by moving fluid in a tube decreases as its velocity (kinetic energy) increases [2, 11, 12]. Inspiration generates negative (relative to the atmospheric) intrapleural pressure, which in continuum is applied to the external surface of the extrathoracic airway wall. In normal individuals, this results in minimal collapse which is not clinically important. If the airway is partially obstructed, there is a disproportionally larger drop in the intraluminal pressure as a consequence of the function of the inspiratory muscles in order to overcome the obstruction. This pressure drop is further augmented by the turbulent flow through the "constricted" laryngeal/tracheal tube due to the Bernoulli principle, causing further deterioration of the narrowed airway. It is evident that a "floppy" extrathoracic airway will deteriorate the collapse even further. The Bernoulli effect, which also contributes to the intraluminal pressure drop, is most likely of primary importance to the dynamic consequences of this phenomenon, i.e., the vibrations of the airway wall that are responsible for the creation of this particular sound. On the other hand, expiration induces a positive intraluminal pressure in the extrathoracic airway, which tends to distend the extrathoracic airway, alleviate the tracheal obstruction, and reduce expiratory flow resistance. These mechanisms explain why stridor is predominantly inspiratory; however, it can also be present during expiration if the obstruction is severe enough. They also make evident the reason why stridor is more common in infants and young preschoolers, whose airways are more collapsible than those of adults.

Assessment: The history and physical examination should seek information on past manipulation of the extrathoracic airway (intubation, tracheotomy, etc.), persistence of stridor (chronic vs. acute), type of onset (abrupt vs. gradual), timing during the respiratory cycle, accompanying symptoms (fever, coryza), hoarse and/or weak cry, cyanotic episodes, positional differences in the intensity of noise, interval symptoms between episodes, and severity of respiratory distress [2, 11, 12].

Common causes of stridor in adults and children are shown in Table 3.1. In children, the most common cause of acute stridor is viral croup, which usually presents at the age range of 6 months to 6 years with stridor accompanied by hoarseness, dry barking cough, and respiratory distress. It is usually preceded by coryza and improves within a few days. It accounts for more than 90% of all cases of stridor in children. Most episodes are mild, and only a minority of children require hospitalization. The airway obstruction is due to subglottic edema, and, on most occasions, stridor is audible only during inspiration, although it can be biphasic in severe

Table 3.1 Clinical relevance of stridor

1. *Inspiratory* (Extrathoracic lesion: rhinopharyngeal, oropharyngeal, laryngeal, tracheal):
• Acute obstruction (viral croup, supraglottitis, bacterial tracheitis, anaphylaxis)
• Congenital nasal, nasopharyngeal atresia/stenosis, congenital subglottic stenosis, laryngeal web, laryngeal cleft
• Enlarged adenoids, tumor (polyp, cyst/cystic hygroma, glossal thyroid gland, teratoma, papilloma, neurofibroma, sarcoma)
• Foreign body
• Trauma, posttraumatic (tracheostomy) granuloma, post-extubation subglottic stenosis
• Vocal cord paralysis
• Malacia (laryngo-, tracheo-)
• Gastroesophageal reflux/aspiration
• Vocal cord paralysis, hypocalcemic tetany, generalized hypotonia
2. *Expiratory* (Intrathoracic large airway lesion: tracheal, bronchial; mimics asthma):
• Intrinsic airway obstruction (tumor, foreign body)
• Extrinsic compression (enlarged lymph node, tumor, arterial vessel, or vascular ring)
• Malacia (traceo-, broncho-)
3. *Biphasic* (glottic/subglottic lesion, severe fixed obstruction)
• Laryngeal masses
• Bilateral VC paralysis
• Vocal cord dysfunction
• Subglottic stenosis (e.g., post-extubation, hemangioma)

disease. Other quite exceptional infectious causes of acute stridor are epiglottitis and bacterial tracheitis [2, 11, 12].

Foreign body aspiration should always be suspected whenever the beginning of stridor is abrupt, does not occur as part of viral airway illness, and is accompanied by severe respiratory distress. Rigid bronchoscopy is used for the visualization of the airways but also for the removal of the foreign body [2, 11, 12].

The most common cause of chronic stridor in infancy is laryngomalacia and/or tracheomalacia of the extrathoracic trachea. It usually manifests weeks after birth (only severe cases present within few days postpartum), and symptoms usually resolve by 12–18 months. The noise varies in intensity depending on the respiratory effort and varies with the position of the patient. The obstruction is due to the prolapse of the epiglottis or the loose mucosal tissue overlying the arytenoid cartilages into the laryngeal inlet. Laryngeal walls collapse due to the subatmospheric pressure generated during inspiration. On expiration, the positive luminal pressure overcomes the obstruction, thus keeping the airway open; therefore, if there is expiratory stridor, an alternative diagnosis needs to be sought [2, 11, 12].

Intermittent, sudden-onset, daytime episodes of stridor in school-aged children, adolescents, and young adults may indicate vocal cord dysfunction (VCD). In this condition the vocal cords assume a paradoxical, adducted (instead of abducted) position during inspiration. Patients may present with significant inspiratory stridor and respiratory distress. Symptoms usually appear during exercise, especially in highly competitive young athletes, but may also appear without any identifiable cause. Spirometry should include an inspiratory maneuver, which may reveal "truncated" inspiratory and expiratory flow-volume loops. Definitive diagnosis can be set only by witnessing the paradoxical movement of the vocal cords during laryngoscopy or bronchoscopy [2, 11, 12].

For acute episodes of stridor that are typical of croup, there is no need for investigations other than clinical evaluation. However, children who have unusually prolonged or recurrent episodes or are not completely asymptomatic between episodes and children younger than 6 months of age require evaluation with laryngoscopy or bronchoscopy (Table 3.1) [2, 11]. In infants with chronic inspiratory stridor who are thriving and do not have significant respiratory distress, cyanotic episodes, chronic cough, hoarseness, or weak cry, the most likely diagnosis is laryngomalacia, and there is no need for further investigations. However, if any of the above characteristics is present, a more thorough investigation is in order. Direct visualization with a laryngoscope will reveal the presence of structural abnormalities in the upper airways. Furthermore, since abnormalities of the upper airways often coexist with lower airway pathology, bronchoscopy of the trachea and the bronchial tree is considered to be an essential part of the investigation.

3.3.1.2 Wheeze

Wheeze is probably the respiratory sound term most widely used by physicians and the general public, albeit with dismal specificity. From the physics point of view, it is characterized by periodic waveforms, i.e., it is continuous and of musical quality (Fig. 3.1). Although wheeze may entail a wide range of frequencies, in clinical practice it implies a musical sound with a high dominant frequency. Lower-frequency wheezes have different pathogenesis and are often termed rhonchi (see below). In general, wheezes are louder than normal breath sounds and may be audible at the patient's mouth or without a stethoscope, at a distance. They are better transmitted through the airways rather than through the lung to the thoracic surface, and their higher frequencies are better or solely transmitted over the trachea [3–6].

Wheeze is of great clinical value as it is most commonly associated with airway obstruction due to various mechanisms, e.g., bronchoconstriction, airway wall edema, intraluminal obstruction (e.g., foreign body, mass), external compression (e.g., mass, anomalous arterial vessel), or dynamic airway collapse; the latter is termed tracheo- or bronchomalacia and is most often encountered in infants and young preschoolers. Prediction models, particularly "the fluid dynamic flutter theory," have shown that expiratory wheeze in healthy subjects during forced expiration always signifies flow limitation resulting in the vibration of the airway wall at the site of airflow limitation due to the dissipation of conserved energy when the driving pressure gradient exceeds that required to achieve maximal flow. However, its absence does not preclude airflow limitation [11, 13–15]. The mechanism of generation of inspiratory wheezes, often associated with more pronounced obstruction, is even less clear. The mechanics of interdependence in inhomogeneous regional lung emptying are discussed elsewhere [16]. It appears that wheeze may also be produced by turbulent flow-induced airway wall vibration, without flow limitation [5].

Although, in theory, wheezing can arise from all conducting airways, it requires a minimum airflow which practically restricts the site of its production to the large- and medium-sized airways. It is common experience that wheezing is audible in cases of diffuse extensive airway narrowing, as is the case with asthma. This is most likely the result of high pleural pressures generated during expiration in order to overcome the narrowing of the small airways and the resultant air trapping; such large pressure gradients cause—via this indirect mechanism—collapse of larger intrathoracic airways with unstable airway wall geometry (e.g., bronchomalacia). Since the sound is produced by a multitude of airway walls throughout the lungs, the wheeze consists of a wide range of distinct harmonics (of differing acoustic characteristics) and is therefore termed "polyphonic." Conversely, when the musical sound is generated by one or few, at the most, large airways (e.g., stenosis, foreign body), it consists of a much more limited number of harmonics and is termed "monophonic." The "focal" nature of the generation of the monophonic wheeze may explain the decrease of its loudness with increasing distance between the site of auscultation and the sound source (i.e., obstruction). It is obvious that the qualitative distinction of wheezes into polyphonic and monophonic may prove of great value in orienting the physician as to the cause of airway obstruction [12].

Assessment: Wheeze is the most common term reported by patients (or guardians of young children) to describe noisy breathing when obtaining medical history [17, 18] and in questionnaire surveys [19–25]. Acoustic analysis of breath sounds [26, 27] and the differential response of wheezes and coarse crackles to ipratropium bromide have verified that these two types of breath sounds are quite distinct and should, therefore, be recognized as such by physicians and epidemiologists [28]. Interestingly, the vagueness of the meaning of the word "wheeze" seems to be deeply rooted in linguistic lineages since both the words "cough" and "wheeze" probably stem from the Indo-European root *kwes*, which also means "to pant" and was passed on to Middle English (1150–1550 AD) as *whesen*. *Kasa*, the Sanskrit word for cough, apparently also stems from *kwes*, thus linking etymologically wheeze with cough [29].

The most common cause of intermittent episodes of polyphonic wheeze is asthma. A prompt response to bronchodilators, as well as a personal and/or family history of atopy, may help to differentiate viral wheeze from asthma. Simple noninterventional studies like chest X-ray, allergy testing, and spirometry may be useful, while more elaborate studies are usually not necessary [11].

Acute onset of monophonic wheeze raises the possibility of foreign body aspiration. In young children, the absence of a choking event does not rule out foreign body aspiration since in about 15% of cases a clear history of such an episode is not reported. Monophonic progressive wheeze implies either a focal endobronchial lesion (endobronchial TB, adenoma) or extraluminal compression of central airways due to lymph node or other mass and should always prompt further investigation [2, 11, 12]. In general, monophonic wheeze needs a thorough investigation with chest X-ray, flexible bronchoscopy, and/or CT scan. If foreign body aspiration is a strong possibility, urgent rigid bronchoscopy should be carried out, while mere suspicion should prompt investigation of the airways with the flexible bronchoscope. Nevertheless, some interventional bronchoscopists opt for the use of the flexible instrument to extract foreign bodies from the airways, particularly of adults and older children.

There is a loose positive correlation between the proportion of wheeze detected through the respiratory cycle and the severity of obstruction. In adult asthmatic patients, biphasic wheeze of high pitch and moderate to high intensity was associated with decreased peak expiratory flow (PEF) values; however, these clinical characteristics cannot substitute for objective spirometry parameters in the evaluation of such patients [30]. Others have shown that patient-reported wheeze in combination with duration of smoking, when associated with wheeze auscultated on physical examination, can adequately predict diagnosis of obstructive airways disease [31, 32]. Studies in adults also reveal that breath sound intensity scoring may be useful in the detection and quantification of airflow obstruction [33], while auscultation of wheeze in adults [34] and children [35–37] may be useful, alone or in combination with other respiratory signs, in the interpretation of airway challenge testing. More accurate identification by acoustic analysis of wheeze and breath sound intensity scoring has confirmed the agreement between auscultated wheeze and sound recordings and can help to simplify bronchial provocation testing and to further improve its positive predictive value [38, 39]. On the other hand, it should be remembered that wheezing is only of relative importance in the clinical severity scoring of asthma exacerbation and acute bronchiolitis [40, 41]. Common causes of wheeze sounds in adults and children are shown in Table 3.2.

3.3.1.3 Rhonchus

A *rhonchus* (plural: *rhonchi*) is a low-pitched continuous (musical) sound that phonographically consists of rapidly dampened sinusoids. It is a variant of wheeze, often termed low-pitched wheeze [9, 10]. Its mechanism of production is similar to that of wheezes, but on occasion it disappears after coughing and clearing of airway secretions. However, the term has also been used for expiratory "gurgling or

Table 3.2 Clinical relevance of wheeze

1. *Generalized*
• Asthma
• COPD
• Bronchiectasis
• Heart failure
• Infections (e.g., croup, whooping cough, tracheobronchitis)
• Bronchorrheal states (e.g., cystic fibrosis, primary ciliary dyskinesia, protracted bacterial bronchitis)
2. *Localized*
• Fictitious asthma
• Foreign body
• Tumor

bubbling sounds" originating in the large airways (i.e., what most authorities would term "coarse expiratory crackles" (see below) [3, 8]; therefore, when used, it should be done so with caution.

3.3.2 Non-musical Sounds

3.3.2.1 Crackles

Crackles (other terms in use are "rales" and "crepitations") are adventitious discontinuous (non-musical) sounds that may be auscultated in the two phases of the respiratory cycle that represent local phenomena. Crackles are classified according to their waveform, duration, and timing in the respiratory cycle [9, 10]. Fine crackles (also known as "crepitant" crackles) are short explosive sounds characterized by high pitch, low intensity, and short duration (Fig. 3.1). Inspiratory fine crackles are caused by the explosive opening of small airways collapsed by surface forces (increased elastic lung recoil pressure or inflammation/edema in the lung). The currently prevailing theory holds that the pressure gradient applied across collapsed airway walls at the beginning of inspiration causes them to "snap open," thus causing rapid pressure equalization and propagation of a pressure wave [42]. This theory is supported by measurements, which show that the timing of any individual crackle is closely correlated with a particular transpulmonary pressure [43]. Further support—albeit through different reasoning—is offered by the mathematical "hypothesis of stress relaxation quadruples" [44]; this concept postulates that it is the dynamic events in the airway wall and their surroundings—and not pressure gradients—that generate the sound waveform of a crackle which then propagates away from its site of origin. The stress-relaxation quadruples hypothesis predicts the existence of both inspiratory and expiratory crackles, that the energy of expiratory crackles should be substantially smaller than that of inspiratory crackles, that the polarity of the acoustic signal of the crackles should be both positive and negative in both phases of respiration, and, finally, that negative polarity crackles should heavily predominate during inspiration, while positive polarity crackles should predominate during expiration. These predictions of the stress-relaxation quadruples hypothesis have been tested and found to be true [45]. At any event, crackles occur in case of an increase in the elastic recoil of the lung or when there is edema/inflammation of the airway wall; smaller airways appear to produce crackles of shorter duration. Fine crackles are gravity dependent, and the sound is rarely transmitted to the mouth.

Coarse (termed by some "subcrepitant") crackles are sounds of low pitch, high intensity, and long duration. They are more scanty than fine crackles, gravity independent, and usually audible at the mouth. They are generated by a different mechanism than that of fine crackles, i.e., by the movement of thin secretions in the bronchi or the bronchioles. They start early and continue until mid-inspiration but may also be heard during expiration [3, 46]. Fine and course crackles may coexist.

Assessment: Fine late inspiratory crackles are typical of interstitial/fibrotic lung disease. They may also be present in normal subjects who inhale slowly from residual lung volume, which can be explained by the mechanism of their generation, as

Table 3.3 Clinical relevance of crackles

• Pulmonary fibrosis
• Sarcoidosis
• Asbestosis
• Congestive heart failure
• Chronic obstructive pulmonary disease (COPD)
• Pneumonia
• Bronchorrheal states, bronchiectasis

already described. However, in this case the crackles disappear after a few deep breaths [4, 42–46]. The typical example of coarse crackles is bronchiectasis and chronic airway obstruction (e.g., cystic fibrosis) [2, 3, 11, 12]. Similar auscultatory findings can be found focally early in pneumonia; however, they eventually shift toward end-inspiratory crackles of variable duration that progress to fine crackles during recovery. Acoustic analysis has characterized the crackles of cardiac failure as coarse, of long duration during inspiration, and appearing late in the course of the disease [2]. Common causes of crackles are shown in Table 3.3.

Community-acquired pneumonia is an important cause of respiratory symptoms. Distinguishing pneumonia from acute bronchitis and upper respiratory tract infection is an important but often difficult task, and there are no clinical findings which, individually or in combination, can rule in the diagnosis in a patient suspected of having pneumonia [47–49]. In a prospective study of adult patients with symptoms of lower respiratory tract infection, unilateral crackles and crackles in the lateral decubitus position stood out as the most valuable clinical findings in detecting pneumonia [50]. In children, especially infants and preschoolers with lower respiratory tract illness, there is better doctor agreement on signs that can be observed (retractions, respiratory rate, color, attentiveness) than auscultatory findings; normal clinical signs (respiratory rate, auscultation, work of breathing) render the radiographic diagnosis of pneumonia unlikely [51]. Research with computerized respiratory sound analysis (CORSA) of crackles, which includes calculation of crackle transmission coefficient and observes the CORSA guidelines, showed crackles' characteristics that appear promising in eventually achieving acoustic differentiation of patients with pulmonary fibrosis, pneumonia, and heart failure [52, 53].

3.3.3 Mixed Sound

The squawk is a "composite" short inspiratory wheeze that is preceded by a crackle. It is thought to result from the vibrations set in motion by the sudden opening of a collapsed airway. Squawks were first described in hypersensitivity pneumonitis, but they are not pathognomonic of this condition and can be found in any pulmonary fibrosing disease, including various causes of "autoimmune" interstitial fibrosis, radiation pneumonitis, and, of course, hypersensitivity pneumonitis. They can also be present in cases of pneumonia; they tend to be audible (but not exclusively) at the site of radiographic opacity and have actually been described to predate the radiographic lesion. In general, squawks are not associated with airway obstruction; however, they have occasionally been described in asthmatic patients [3, 54].

3.3.4 Pleural Friction Rub

The pleural friction rub resembles coarse crackles (often described as "leathery"); however, on occasion, its non-musical components are abundant and the accoustic impression may be that of a continuous sound. It is generated by the friction of inflamed parietal and visceral pleura causing vibration of the chest wall and local pulmonary parenchyma. It can be auscultated during inspiration or in both phases of breathing. Pleural friction rub usually precedes pleural effusion and disappears when fluid is formed. The "rub" is synchronous to breathing and does not disappear with cough but is modified by the breathing pattern and posture [2, 3].

3.4 Voice-Transmitted Sounds

Voice sounds are auscultatory sounds obtained when the individual who is being evaluated is asked to voice words or particular vowels. In normal condition, the peaks in the harmonic spectrum of the vowels—termed formants—are filtered by the lung parenchyma so that speech becomes indistinct (i.e., perceived as an incomprehensible "mumble") when auscultated over the chest. When there is underlying consolidation or compression, this filtering effect disappears, and the higher frequencies of the vowels formants are effectively transmitted. By consequence, normally spoken syllables become distinct during auscultation; this is termed *bronchophony*. *Whispered pectoriloquy* is an unusually clear transmission of whispered sounds during auscultation in cases of severe consolidation or compression. *Egophony* is a similar change in transmission but has a nasal quality with a change of "e" sound to "a" [3, 8].

3.5 Noisy Breathing

Noisy breathing is a loose term which refers to adventitious sounds heard from a distance (rather than through the stethoscope). It includes stridor and wheezing (already described above) and other "abnormal" breathing sounds such as grunting, snuffling, ruttling, and snoring.

3.5.1 Grunt

It is an expiratory sound produced by vocal cord adduction in children, thus creating a natural form of continuous positive airway pressure (CPAP) aimed at improving oxygenation in the presence of airway distress [11, 12]. It is considered to be the equivalent of "pursed-lip breathing" in adults with serious chronic respiratory disease. Grunting signifies extensive alveolar pathology and is particularly seen in hyaline membrane disease in neonates and in serious bacterial disease, particularly pneumonia, in previously healthy children older than 3 months [11, 12, 55].

3.5.2 Snuffle

Snuffle (or snort) is the noise produced by (partially) blocked nasal passages throughout the entire breathing cycle. Thus, it is often used to refer to the common cold or simply a runny nose and is often associated with visible nasal secretions. Other than upper respiratory tract infection, snuffle may also indicate allergic rhinitis or, on a rare occasion, primary ciliary dyskinesia (especially when present within the first hours of life) and nasal polyps as in cystic fibrosis (particularly when present before the age of 12 years) [11, 12].

3.5.3 Ruttle

Ruttles (or rattles) are the non-auscultatory equivalent of coarse crackles heard by the physician or reported in the medical history. They are characterized by a "ruttling" noncontinuous quality, are usually accompanied by chest wall vibrations that are easily detectable by feeling the patient's chest, and may occur during both inspiration and expiration [2, 11, 12]. Ruttles are found quite often in infants and toddlers, and although there is paucity of data in the literature regarding the underlying mechanism, they are believed to be created by excessive secretions which move during normal airflow within the central, including the extrathoracic, airways. The mislabelling of a ruttle as wheeze results in overdiagnosis [17, 18, 26–28] and consequently in overtreatment of asthma [17–24, 26], particularly in children [2, 11, 12]. The most common cause of ruttles is acute viral bronchitis and, in young children, upper airway viral infection. Ruttle can be heard for a few days or weeks and usually subsides after the removal of secretions from cough and mucociliary clearance. Chronic ruttling sound is often related to chronic aspiration in patients with various neuromuscular diseases [2, 11, 12].

3.5.4 Snore

Snore is the most usual symptom linked to the obstructive sleep apnea-hypopnea syndrome (OSAHS) which, in turn, is associated with significant morbidity, including daytime somnolence, behavioral and personality changes, hypertension, cor pulmonale, and cerebrovascular morbidity in adults. Its prevalence climbs to 63% in males and 44% in females after the age of 40 years, and its presence may in fact represent the first stage of the OSAHS [56, 57]. Although absence of a history of snoring does not exclude a diagnosis of OSAHS, virtually all patients with this diagnosis snore [57]. Up to 50% of children will experience a sleep problem, but only 1–5% of them will be diagnosed with OSAHS; the reported prevalence of snoring ranges 5–20% [58–60].

Snore is a sound that is produced during sleep from the increase in resistance to the airflow in the upper airways in the region of the nasopharynx and oropharynx and more specifically from the vibration of the soft palate and adjacent tissues [61, 62];

indeed, flow oscillation during simulated snoring has been demonstrated [61]. The cross-sectional area of the oropharynx, which is the most usually collapsible segment, mainly determines upper airway patency during sleep, but the nose/nasopharynx and the tongue also contribute. Three constrictor and two dilator pharyngeal muscles (the muscles of the soft palate, the muscles of the posterior tongue, and the pharyngeal uvular muscles) regulate the "pharyngeal duct patency." Snoring is a function of five contributing factors: sleep, flow limitation, vibrating structures, reduced upper airway cross-sectional area, and effective respiratory pump [62].

During rapid eye movement (REM), sleep pharyngeal muscle tone is reduced, thus resulting in the increase of the frequency and severity of obstruction [11, 12]. Snoring is more pronounced on inspiration, but it can also be audible during expiration. Using acoustic analysis characteristics of snores, attempts have been made to differentiate snoring patients with occlusive sleep apnea from those without (i.e., "primary snoring") [63]. Thus, the severity of snoring ranges from primary snoring with no evidence of ventilation abnormalities to severe obstructive sleep apnea-hypopnea syndrome (OSAHS) with disordered gas exchange, which leads to hypoxemia and/or hypercapnia with frequent nocturnal arousals [11, 12, 64]. The spectrum of these disorders is characterized as obstructive sleep-disordered breathing (SDB) [11, 58, 65]. Children who snore tend to have more collapsible airways and increased size of adenotonsillar tissue [56–58, 65].

Assessment: The main concern in the evaluation of snoring is to define those patients who may suffer health consequences related to the pathology underlying this breath sound; however, this may prove to be difficult both in adults [64] and in children [11, 59, 65]. OSAHS cannot be diagnosed simply on the grounds of a history of snoring since not all patients who snore have OSAHS. On the other hand, the absence of snoring is not sufficient to exclude OSAHS as the partners or the parents may not have noticed the snoring of the patient in question. Furthermore, there is some evidence suggesting that the so-called primary snoring, i.e., heavy snoring without objective evidence that fulfills the requirements to diagnose OSAHS, may not be completely benign [56, 58].

A detailed history can be very helpful. Patients who suffer from OSAHS snore almost every night, their snoring usually persists throughout night sleep, and there are frequent apneic episodes followed by loud snorts and changes in position. They may suffer from daytime tiredness, poor concentration, and enuresis. Behavior and learning problems (including attention-deficit hyperactivity disorder) are not unusual in children. Obesity and craniofacial anomalies in adults and children, prematurity, and family history of snoring are all well-known risk factors for OSAHS [11, 58–60, 64, 65]. In children, clinical examination may reveal adenoidal facies, enlarged tonsils, or hyponasal speech [11, 58–60, 65]. However, history and clinical examination are not sufficient to reliably diagnose or rule out OSAHS, and definitive diagnosis relies on polysomnography, which is considered the gold standard for evaluating children for obstructive SDB [11, 58–60, 64, 65]. Unfortunately, this method is complex, expensive, and time-consuming, and these drawbacks restrict its usefulness to a rather limited number of specialized centers.

3.6 Clinical Cases

Case 1: Silence May Not Be Golden

History: A 27-year-old, non-smoking woman with a history of moderate, persistent asthma presents to the emergency room with progressive worsening of shortness of breath, wheezing, and cough over the past 3 days. Her symptoms worsened considerably despite increased use of her rescue inhaler. Her current medication includes salbutamol *prn* and an inhaled corticosteroid for maintenance therapy.

Clinical examination

Parameter	Arrival	20′ later
Dyspnea	++	+++
Talks in	Phrases	Words
Alertness	Agitated	Drowsy; sweaty
RR breaths/min	20	33
Pulse/min	110	140
AM; SS retraction	Yes	Usually
PEFR L/min (% predicted)	246 (50%)	Not measurable
SpO_2%	88% RA	90% 4 LO_2/min
Breath (vesicular) sounds	Diminished	Silent
Adventitious sounds	Wheezes	Silent

Comment: This case illustrates the importance of lung auscultation in the acute setting. Upon arrival, this patient had diminished breath sounds (vesicular murmur) accompanied by inspiratory and expiratory wheezes scattered over the chest. This finding is consistent with diffuse airway obstruction. Twenty minutes later, despite treatment, her condition deteriorated considerably. The disappearance of wheezes combined with the severe decrease of breath sound intensity is an ominous sign indicating severe airway obstruction necessitating prompt medical intervention. The reappearance, 2 h later, of wheezes, along with an increase in breath sound intensity during inspiration, indicated improvement in airway ventilation with decrease of airflow obstruction.

Case 2: All that Wheezes Is Not a Wheeze

History: A 35-year-old woman presented to the emergency room with a history of acute respiratory distress for 48 h. For the past 8 years, she was on salbutamol and inhaled corticosteroids because of asthma. Over this time, she took frequent short courses of oral corticosteroids for asthma exacerbation. In addition, she reported a history of three hospital admissions for respiratory distress attributed to asthma.

Clinical examination: On examination, she was apprehensive, sitting upright, and using the accessory muscles of respiration. Her pulse rate was 120 bpm, BP 140/80 mmHg, and SpO_2 93% on RA. A physical sign prompted the request of a flow-volume curve.

Comment: The sign was an inspiratory stridor, well heard without the stethoscope. The intensity of breath sounds over the chest was normal. The flow-volume curve depicted below displays an inspiratory plateau typical of variable extrathoracic obstruction. Upon fibroscopy, a paradoxical closure of vocal cords was seen in inspiration compatible with the diagnosis of vocal cord dysfunction. The patient was referred for speech therapy, and deep breathing techniques and asthma treatment were discontinued.

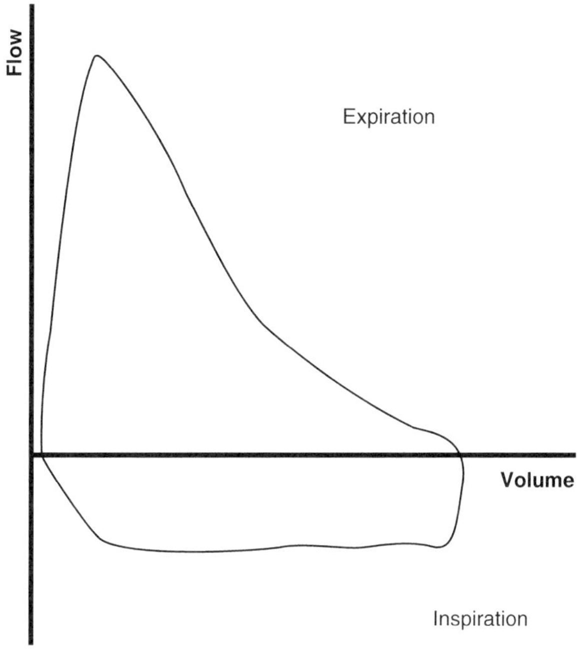

Case 3: All that Wheezes Is Not Asthma

History: A 10-year-old boy presents to the emergency room with acute respiratory distress which started at school 1 h ago. He reports sudden cough and shortness of breath while attending his class. He has been diagnosed with asthma, which is well controlled on low-dose inhaled corticosteroids.

Clinical examination: The patient appears frightened. He is tachypneic (45 breaths per min) with a heart rate of 110 beats per min and SpO_2 92%. On auscultation he has monophonic wheeze audible over the right lung. His chest X-ray (shown below) demonstrates hyperinflation of the right lung. He was referred to ENT, and the small plastic top of a ballpoint pen was removed from the right main stem bronchus by rigid bronchoscopy.

Comment: This case highlights the importance of differentiating monophonic from polyphonic wheeze. The latter is typical of diffuse airway obstruction, which is consistent with the diagnosis of asthma. Conversely, monophonic wheeze, especially when unilateral, signifies obstruction of a large intrathoracic airway. Upon repeat questioning of the child, it was revealed that he had a choking episode while chewing on his pen.

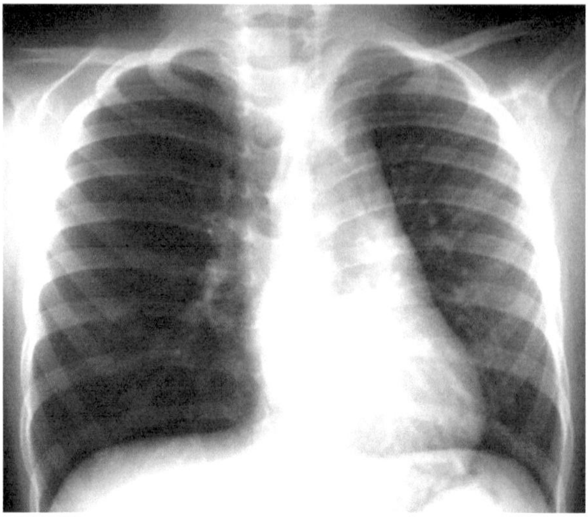

Case 4: Mind the... Heart

History: A 6-year-old Caucasian boy is referred for persistent wet cough for 9 weeks. His mother reports similar episodes in the past 3–4 years, mostly during the cold months, which have been treated with short courses of inhaled bronchodilators and corticosteroids and occasionally with antibiotics. She also reports "continuous ruttling over the chest and stuffy nose" as well as multiple episodes of acute otitis media. A recent sweat test showed normal chloride levels.

Clinical examination: On chest auscultation diffuse coarse crackles were noted over both lung fields. Notably, the heart sounds were loudest on the right side. The chest X-ray (shown below) revealed situs inversus and diffuse peribronchial thickening bilaterally ("dirty lung") with scant small consolidations at the base of the upper lobe on the left.

Comment: This is a case of primary ciliary dyskinesia with situs inversus (Kartagener's syndrome). Episodes of persistent wet cough with ruttling and coarse crackles in a child should alert the physician on the possibility of a serious underlying disease. In this case, careful auscultation of the chest—including the auscultation of heart sounds—would have led to the prompt diagnosis of this rare disorder. Also, attention should be paid to the proper right-left orientation of the chest film.

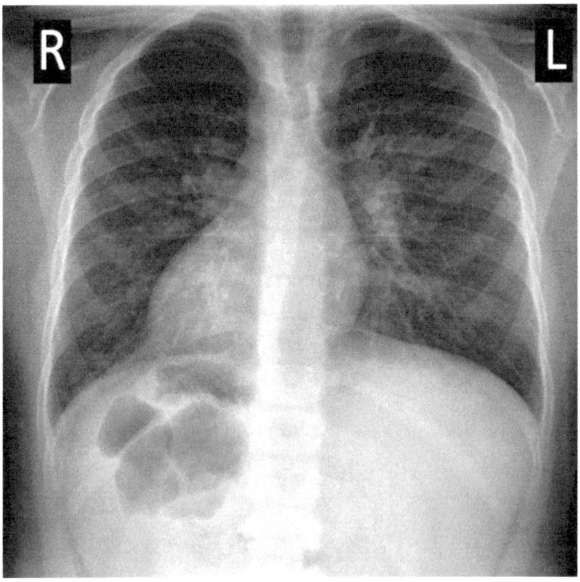

References

1. DeGowin EL (ed) (1987) Bedside diagnostic examination: a comprehensive pocket textbook. Macmillan, New York
2. Brown AM, von Mutius E, Morgan WJ (2008) Clinical assessment and diagnostic approach to common problems. In: Taussig LM, Landau LI, LeSouëf PN, Martinez FD, Morgan WJ, Sly PD (eds) Pediatric respiratory medicine, 2nd edn. Mosby-Elsevier, Philadelphia, pp 491–499
3. Anthracopoulos MB, Douros K, Priftis KN (2013) History and physical examination. In: Eber E, Midulla F (eds) ERS handbook paediatric respiratory medicine. HERMES ERS, Lausanne, pp 33–43
4. Bohadana A, Izbicki G, Kraman SS (2014) Fundamentals of lung auscultation. N Engl J Med 370(8):744–751
5. Pasterkamp H, Kraman SS, Wodicka GR (1997) Respiratory sounds: advances beyond the stethoscope. Am J Respir Crit Care Med 156(3 Pt 1):974–987
6. Pasterkamp H (2012) The history and physical examination. In: Wilmott RW, Boat TF, Bush A, Chernick V, Deterding RR, Ratjen F (eds) Kendig and Chernick's disorders of the respiratory tract in children, 8th edn. Elsevier-WB Saunders, Philadelphia, pp 110–130
7. Dalmay F, Antonini MT, Marquet P, Menier R (1995) Acoustic properties of the normal chest. Eur Respir J 8(10):1761–1769
8. Sovijärvi AR, Dalmasso F, Vanderschoot J, Righini G, Stoneman SA (2000) Definition of terms for applications of respiratory sounds. Eur Respir Rev 10(77):597–610
9. Pasterkamp H, Brand PL, Everard M, Garcia-Marcos L, Melbye H, Priftis KN (2016) Towards standardisation of lung sound nomenclature. Eur Respir J 47(3):724–732
10. Melbye H, Garcia-Marcos L, Brand P, Everard M, Priftis K, Pasterkamp H (2016) Wheezes crackles and rhonchi: simplifying description of lung sounds increases the agreement on their classification: a study of 12 physicians' classification of lung sounds from video recordings. BMJ Open Respir Res 3(1):e000136

11. Priftis KN, Douros K, Anthracopoulos MB (2013) Snoring hoarseness, stridor and wheezing. In: Eber E, Midulla F (eds) ERS handbook paediatric respiratory medicine. HERMES ERS, Lausanne, pp 57–64
12. Mellis C (2008) Respiratory noises: how useful are they clinically? Pediatr Clin N Am 56(1):1–17
13. Meslier N, Charbonneau G, Racineux JL (1995) Wheezes. Eur Respir J 8(11):1942–1948
14. Grotberg JB, Gavriely N (1989) Flutter in collapsible tubes: a theoretical model of wheezes. J Appl Physiol 66(5):2262–2273
15. Sly PD, Collins RA (2006) Physiological basis of respiratory signs and symptoms. Paediatr Respir Rev 7(2):84–88
16. Solway J, Fredberg JJ, Ingram RH, Pedersen OF, Drazen JM (1987) Interdependent regional lung emptying during forced expiration: a transistor model. J Appl Physiol 62(5):2013–2025
17. Elphick HE, Sherlock P, Foxall G et al (2001) Survey of respiratory sounds in infants. Arch Dis Child 84(1):35–39
18. Davies MJ, Cane R, Ranganathan S, McKenzie SA (1998) Cough, wheeze and sleep. Arch Dis Child 79(5):465
19. Cane RS, Ranganathan S, McKenzie SA (2000) What do parents of wheezy children understand by "wheeze"? Arch Dis Child 82(4):327–332
20. Cane RS, McKenzie SA (2001) Parents' interpretations of children's respiratory symptoms on video. Arch Dis Child 84(1):31–34
21. Chong Neto HJ, Rosario N, Dela Bianca AC, Solé D, Mallol J (2007) Validation of a questionnaire for epidemiologic studies of wheezing in infants. Pediatr Allergy Immunol 18(1):86–87
22. Lowe L, Murray CS, Martin L et al (2004) Reported versus confirmed wheeze and lung function in early life. Arch Dis Child 89(6):540–543
23. Michel G, Silverman M, Strippoli MP et al (2006) Parental understanding of wheeze and its impact on asthma prevalence estimates. Eur Respir J 28(6):1124–1130
24. Anthracopoulos MB, Liolios E, Panagiotakos DB, Triantou K, Priftis KN (2007) Prevalence of asthma among schoolchildren in Patras, Greece: four questionnaire surveys during 1978–2003. Arch Dis Child 92(3):209–212
25. Asher MI, Keil U, Anderson HR et al (1995) International study of asthma and allergies in childhood (ISAAC): rational and methods. Eur Respir J 8(3):483–491
26. Elphick HE, Ritson S, Rodgers H, Everard ML (2000) When a wheeze is not a wheeze: acoustic analysis of breath sounds in infants. Eur Respir J 16(4):593–597
27. Elphick HE, Lancaster GA, Solis A, Majumdar A, Gupta R, Smyth RL (2004) Validity and reliability of acoustic analysis of respiratory sounds in infants. Arch Dis Child 89(11):1059–1063
28. Elphick HE, Ritson S, Everard ML (2002) Differential response of wheezes and ruttles to anticholinergics. Arch Dis Child 86(4):280–281
29. Netuveli G, Hurwitz B, Sheikh A (2007) Lineages of language and the diagnosis of asthma. J R Soc Med 100(1):19–24
30. Shim CS, Williams MH Jr (1983) Relationship of wheezing to the severity of obstruction in asthma. Arch Intern Med 143(5):890–892
31. Holleman DR, Simel DL, Goldberg JS (1993) Diagnosis of obstructive airways disease from the clinical examination. J Gen Intern Med 8(2):63–68
32. Badgett RG, Tanaka DJ, Hunt DK et al (1994) The clinical evaluation for diagnosing obstructive airways disease in high-risk patients. Chest 106(5):1427–1431
33. Bohadana AB, Peslin R, Uffholtz H (1978) Breath sounds in the clinical assessment of airflow obstruction. Thorax 33(3):345–351
34. Purohit A, Bohadana A, Kopferschmitt-Kubler MC, Mahr L, Linder J, Pauli G (1997) Lung auscultation in airway challenge testing. Respir Med 91(3):151–157
35. Yong SC, Smith CM, Wach R, Kurian M, Primhak RA (1999) Methacholine challenge in preschool children: methacholine-induced wheeze versus transcutaneous oximetry. Eur Respir J 14(5):1175–1178

36. Springer C, Godfrey S, Picard E et al (2000) Efficacy and safety of methacholine bronchial challenge performed by auscultation in young asthmatic children. Am J Respir Crit Care Med 162(3 Pt 1):857–860
37. Godfrey S, Uwyyed K, Springer C, Avital A (2004) Is clinical wheezing reliable as an endpoint for bronchial challenges in preschool children? Pediatr Pulmonol 37(3):193–200
38. Bohadana AB, Peslin R, Uffholtz H, Pauli G (1995) Potential for lung sound monitoring during bronchial provocation testing. Thorax 50(9):955–961
39. Bohadana AB, Michaely JP (2006) Does the inclusion of wheeze detection as an outcome measure affect the interpretation of methacholine challenge tests? A study in workers at risk of occupational asthma. Lung 184(3):151–157
40. Global Initiative for Asthma (GINA) (2016) Global strategy for asthma management and prevention. http://ginasthma.org/wp-content/uploads/2016/04/GINA-2016-main-report_tracked.pdf
41. National Institute for Health and Care Excellence (NICE) (2016) Bronchiolitis in children: diagnosis and management. NICE guideline. Published: 1 June 2015. https://www.nice.org.uk/guidance/ng9/resources/bronchiolitis-in-children-diagnosis-and-management-51048523717
42. Piirilä P, Sovijärvi AR (1995) Crackles: recording, analysis and clinical significance. Eur Respir J 8(12):2139–2148
43. Nath AR, Capel LH (1974) Inspiratory crackles and mechanical events of breathing. Thorax 29(6):695–698
44. Fredberg JJ, Holford SK (1983) Discrete lung sounds: crackles (rales) as stress-relaxation quadruples. J Acoust Soc Am 73(3):1036–1046
45. Vyshedskiy A, Alhashem RM, Pciej R et al (2009) Mechanism of inspiratory and expiratory crackles. Chest 135(1):156–164
46. Munakata M, Ukita H, Doi I et al (1991) Spectral and waveform characteristics of fine and coarse crackles. Thorax 46(9):651–657
47. Metlay JP, Kapoor WN, Fine MJ (1997) Does this patient have community-acquired pneumonia? Diagnosing pneumonia by history and physical examination. JAMA 287(17):1440–1445
48. Lim WS, Baudouin SV, George RC et al (2009) BTS guidelines for the management of community-acquired pneumonia in adults: update 2009. Thorax 64(Suppl 3):iii1–iii55
49. Bradley JS, Byington CL, Shah SS et al (2011) Executive summary: the management of community-acquired pneumonia in infants and children older than 3 months of age: clinical practical guidelines by the Pediatric Infectious Diseases Society of America. Clin Infect Dis 53(7):617–630
50. Wipf JE, Lipsky BA, Hirshmann JV et al (1999) Diagnosing pneumonia by physical examination: relevant or relic? Arch Intern Med 159(10):1082–1087
51. Margolis P, Gadomski A (1998) Does this infant have pneumonia? JAMA 279(4):308–313
52. Vyshedskiy A, Bezares F, Paciej R, Ebril M, Shane J, Murphy R (2005) Transmission of crackles in patients with interstitial pulmonary fibrosis, congestive heart failure, and pneumonia. Chest 128(3):1468–1474
53. Ponte DF, Moraes R, Hizume DC, Alencar AM (2013) Characterization of crackles from patients with fibrosis, heart failure and pneumonia. Med Eng Phys 35(4):448–456
54. Paciej R, Vyshedskiy A, Bana D, Murphy R (2004) Squawks in pneumonia. Thorax 59(2):177–178
55. Bilavsky E, Shouval DS, Yarden-Bilavsly H, Ashkenazi S, Amir J (2008) Are grunting respirations a sign of serious bacterial infection in children? Acta Paediatr 97(8):1086–1089
56. Beck R, Odeh M, Oliven A, Gavriely N (1995) The acoustic properties of snores. Eur Respir J 8(12):2120–2128
57. Jennum P, Riha RL (2009) Epidemiology of sleep apnoea/hypopnoea syndrome and sleep-disordered breathing. Eur Respir J 33(4):907–914
58. Witmans M, Young R (2011) Update on pediatric sleep-disordered breathing. Pediatr Clin N Am 58(3):571–589

59. Au CT, Li AM (2009) Obstructive sleep breathing disorders. Pediatr Clin N Am 56(1):243–259
60. Li Z, Celestin J, Lockey RF (2016) Pediatric sleep apnea syndrome: an update. J Allergy Clin Immunol Pract 4(5):852–861
61. Liistro G, Stanescu D, Veriter C (1991) Pattern of simulated snoring is different through mouth and nose. J Appl Physiol 70(6):2736–2741
62. Dalmasso F, Prota R (1996) Snoring: analysis, measurement, clinical implications and applications. Eur Respir J 9(1):146–159
63. Perez-Padilla JR, Slawinski E, Difrancesco LM, Feige RR, Remmers JE, Whitelaw WA (1993) Characteristics of the snoring noise in patients with and without occlusive sleep apnea. Am Rev Respir Dis 147(3):635–644
64. Riha RL (2015) Diagnostic approaches to respiratory sleep disorders. J Thorac Dis 7(8):1373–1384
65. Kaditis AG, Alonso Alvarez ML, Boudewyns A et al (2016) Obstructive sleep disordered breathing in 2- to 18-year-old children: diagnosis and management. Eur Respir J 47(1):69–94

Breath Sounds in Epidemiology

4

Patricias W. Garcia-Marcos, M. Innes Asher, Philippa Ellwood, and Luis Garcia-Marcos

4.1 Introduction: A Bibliographic Exercise

In the approach to a quite original chapter of the epidemiology of breath sounds, one invariably looks for references in the literature. The first problem is choosing the right keywords to introduce in your reference manager software (as you intend to keep those references in a safe place). For example, if you introduce the following search strategy in Reference Manager V10 (Thomson Reuters, New York, USA): [(wheeze*) OR (rale) OR (crackle) OR (rhonch*) OR (breath sound) AND (Epidemiology)] for years 2000 and over, 3193 records are retrieved. This is mainly noise coming from any article which includes any of those sounds and deals with the epidemiology or a specific disease, which is different from a true epidemiological study on breath sounds. For instance, if the term "rale*" is looked for in the nonindexed text fields (NIT) (including abstract) of all those 3193 papers, only 26 articles are retrieved, and none of them is actually related to the epidemiology of "rales". Repeating the same procedure for "crackle" and "rhonch*", the corresponding number is 25 and 12, with again, no actual relationship with crackles or rhonchi except for one paper entitled "Wheezes, crackles and rhonchi: simplifying

P. W. Garcia-Marcos
Department of Paediatrics, "Santa Lucia" University General Hospital, Cartagena, Spain

M. I. Asher · P. Ellwood
Department of Paediatrics: Child and Youth Health, University of Auckland, Auckland, New Zealand
e-mail: i.asher@auckland.ac.nz; p.ellwood@auckland.ac.nz

L. Garcia-Marcos (✉)
Respiratory and Allergy Units, Arrixaca Children's University Hospital, University of Murcia, Murcia, Spain

IMIB Bio-health Research Institute of Murcia, Murcia, Spain
e-mail: lgmarcos@um.es

K. N. Priftis et al. (eds.), *Breath Sounds*, https://doi.org/10.1007/978-3-319-71824-8_4

description of lung sounds increases the agreement on their classification: a study of 12 physicians' classification of lung sounds from video recordings" [1].

The message seems to be quite clear: there is no information about the epidemiology of rales, crackles or rhonchi when the specific breath sound is the end point of a survey. This makes quite a lot of sense if one considers that rales and crackles are usually associated to lung conditions where other signs (fever, for instance) or symptoms (e.g. malaise) are as important as the breath sound itself and, at least in some societies in which pneumonia is diagnosed and treated early, a stethoscope is needed to hear those sounds. Nevertheless, it does not seem feasible that a person with audible (without stethoscope) and actual rales or crackles (representing any pathological condition) is at work, on a street or at school, where proper epidemiological studies are carried out. Thus, while the epidemiology of pneumonia sounds perfectly right, the epidemiology of rales or crackles does not. Briefly speaking crackles or rales are not a kind of synonym for pneumonia or have not been used (quite wisely) as markers of pneumonia in epidemiological studies.

The case of a rhonchus might be a different matter as rhonchi are usually associated with wheezes and probably "hidden" in them. The term "wheezing" is included in the abstract of 1018 papers of our original dataset of 3193, which is much big different from crackles and rales. The explanation might well be that "wheezing" has become a marker for asthma and can be more easily be heard than crackles or rales without a stethoscope. In fact the terms "infant wheeze", "severe wheeze" and "recurrent wheeze" are concepts that refer to specific conditions in itself, no matter whether they are real asthma or not. "Wheezing" has also been used as a keyword in asthma surveys, particularly in the International Study of Asthma and Allergies in Childhood (ISAAC) [2]. In contrast with rales or crackles, the epidemiology of wheeze makes sense as it indicates a specific disease (in infancy and young children) and has been demonstrated to be a quite reliable marker of asthma in older ages as shown in this chapter.

The case of cough, an arguable breath sound, is more similar to wheeze than to crackles or rales. On top of being a clinical sign, cough has become a syndrome, and terms such as "chronic cough" have turned into a specific diagnosis. There is a specific chapter on cough in this book, and thus, it will not be considered here.

Taking together the previous data and comments, the authors believe that the rest of the present chapter should be focused on the value of just one adventitious breath sound, i.e. wheeze. As this is not a book on asthma but on breath sound, the chapter needs to be focused on the ability of the term "wheeze" to diagnose the disease to which it is associated, i.e. asthma. Also, and as epidemiological studies are performed in many languages, some comments dedicated to the interchangeability of the translation of wheeze between different languages are warranted. The epidemiology of cough, not and adventitious sounds, is covered in a different chapter of this book.

4.2 What Does Wheeze Mean?

For non-English-speaking doctors, "wheezing" may be a startling word which does not have a good equivalent in many languages. For one of the authors, after using and reading the term in relation to the lung for years, it was an amazing experience to read the following sentence in the chapter "Immediate Experience" of the famous novel *Ulysses* by James Joyce: "I pull the wheezy bell of their shuttered cottage: and wait". Thus, it seems that wheezing does not necessarily relate to all instances to the sound that air can make when flowing through a tube. Anyhow, the definition of "wheeze" in the *Oxford Dictionary* is "Breathe with a whistling or rattling sound in the chest, as a result of obstruction in the air passages", although the sound can be applied to other situations in which a sound is similar to that of wheeze, as in the *Ulysses* sentence. The *Merriam-Webster Dictionary* more specifically defines wheeze as "to breathe with difficulty usually with a whistling sound". What it is of interest to the epidemiology of wheeze is to what extent this is a precise term in English and how well it can be translated to other languages.

In epidemiological studies, it is crucial that the outcome variable is well defined in order to avoid misclassification bias. This bias, as its name indicates, relates to the classification of cases as healthy and the other way around. Usually, as misclassification is random, the effect is towards the null hypothesis, and thus the study would conclude that there is no difference between the group of cases and the group of healthy population.

4.3 How Well Parents Report Wheezing in Their Infant Children

The validation study [3] of the "Estudio Internacional de Sibilancias en lacantes" (EISL) (International Study of Wheezing in Infants) questionnaire, carried out in Cartagena (Spain) and Santiago (Chile), correctly detected infants who have suffered from wheezing during their first year of life, independently of the settings and countries in which it was applied. Furthermore, this ability was maintained in international comparisons between centres of different sociocultural background. The gold standard for this study was the previous diagnosis by a paediatric pulmonologist. For criterion validity, and since there is no gold standard test which can be used to categorise infants into wheezers and non wheezers to compare the questionnaire to, the opinion of the paediatric pulmonologist was chosen as the standard. They are more aware of the different wheezing phenotypes at this age, and despite certain variability among them, it appears much more reliable as the "gold standard" than any laboratory test available at present. The Youden index (Y-index) found for the question "Has your baby had wheezing or whistling in the chest during his/her first 12 months of life?" (which was the same question as in the ISAAC study, except for the time frame) was quite high (75% in Cartagena and 67% in Santiago). The greater agreement found in Cartagena as compared to Santiago was explained by the authors on the bases of the differences in socioeconomic and cultural status between both city areas where the study was carried out. This different diagnostic power seemed to result from an overreporting of parents in Santiago. However, specificity was quite high and similar in both cities, approaching 90%. As specificity is the most important validity measure in studies where the relative risk is the way of measuring an effect, it is likely that the results obtained with the aforementioned question would approach the true value.

Moreover, in a very different setting such as in the emergency room, this question reliably identified wheezing in infants by their parents at the moment the symptom is occurring, with a high specificity and sensitivity [4, 5].

Previously, several British studies had addressed the issue of parents reporting wheezing in infants. In the first one, the main objective was to assess whether parents, clinicians and epidemiologists understood "wheeze" in the same way. Cane et al. [6] performed a study in two different settings with two similar aims: to know what parents who reported wheeze understood by wheeze and to compare parents' reports of wheeze in children brought to the emergency department with the doctors' findings. For the first aim, the authors developed a 12-item questionnaire, which was also translated into Urdu, Bengali and Turkish. Very interestingly, "wheeze" was translated as "squeaking" in the Asian languages, although the number of parents in this category was negligible. Most parents described "wheeze" as a sound only or as a sound with difficulty of breathing. The sound, however, has been termed in different ways such as "hissing", "squeaking", "whistling" or "rasping". Only 11% included the word "whistle" in their idea of "wheeze". With respect to the agreement between parents and clinicians, the agreement was quite low (45%), although parents described what doctors diagnosed as wheezing in other words such as "difficulty of breathing" or "noisy breathing" in 39% of instances. Unfortunately, the power of the study was not high enough to perform a stratified analysis by age group, and there were children from too wide a range of ages from 4 months to 15.5 years (median 2.5 years). Additionally, Cane et al. [6] also performed a reference search to find definitions of wheeze and response options in epidemiological studies coming from the UK between 1983 and 1998. They reported 12 different questions to ask about the presence of wheeze. In the first eight, six studies included a very similar question (with very minor differences) as follows: "Noisy breathing with a whistling sound coming from the chest, not the throat". The last four came from the ISAAC study and actually shared the same wording of the question, which included "wheezing or whistling in the chest". It is important to underline that those epidemiological studies were designed to study asthma prevalence, using the different questions or wording as a marker of the presence of the disease. The idea of wheeze as a whistling sound coming from the chest seems quite consistent in all definitions and probably reflects the idea of most clinicians and epidemiologists, many of whom have learned the term by means of the stethoscope. This is also in keeping with the standard definitions from two of the most important English dictionaries, but is in contrast with the low frequency in which parents include the word "whistle" in their concept of wheeze in the study by Cane et al. [6]. However, the much better agreement between parents and paediatric pulmonologists in the Spanish-Chilean study [3] speaks of better understanding of the definition when including "whistling in the chest". Of course, there are important differences between both studies, including the design, the settings, the language, the culture, the age groups and the time in which they were carried out.

Another early British study on infants under the age of 18 months recruited children from inpatients ($n = 44$) and outpatients ($n = 19$) from a children's hospital and also from the community ($n = 29$). All of them had noisy breathing. Parents were asked to choose from a list of ten words to describe their child's condition, and 65% chose the word "wheeze". The point raised by the authors in this case is that noisy breathing is quite common in infancy (in many instances coming from the upper airways) and that wheezing was used too freely by parents, describing conditions far from that of asthma or asthma-like symptoms. Again, only a low proportion of parents used the term "whistling" to qualify wheeze. However, the design of this study does not allow finding out how well a specific question or word defines an asthma-like condition.

The last early British study [7] dealing with the issue of parents diagnosing their infants' wheezing condition is a proper validation study. The questionnaire used in the study was based on previous questionnaires used in older populations, mainly the ISAAC one, but was translated into a score system. The authors felt that recall bias was very likely if symptoms were asked for in a period longer that the previous 3 months. The gold standard was the consultant respiratory specialist opinion, and the analysis could be performed in 114 repeated pairs of questionnaires. However, for the purpose of comparing how scores were able to distinguish asthmatic children from non-asthmatic ones, the analysis was made on 20 asthmatics against 72 with no or minimal symptoms. Although the mean age of those 92 children is not reported, according to the whole cohort of 114, it would have been between 10 and 13 months. With respect to the activity wheeze and rattle score, the difference was quite substantial (mean [95% CI], 4.6 (2.7–6.4) vs. 14.4 (9.6–19.1)). The authors report a high sensitivity of all scores used but unacceptable specificity in some of them. Unfortunately, they did not report the exact numbers for each score; thus, the values for the wheezing score cannot be known. In summary, this study does not seem to be very useful to give information about how well parents "diagnose" their infant wheeze.

It is quite remarkable that in two of the aforementioned British studies, "whistling" was not helpful to qualify the term "wheezing", especially when many languages which do not have a direct translation for wheeze actually use their word for "whistling". This was the case of the EISL questionnaire in Spanish and Portuguese: in both languages, the core question included a direct translation for "whistling" ("pitos"/"pieira") and a more technical synonym ("silbidos"/"sibilância") which might be closer to "wheeze", especially when specifying "in the chest". In the end, it is quite probable that such questions, either in the two Latin languages or in English, are identifying "noisy breathing", the noise coming from the chest. To what extent a language can modify the results of an asthma survey will be discussed below.

Some new data does not seem to add some light on the matter. A recent study [8] compared two very similar cohorts of children based in Leicester, United Kingdom (UK), in terms of phrasing of the questions related to wheeze. In one of the cohorts ($n = 534$), the question on "ever wheeze" was: "Has your child ever had attacks of wheezing?"; and in the other one ($n = 2859$), the equivalent question was the same as in the ISAAC study as follows: "Has your child ever had wheezing or whistling in the chest at any time in the past?" The questionnaire also included common questions for both cohorts when referring to the past 12 months (current wheeze). In particular the authors state that those questions were worded as in the ISAAC study, namely: "Has your child had wheezing or whistling in the chest in the past 12 months?". The study included three time points at 1, 4, and 6 years of age of the children, meaning that in the first time point the lifetime question and the question referred to "current" wheeze extended for the same time frame, i.e. from birth. As it might be expected, the ISAAC phrasing both referred to "ever" and to the "past year" obtained very similar values of wheezing prevalence (39.6% vs. 37.4%; $p = 0.04$) in one of the cohorts. With respect to the cohort which used "attacks of wheeze ever" and "wheezing or whistling in the past year", the wheezing prevalence was respectively 31.8% and 33.7%, the difference not being statistically significant ($p = 0.55$). Thus, although the authors concluded that the prevalence of wheeze was statistically different between "attacks of wheeze" and "wheeze/whistling ever" (31.8% vs. 39.6%, $p < 0.001$), what is of more interest from our point of view is that there was no difference between "attacks" and "wheezing/whistling in the past 12 months" within the same cohort, as indicated previously. This lack of difference may indicate that the word "whistling" does not add much to "wheezing" in English, at least in infancy. Maybe a validation study in an English-speaking population of two different questions one including just "wheeze" and the other one just including "whistling" could clarify the issue.

4.4 A Historic Perspective of Questionnaires on Wheeze to Diagnose Asthma in Children and Adults

The investigation of asthma prevalence in populations identified the need to establish reliable and valid measurement instrument which was applicable to large numbers of individuals. Obviously asking individuals about suffering from asthma or about having symptoms of asthma is the easiest and cheapest way. This is probably the reason why the first known asthma questionnaire was constructed by the Medical Research Council (MRC) in the UK. There are at least three different versions of this questionnaire, those of 1960, 1966 and 1986 as reviewed by Toren et al. [9] in 1993. The three questionnaires include the words "wheezing" and "whistling" coming from the chest as part of the question related to asthma. The phrase "shortness of breath" was included in the 1966 version and also in the 1986 one. A specific time frame of "the last 12 months" was only included in the last version. With respect to the diagnosis of asthma, no such word is included in any of the questions of the earlier questionnaire, but it appears afterward, although with a slightly different phrasing: "Have you ever had bronchial asthma?" (1966) and "Have you ever had, or being told you have bronchial asthma" (1986).

In 1962 the first version of the European Coal and Steel Community (ECSC) questionnaire on respiratory symptoms appeared. This questionnaire was mainly a repetition of the MRC questionnaire including some items related to occupational asthma [10]. This questionnaire was further revised in 1967 [11] and 1987 [12]. In this last version, it includes a direct question on an asthma diagnosis made by a doctor in this question: "Has a doctor ever told you that you have asthma?"

Following the steps of the MRC, the Division of Lung Diseases of the National Heart and Lung Institute (NHLI) of the USA produced the NHLI questionnaire in 1971 and further refined in 1978 which was the questionnaire recommended by the American Thoracic Society and the Division of Lung Diseases (ATS-DLD) [13]. As reviewed by Toren et al. [9], the main questions related to asthma were (again playing with the same terms): "Does your chest ever sound wheezy or whistling?"; "Have you ever had an attack of wheezing that has made you feel short of breath?"; and "Have you ever had asthma?". The combination of "shortness of breath" and "wheezing" in the same sentence had been previously included in the 1966 MRC questionnaire.

There is a questionnaire that was specifically developed for the Tucson cohort and which focused only on asthma which integrates both MRC and ATS-DLD questionnaires in four different questions combining wheezing and whistling, wheezing and shortness of breath and asthma diagnosis (either confirmed or not by a doctor) [14].

Some years afterwards, in 1984, the International Union Against Tuberculosis and Lung Diseases (IUATLD) developed its own questionnaire on respiratory symptoms, including symptoms of asthma [15]. It was used firstly in the UK and later in several EU countries [16] with apparently good performance in the translations to Finnish, French and German. There is a short version of this questionnaire produced in 1986 known as "the IUATLD (1986) Bronchial Symptoms Questionnaire". Interestingly, as it was developed to find the best combination to diagnose asthma, it did not include any question on asthma diagnosis.

The European Community Respiratory Health Survey (ECRHS), launched in 1994, is a milestone in the surveys on asthma symptoms in adults. The initial phase was carried out in various EU countries and several others out of the EU. It included the IUATLD 1984 questionnaire [17] which had been previously validated (see below). After ECRHS most adult surveys have used it in different countries and times, and the questionnaire has been validated in other languages than those of the four original ones [18].

A really unique case in the area of asthma symptoms surveillance using questionnaires and starting in 1992 is that of the International Study of Asthma and Allergies in Childhood. Due to its impact in the way asthma surveys have been performed in the last two decades, this study deserves a special section in its own right.

After ECRHS and ISAAC, there have been some new questionnaires either with a limited impact [19–23] or focused on areas which the two aforementioned studies did not cover, i.e. very young children or specific populations. One of those post-ISAAC questionnaires, including also a question on wheezing, has its own original touch, as it was validated against a population-based prescription database [24].

Another two of those post-ISAAC questionnaires, based on it, are the Brief Pediatric Asthma Screen (BPAS) [25, 26] and the Brief Pediatric Asthma Screen Plus (BPAS+) [27], which were built to screen communities with a mixture of English- and Spanish-speaking children. Apart from a direct question on an asthma diagnosis by a doctor or a nurse, this questionnaire has a specific question on wheeze as follows: "Does your child EVER wheeze (have whistling in the chest)?". It is of interest that both wheeze and whistling are translated to Spanish using the same word "respiración silbante (silbidos en el pecho)" omitting a more common word—at least in Spain and in certain Latin American countries, such as "pitos"—which is included in the ISAAC instrument.

Other post-ISAAC questionnaires are the ones used in the "Breathmobile Case Identification Survey" (BCIS) [28] and in the "Easy Breathing Survey". The last one was based in the IUATLD questionnaire [16]. The BCIS has been used in preschool and school-age children and has used an asthma case-detection tool in which the key question of which is "During the last 2 years, has your child had repeated episodes of any of the following conditions: Asthma; Cough; Trouble breathing; Chest tightness; Bronchitis?". No question on any sound such as wheezing or whistling was included in this questionnaire [29–32].

Yet another post-ISAAC questionnaire is named Brief Respiratory Questionnaire (BRQ). This one includes the same question for wheezing ever as in the ISAAC one ("Has your child ever had wheezing or whistling in the chest at *any time in the past*?") and adds another one as follows: "*In the past 12 months*, has your child had any of these three symptoms: wheezing or whistling in the chest, a cough that lasted more than a week, or other breathing problems?" [33].

In 2012 the Global Initiative for Asthma (GINA) included in its asthma guideline a very short set of questions to diagnose asthma (as reviewed by Lim et al. [34]). Two out of five questions include the term "wheeze" as follows: (1) *Has the patient had an attack of wheezing?* and (2) *Does the patient have wheeze or dyspnoea after exercise?* Note that the questions are not designed for epidemiologic studies but to screen referred patients with suspected asthma in order to discriminate those asthmatics from those who are not. However, the wording of the two questions is quite similar to those previously discussed.

4.5 The International Study of Asthma and Allergies in Childhood (ISAAC) and the Global Asthma Network (GAN)

ISAAC was launched in 1991, and according to its website (http://isaac.auckland.ac.nz/), "ISAAC has become the largest worldwide collaborative research project ever undertaken, involving more than 100 countries and nearly two million children and its aim is to develop environmental measures and disease monitoring in order to form the basis for future interventions to reduce the burden of allergic and non-allergic diseases, especially in children in developing countries". This study was closed in 2012 and the "Global Asthma Network" (GAN) (www.globalasthmanetwork.org) established the same year, a collaboration between some individuals of ISAAC and the IUATLD.

The ISAAC study has had an incredible impact in the epidemiology of asthma symptoms all over the world, and its questionnaire has become a standard for a great majority of surveys carried out in children and adolescents. The specific instruments, including the questionnaires, for each of the three main phases related to asthma symptoms (1992–1996, 1999–2002, 2002–2006) can be found in the study website. The age groups for which the ISAAC questionnaire has been designed were 13–14-year-olds (self-completed questionnaires) and 6–7-year-olds (parent-completed questionnaires). It was also used in ISAAC Phase II, in children 9–12 years of age.

4.5.1 Written Questionnaires

The core questionnaire on asthma has been the same from the beginning and included three main questions about asthma [35]: "Have you (has your child) ever had wheezing or whistling in the chest at any time in the past?"; "Have you (has your child) had wheezing or whistling in the chest in the last 12 months?" and "Have you (has your child) ever had asthma?" According to the Phase One manual (http://isaac.auckland.ac.nz/phases/phaseone/phaseone.html), the first question "is based on the IUATLD questionnaire" [16]. It does not mention "attacks" of wheezing, in order to identify children with persistent symptoms which are not obviously characterised as episodes or attacks. This is seen as a very sensitive question. With respect to the second question, the manual states that "Limitation to a 12 month period reduces errors of recall and (at least in theory) should be independent of month of completion. This is considered to be the most useful question for assessing the prevalence of wheezing illness". The rationale for the third question is "All respondents are asked about diagnosed asthma, as occasionally asthma may be diagnosed in the absence of wheeze (on the basis of recurrent nocturnal cough etc.)". As in other questionnaires, the diagnostic questions can be qualified by frequency and severity questions.

The three core questions are also included in the GAN questionnaire which is currently in use for GAN Phase I. In the Phase I GAN Manual, there is some qualification of the reason for including the second question (past 12 months) as follows: "Limitation to a 12 month period reduces errors of recall [36] and is believed to be independent of month of completion" [37]. The third question is justified in GAN as follows:

This is the first time in the questionnaire that 'asthma' is mentioned. It is deliberately asked after the questions on asthma symptoms. The asthma label is affected by many factors such as awareness of asthma, medical training and experience, cultural and societal factors. Occasionally asthma may be suggested in the absence of wheeze (on the basis of recurrent nocturnal cough etc.). This question was used in all phases of ISAAC. It has not been clear whether the answer represents the opinion of the adolescent, or was a label given by a doctor. In GAN the same question will be used, followed by a clarification question.

This clarification question is "Was asthma confirmed by a doctor?" (http://www.globalasthmanetwork.org/surveillance/manual/-manual.php). Very interestingly, GAN includes also modules for parents of the children, including the same four questions on asthma symptoms and asthma diagnosis.

4.5.2 Video Questionnaire

As a way to better qualify the diagnosis of asthma from the written questionnaire, ISAAC launched a video questionnaire which was used in Phases I and III and is being used in GAN Phase I. The video has five different scenes: (1) a girl sitting at a table with audible wheezing and whistling and mild dyspnoea, (2) a boy who is running and has to stop due to wheezing, (3) a boy waking at night with wheeze and dyspnoea, (4) a girl waking at night with a cough attack and (5) a severe attack of asthma with important dyspnoea and wheeze but no whistling. Each of the five scenes is followed by questions read in the local language by a narrator, "Has your breathing been like this, at any time in your life?", with the same possible three different answers—(1) "...at any time of your life", (2) "If yes: has this happened in the past year?" and (3) "if yes, has this happened one or more times a month?" The video questionnaire is only for use in children 13–14 years of age.

4.6 How Well Questionnaires on Wheeze Perform

From the beginning, validation of asthma questionnaires has been a key issue. As there is no clear gold standard for asthma, three main methods have been used: (1) test the questions against clinical diagnosis and objective measurement such as non-specific bronchial challenge tests; (2) obtain clinical diagnosis of asthma by experienced doctors; and (3) compare new questionnaires with old ones. In the lines that follow, this chapter will focus on the validation against clinical diagnosis and hyperresponsiveness.

4.6.1 Validation Against Clinical Diagnosis of Asthma

The key review by Toren et al. [9] includes several early studies, starting in 1971 in which the question "Have you ever had asthma" was assessed. Edfors-Lubs [38] and Kiviloog et al. [39] found very high values (close to 100%) both in sensitivity and specificity. In the first one only 39 patients were included; and in the second there were 95 potential cases and 299 potential controls. In a more recent study, and more interestingly as the investigators included four centres in four different EU countries as previously quoted, they tested the same question of the IUATLD 1984 questionnaire [16] and found variable validity between centres: sensitivity ranged from 48% to 75% and specificity from 77% to 100%. The Y-indexes ranged from 48% (British centre) to 63% (Finnish centre). ECRHS groups have validated this questionnaire in other languages [40] and specific populations such as the health workers [41].

Specifically in children, there are several studies validating asthma questionnaires against the clinical diagnosis of asthma, including at least clinical history and physical examination. In children 7–12 years of age, Remes et al. [42] defined asthma as a positive answer to either one of three questions—doctor diagnosis of asthma ever, attacks of "wheezing" or episodes of "breathlessness" in the last 12 months—and achieved a sensitivity of 88%, a specificity of 97% and a Y-index of 85%. Using the doctor diagnosis of asthma ever, the corresponding figures were 82%, 99% and 81%. In the same age group, Steen-Johnsen et al. [43] asking about "asthma ever" obtained a sensitivity of 63%, a specificity of 99% and a Y-index of 62%. Wolf et al. [25] found a sensitivity and specificity of 65% and 88% (Y-index 53%) for the question of a wheezing episode among parents of children in elementary schools (5–13-year-olds). More recently the same group has updated their questionnaire (Brief Paediatric Asthma Screen, BPAS) to BPAS+ and has included additional questions to detect allergy as well as asthma [26]. In the same age group, parents reached 73% sensitivity and 74% specificity (Y-index 47%) when answering positively to any of four items (wheeze, persistent cough, night cough and response to change in air temperature).

In younger children (grades kindergarten through 6 years), also using clinical diagnosis as the "gold standard", and referring to the past year, Redline et al. [44] reached a sensitivity of 80% and a specificity of 75% (Y-index 55%) when considering the presence of cough (sometimes or more) and/or breathing problem (rarely or more). Similar results have been obtained by the same authors in children 7–13 years of age [45]. The "Easy Breathing Survey" [28], in its validation study performed in children 0–17 years old (including 40% of 0–4-year-olds), found a sensitivity of 73% (newly diagnosed) or of 82% (previously diagnosed) and a specificity of 83% for the question about wheezing based on the IUATLD questionnaire [16]. Other questions obtained poorer results in the diagnostic tests, and the combination of any of four questions improved sensitivity but decreased specificity. The best Y-index was obtained with the question about wheezing (65% among those previously diagnosed and 56% among those newly diagnosed). As said in a previous section, this questionnaire was the base for the ECRHS, ISAAC and GAN questionnaires.

A validation study with the ISAAC questionnaire was carried out and published by Jenkins et al. in 1996 [46]. From a cohort of 2845 children aged 13–14 years from 25 schools randomly selected, 361 children were invited to complete the ISAAC core questionnaire. A total of 345 children completed the questionnaire, 123 of whom had wheezed during the past year. Additionally 40 had wheezed in the past but not in the last year. From the "never wheezers", 128 nonsymptomatic children were selected as controls. Children were interviewed by a paediatric respiratory physician and also underwent pulmonary function tests and a BHR test with hypertonic saline. The questionnaire achieved high values both in sensitivity (85%) and specificity (81%), with a Y-index of 66%, which is even higher than the best obtained in the ECRHS validation study in Finland. The questions validated where the two first questions of the ISAAC questionnaire which includes "wheeze ever" and "wheeze in the past year" but not "asthma". The authors considered current wheezers those children answering positively to both questions. The Spanish version of the ISAAC questionnaire, the language with more centres in Phase III (48 Spanish-speaking vs. 47 English-speaking centres in the older age group and 36 vs. 26, respectively) [35], has been also validated against asthma diagnosis by a physician with comparable results: sensitivity 65%, specificity 92% and Y-index 57% [47].

The ISAAC questionnaire has been validated in other languages [48–53] and in special populations, such as in anthroposophic children [54]. It has also been validated in a shortened version [55].

The BCIS questionnaire (answered by parents) was validated against an asthma evaluation (history, physical examination and spirometry) by an asthma specialist (blinded with respect to the questionnaire) in a multiethnic population of children 5–11 years old. The question on asthma (repeated episodes of asthma in the last 2 years) obtained a Y-index of 48% [56].

The BRQ questionnaire was validated against administered validation interviews by trained interviewers with and had a high agreement value (Kappa = 0.73) and a remarkable Y-index of 90% [33].

The BPAS+ questionnaire for use in Hispanics [27] obtained interesting results as the Y-index for the wheezing question was higher for the Spanish (38%) than for the English questionnaire (20%) due to a lower sensitivity in the second (25%) as compared with the first one (40%).

The GINA questionnaire has been recently validated against clinical diagnosis of asthma and has achieved similar results as the previous questionnaires, with a quite poor Y-index of 17% in the question about wheeze. This index was similar (19%) when wheezing was put in relation to exercise [34]. A summary of the results of the validation of the aforementioned studies is shown in Table 4.1.

4.6.2 Validation Against Bronchial Hyperresponsiveness

There has been some debate as to whether asthma questionnaires designed for epidemiological studies correctly detect asthma cases as compared to bronchial hyperresponsiveness (BHR) [57, 58]. Most of the current evidence suggests that for both children and adults, symptom questionnaires are better than BHR tests for the purpose of identifying asthma prevalence. Furthermore, BHR and other lung function tests are difficult to perform and interpret in young children, particularly in infants, and there is no information comparing wheezing questions with any specific pulmonary function test in children during their first year of life.

Nevertheless, and as the early questionnaires were designed for the adult population, validation against nonspecific BHR was carried out in several studies. It is of great interest that when compared to physician-diagnosed asthma, BHR had very high specificity (99% in two early studies) but unacceptable poor sensitivity (38% and 10%) [59, 60] with Y-indexes of 37% and 9%, respectively (very far from that of questionnaires). In the second of those studies [60], which included also self-reported asthma, this has the same Y-index (9%) as physician-diagnosed asthma.

Several early studies compared BHR with self-reported asthma and found also low values of Y-index in the range of 4–21% [15, 61, 62]. However, in the multinational study by Burney et al. in which they tested the validity of the IUATLD 1984 questionnaire, the figures of that index were substantially better, ranging from 26% (Berlin, Germany) to 65% (military recruits from several areas of Finland). It is of interest that in three cities (Berlin, Paris and Nottingham), the study population

Table 4.1 Validation of the question on wheeze against clinical diagnosis of asthma in selected studies

Study	Year	*N*	Age range (years)	Sensitivity (%)	Specificity (%)	Y-index
Edfors-Lubs [38]	1971	39	–	88	97	85
Kiviloog et al. [39]	1974	299	35–54	100	97	97
Burney et al. [16]	1989					
Overall		175	16–66	62	91	53
Finland		42	17–24	68	95	63
Germany		42	16–60	56	100	56
France		51	20–66	75	77	52
England		40	21–64	48	100	48
Remes et al. [42]	1994	247	7–12	88	97	85
Steen-Johnsen et al. [43]	1995	369	7–13	96	88	84
Jenkins et al. [46]	1996	168	13–14	85	81	66
Bonner et al. [33]	1999	200	Preschoolers	93	97	90
Wolf et al. [25]	1999	81	4–13	65	88	53
Hall et al. [28]	2001	197	0–17	73	82	55
Wolf et al. [26]	2003	129	6–12			
Six items				71	77	48
Four items				73	74	47
Redline et al. [44]	2003	107	4–13	80	75	55
Galant et al. [56]	2004	401	5–11	50	98	48
Mata Fernández et al. [47]	2005	366	3–17	65	92	57
Berry et al. [27]	2005					
Spanish		145	4–13	74	86	60
English		78	4–13	61	83	44
Delclos et al. [41]	2006	118	18–65	79	98	77
Lim et al. [34]	2014	164	20–64	51	66	17

came from outpatients (nonrespiratory) from hospitals, which might be different from the general population. Nevertheless those figures are not better than the ones obtained when comparing self-reported asthma with physician-diagnosed asthma [16]. In an Australian study, the IUATLD 1984 questionnaire was used in a sample of 809 workers of an aluminium smelter, and the Y-index for self-reported asthma against a methacholine test was not as high (25%) [63].

A question about wheezing was compared also to BHR in most of the previous studies, this question, as reviewed by Toren et al. [9], having a Y-index ranging from 12% to 69%. It is of interest that the highest values were found in the international validation study [16] (69% in Finland) and that the high value obtained in Nottingham (UK) (52%) was almost repeated by the same group in a subpopulation of non-smoking individuals from Hampshire and Dorset (UK) (51%) [15].

With respect to the ISAAC questionnaire, the study by Jenkins et al. [46] previously quoted observed a greater sensitivity (85% vs. 54%), a slightly lower specificity

(81% vs. 89%) and a substantially higher Y-index (66% vs. 43%) when asthma was diagnosed by the ISAAC questionnaire as compared to a BHR test with hypertonic saline (with the gold standard being physician-diagnosed asthma). A positive answer to the questionnaire plus a positive BHR test substantially increased the specificity to 94% but decreased the sensitivity to 47%, thus reducing the Y-index to 41%. In children 7 years of age, the ISAAC questionnaire performed quite well as compared to an exercise BHR test: using a 12% or greater fall in FEV1 postexercise as a positive test response, the exercise challenge had sensitivity and specificity estimates for current asthma and exercise-induced wheeze (as reported by parents) of 58% and 77% and 60% and 77% corresponding to Y-indexes of 18% and 54% [64].

The ISAAC video questionnaire was compared with the written one in a population of adolescents from a mixed ethnic background in Sydney (Australia) recruited from four secondary schools (mean age 13.5 ± 1.3 years). The aims of the study were to compare the video questionnaire with a written questionnaire in the detection of BHR to hypertonic saline. The area in which the study was performed contained a considerable proportion of non-English-speaking population. A subgroup of 127 children (out of 475 who completed the video questionnaire) took the written questionnaire and the hypertonic saline inhalation challenge. The reproducibility of the questionnaire was evaluated by administering the questionnaire to a subsample of students 2 weeks later. The two questionnaires and the BHR test were completed by 169 children. There was moderate agreement between the questionnaires for wheeze (80% of concordant classification, kappa 0.42). Questions on the written questionnaire concerning wheezing had good sensitivity (88%) and specificity (66%) for BHR (Y-index 54%). The corresponding figures for the video questionnaire were 75%, 68% and 58%. The video questionnaire was reproducible (kappa 0.82) and had good internal consistency (Cronbach's alpha 0.81), and each question pertained to a single construct explaining 58% of the variance in total score [65]. In previous studies, the concordance between the written and the video questionnaire ranged from 74% to 88% and the agreement (kappa) between 0.30 and 0.68 [66–69].

Additionally IUATLD and ISAAC (written and video) questionnaires were compared in predicting BHR. The sensitivity and specificity for predicting BHR were similar for individual questions from the IUATLD and video questionnaires. The video questions with the highest Y-index related to wheezing at rest (46%), severe wheezing at rest (38%) and nocturnal wheezing (37%). The ISAAC and the IUATLD written questionnaires performed similarly in predicting BHR (27% and 30% Y-indexes, respectively, for the question on wheezing in the last 12 months) [70].

An interesting finding is one from the study on the agreement between the ISAAC video (first video scene) and written questionnaire between centres by region and language groups. Responses to the video questionnaire obtained a lower prevalence than to the written questionnaire, and responses were well correlated. The overall proportion of agreement was high, (0.89) but unbalanced, with good negative agreement but poor positive agreement, thus resulting in only 20 centres having higher than a moderate kappa value (0.4). The contribution of each questionnaire to wheezing prevalence varied between centres and suggests that written questions about wheezing are variably understood and interpreted by 13–14-year-old adolescent [71]. A summary of the results of the validation of the previous studies is shown in Table 4.2.

Table 4.2 Validation of the questions on self-reported asthma[a] and on wheeze against bronchial hyperresponsiveness in selected studies

				Self-reported asthma[a]			Wheeze		
Study	Year	*N*	Age range (year)	Sensitivity (%)	Specificity (%)	Y-index	Sensitivity (%)	Specificity (%)	Y-index
Welty et al. [59]	1984	171	Adults	38	99	77	55	66	21
Enarson et al. [60]	1987	1392	Male adults	10	99	9	29	85	14
Dales et al. [61]	1987	200	Male adults	7	97	4	26	87	13
Rijcken et al. [62]	1987	1905	Adults	13	97	10	16	96	12
Burney et al. [15]	1989	397	18–64	22	99	21	47	92	39
Burney et al. [16]	1989								
Finland		42	17–24	74	91	65	95	74	69
Germany		42	16–60	33	93	26	59	80	39
France		51	20–66	80	74	54	73	65	38
England		40	21–64	53	100	53	89	62	51
Abramson et al. [63]	1991	809	Adults	28	97	25	49	86	35
Shaw et al. [70]	1991	87	13–16						
ISAAC questionnaire							65	62	27
IUATLD questionnaire							69	61	30
Jenkins et al. [46]	1996	168	13–14	54	89	43			
Ponsonby et al. [64]	1996	191	7	58	60	18	77	77	54
Gibson et al. [65]	1999	127	12–15						
Video questionnaire							75	68	58
Written questionnaire							88	66	54
Delclos et al. [41]	2006	118	18–55						
PC20 ≤ 8 mg/ml				71	70	41			
PC20 ≤ 4 mg/ml				61	85	46			
Lim et al. [34]	2014	164	20–64						
PC20 ≤ 25 mg/ml				44	75	19			
PC20 ≤ 50 mg/ml				62	52	14			

[a]Positive question to either having asthma or being told by a doctor to have asthma

As a kind of summary and following Pekkanen and Pearce [58], it could be said that when the aim of an epidemiological study is to compare differences in prevalence between populations, the Y-index is the best single measure of validity. BHR has similar or even higher specificity as compared to diagnosis by a physician, but considerably lower sensitivity, and thus a worse Y-index, than symptom questionnaires. This is clearly shown in the studies by Declos et al. [41] and Jenkins et al. [46]. Consequently, the method of choice for prevalence comparisons is standardised written or video symptom questionnaires. To better explore reasons for the differences in asthma prevalence, and to estimate possible differential symptom reporting, questionnaires might be supplemented with BHR in subsamples of the symptomatic and asymptomatic subjects. However, the results of symptom questionnaires and BHR should usually be analysed separately rather than combined due to the poor agreement between BHR and clinical asthma.

4.7 Internationalization of Questionnaires on Wheezing: How Not to Get Lost in Translation

When performing international surveys of asthma translations of questionnaires and, particularly, translations of the key English words, the term "wheezing" becomes a very important issue as a non-exact translation or good description (when direct translation is not possible) might invalidate the questionnaire in a specific language and/or a different cultural background [72].

There is not much information about standardised translations of questionnaires into different languages, and here, the example of ISAAC is of great interest. In the older age group (13–14 years of age), this study used in its Phase III 49 languages which were used in 201 centres; and the main languages were Spanish (48 centres), English (47 centres), Portuguese (25 centres), Arabic (16 centres), Italian (13 centres) and French (11 centres). In the younger age group (6–7 years of age), 42 languages in 131 centres were used, with the main languages being Spanish (36 centres), English (26 centres), Portuguese (13 centres) and Italian (10 centres) [73].

Early in this survey and previously to Phase I, during a pilot study in Germany, the need for perfect guidelines of translation and back-translation was raised [74] independently of the important fact that the original questionnaire was designed in English by the ISAAC Steering Committee members, representing 12 countries and 10 languages [75]. The back-translation to English by an independent person was considered fundamental, and a very detailed guideline was made which is fully depicted in Ellwood et al. [73].

Each ISAAC centre was asked about several aspects of the methodology followed in their areas, including the process of translation. At the beginning of Phase III, the ISAAC Steering Committee carefully reviewed each back-translation and compared it to the original English questionnaire. Deviations from the original questionnaire were classified as follows: (1) major deviations (changing the meaning of the question), (2) minor deviations (e.g. additional questions included between the ISAAC core questions) and (3) very minor deviations (e.g. changing or adding one or several words without altering the meaning of the questions). Depending on the deviation, the following actions were taken, respectively: (1) exclude the data for the specific questions; (2) include the question and identify the centre in the first worldwide publication; and (3) include the questions without identification. From the 233 centres in the 13–14-year-old group, the number of deviations was 7 major, 24 minor and 12 very minor. The corresponding figures in the 144 centres of the 6–7-year-old group were 3, 13 and 9 [73].

Although some translation errors were detected in the ISAAC study, only a few were major and required data exclusion. According to the ISAAC paper on translation, the rechecking of the questionnaire by an independent translation service and the close contact and information interchange with collaborators seeking their local knowledge could solve most of the issues. They also recommend the implementation of a web-designed database including the keywords for the survey with the translations into other languages together with description terms such as "wheezing" or "whistling" in the case of asthma.

Conclusion

The term "wheeze" is the only adventitious sound of which epidemiology can be spoken of as it has been used in numerous epidemiological studies as a surrogate of asthma. The validity of several sentences including the term "wheeze" is acceptable and probably better (and definitely more convenient and cheaper) than nonspecific BHR tests in epidemiological studies on asthma and related diseases, including infant wheezing. The ISAAC programme and now GAN have shown themselves to be paradigms of the global epidemiology of the breath sound "wheeze".

References

1. Melbye H, Garcia-Marcos L, Brand P, Everard M, Priftis K, Pasterkamp H (2016) Wheezes, crackles and rhonchi: simplifying description of lung sounds increases the agreement on their classification: a study of 12 physicians' classification of lung sounds from video recordings. BMJ Open Respir Res 3:e000136
2. Asher MI, Keil U, Anderson HR, Beasley R, Crane J, Martinez F, Mitchell EA, Pearce N, Sibbald B, Stewart AW (1995) International Study of Asthma and Allergies in Childhood (ISAAC): rationale and methods. Eur Respir J 8:483–491
3. Mallol J, Garcia-Marcos L, Aguirre V, Martinez-Torres A, Perez-Fernandez V, Gallardo A, Calvo M, Rosario FN, Rocha W, Fischer G, Baeza-Bacab M, Chiarella P, Pinto R, Barria C (2007) The International Study of Wheezing in Infants: questionnaire validation. Int Arch Allergy Immunol 144:44–50
4. Chong Neto HJ, Rosario N, Dela Bianca AC, Sole D, Mallol J (2007) Validation of a questionnaire for epidemiologic studies of wheezing in infants. Pediatr Allergy Immunol 18:86–87
5. Bianca AC, Wandalsen GF, Miyagi K, Camargo L, Cezarin D, Mallol J, Sole D (2009) International Study of Wheezing in Infants (EISL): validation of written questionnaire for children aged below 3 years. J Investig Allergol Clin Immunol 19:35–42
6. Cane RS, Ranganathan SC, McKenzie SA (2000) What do parents of wheezy children understand by "wheeze"? Arch Dis Child 82:327–332

7. Powell CV, McNamara P, Solis A, Shaw NJ (2002) A parent completed questionnaire to describe the patterns of wheezing and other respiratory symptoms in infants and preschool children. Arch Dis Child 87:376–379
8. Pescatore AM, Spycher BD, Beardsmore CS, Kuehni CE (2015) "Attacks" or "whistling": impact of questionnaire wording on wheeze prevalence estimates. PLoS One 10:e0131618
9. Toren K, Brisman J, Jarvholm B (1993) Asthma and asthma-like symptoms in adults assessed by questionnaires. A literature review. Chest 104:600–608
10. Brille D, Bolt W, Greve LH, Minette A, Sartorelli E (1962) European Steel and Coal Community (ECSC): high authority questionnaire on the study of chronic bronchitis and emphysema. Louxemburg, ECSC
11. Minette A, Brille D, Casula D, van der Lende R, Smidt U (1967) European Steel and Coal Community (ECSC): high authority questionnaire on the study of chronic bronchitis and emphysema. Lousemburg, ECSC
12. Minette A (1989) Questionnaire of the European Community for Coal and Steel (ECSC) on respiratory symptoms. 1987—updating of the 1962 and 1967 questionnaires for studying chronic bronchitis and emphysema. Eur Respir J 2:165–177
13. Ferris BG (1978) Epidemiology standardization project (American Thoracic Society). Am Rev Respir Dis 118:1–120
14. Lebowitz MD, Burrows B (1976) Comparison of questionnaires: the BMRC and NHLI respiratory questionnaires and a new self-completion questionnaire. Am Rev Respir Dis 113:627–635
15. Burney PG, Chinn S, Britton JR, Tattersfield AE, Papacosta AO (1989) What symptoms predict the bronchial response to histamine? Evaluation in a community survey of the bronchial symptoms questionnaire (1984) of the International Union Against Tuberculosis and Lung Disease. Int J Epidemiol 18:165–173
16. Burney PG, Laitinen LA, Perdrizet S, Huckauf H, Tattersfield AE, Chinn S, Poisson N, Heeren A, Britton JR, Jones T (1989) Validity and repeatability of the IUATLD (1984) Bronchial Symptoms Questionnaire: an international comparison. Eur Respir J 2:940–945
17. Burney PG, Luczynska C, Chinn S, Jarvis D (1994) The European Community Respiratory Health Survey. Eur Respir J 7:954–960
18. Song WJ, Lee SH, Kang MG, Kim JY, Kim MY, Jo EJ, Lee SY, Lee SE, Kim MH, Yang MS, Kim SH, Kang HR, Park HK, Park HW, Chang YS, Kim SS, Lee JM, Min KU, Cho SH (2015) Validation of the Korean version of the European Community Respiratory Health Survey screening questionnaire for use in epidemiologic studies for adult asthma. Asia Pac Allergy 5:25–31
19. Joseph CL, Foxman B, Leickly FE, Peterson E, Ownby D (1999) Sensitivity and specificity of asthma definitions and symptoms used in a survey of childhood asthma. J Asthma 36:565–573
20. Frank TL, Frank PI, McNamee R, Wright T, Hannaford P, Morrison J, Hirsch S, Pickering CA (1999) Assessment of a simple scoring system applied to a screening questionnaire of asthma in children aged 5–15 yrs. Eur Respir J 14:1190–1197
21. Glasgow NJ, Ponsonby AL, Yates RE, McDonald T, Attewell R (2001) Asthma screening as part of a routine school health assessment in the Australian Capital Territory. Med J Aust 174:384–388
22. Kilpelainen M, Terho EO, Helenius H, Koskenvuo M (2001) Validation of a new questionnaire on asthma, allergic rhinitis, and conjunctivitis in young adults. Allergy 56:377–384
23. Sistek D, Tschopp JM, Schindler C, Brutsche M, Ackermann-Liebrich U, Perruchoud AP, Leuenberger P (2001) Clinical diagnosis of current asthma: predictive value of respiratory symptoms in the SAPALDIA study. Swiss Study on Air Pollution and Lung Diseases in Adults. Eur Respir J 17:214–219
24. Wogelius P, Poulsen S, Sorensen HT (2005) Validity of parental-reported questionnaire data on Danish children's use of asthma-drugs: a comparison with a population-based prescription database. Eur J Epidemiol 20:17–22
25. Wolf RL, Berry CA, O'Connor T, Coover L (1999) Validation of the brief pediatric asthma screen. Chest 116:224S–228S

26. Wolf RL, Berry CA, Quinn K (2003) Development and validation of a brief pediatric screen for asthma and allergies among children. Ann Allergy Asthma Immunol 90:500–507
27. Berry CA, Quinn K, Wolf R, Mosnaim G, Shalowitz M (2005) Validation of the Spanish and English versions of the asthma portion of the brief pediatric asthma screen plus among hispanics. Ann Allergy Asthma Immunol 95:53–60
28. Hall CB, Wakefield D, Rowe TM, Carlisle PS, Cloutier MM (2001) Diagnosing pediatric asthma: validating the Easy Breathing Survey. J Pediatr 139:267–272
29. Jones CA, Morphew T, Clement LT, Kimia T, Dyer M, Li M, Hanley-Lopez J (2004) A school-based case identification process for identifying inner city children with asthma: the Breathmobile program. Chest 125:924–934
30. Vargas PA, Magee JS, Bushmiaer M, Simpson PM, Jones CA, Feild CR, Jones SM (2006) School-based asthma case finding: the Arkansas experience. J Sch Health 76:223–226
31. Kachru R, Morphew T, Kehl S, Clement LT, Hanley-Lopez J, Kwong KY, Guterman JJ, Jones CA (2006) Validation of a single survey that can be used for case identification and assessment of asthma control: the Breathmobile Program. Ann Allergy Asthma Immunol 97:775–783
32. Berg J, Brecht ML, Morphew T, Tichacek MJ, Chowdhury Y, Galant S (2009) Identifying preschool children with asthma in Orange County. J Asthma 46:460–464
33. Bonner S, Matte T, Rubin M, Sheares BJ, Fagan JK, Evans D, Mellins RB (2006) Validating an asthma case detection instrument in a Head Start sample. J Sch Health 76:471–478
34. Lim SY, Jo YJ, Chun EM (2014) The correlation between the bronchial hyperresponsiveness to methacholine and asthma like symptoms by GINA questionnaires for the diagnosis of asthma. BMC Pulm Med 14:161
35. Ellwood P, Asher MI, Beasley R, Clayton TO, Stewart AW (2005) The international study of asthma and allergies in childhood (ISAAC): phase three rationale and methods. Int J Tuberc Lung Dis 9:10–16
36. Pearce N, Beasley R, Burgess C, Crane J (1998) Asthma epidemiology. Principles and methods. Oxford University Press, New York
37. Stewart AW, Asher MI, Clayton TO, Crane J, D'Souza W, Ellwood PE, Ford RP, Mitchell EA, Pattemore PK, Pearce N (1997) The effect of season-of-response to ISAAC questions about asthma, rhinitis and eczema in children. Int J Epidemiol 26:126–136
38. Edfors-Lubs ML (1971) Allergy in 7000 twin pairs. Acta Allergol 26:249–285
39. Kiviloog J, Irnell L (1974) The prevalence of bronchial asthma and chronic bronchitis in Uppsala, Sweden. Scand J Respir Dis Suppl 89:35–40
40. Ribeiro M, Angelini L, Robles-Ribeiro PG, Stelmach R, Santos UP, Terra-Filho M (2007) Validation of the Brazilian-Portuguese version of the European Community Respiratory Health Survey in asthma patients. J Asthma 44:371–375
41. Delclos GL, Arif AA, Aday L, Carson A, Lai D, Lusk C, Stock T, Symanski E, Whitehead LW, Benavides FG, Anto JM (2006) Validation of an asthma questionnaire for use in healthcare workers. Occup Environ Med 63:173–179
42. Remes ST, Korppi M, Remes K, Pekkanen J (1996) Prevalence of asthma at school age: a clinical population-based study in eastern Finland. Acta Paediatr 85:59–63
43. Steen-Johnsen J, Bolle R, Holt J, Benan K, Magnus P (1995) Impact of pollution and place of residence on atopic diseases among schoolchildren in Telemark County, Norway. Pediatr Allergy Immunol 6:192–199
44. Redline S, Larkin EK, Kercsmar C, Berger M, Siminoff LA (2003) Development and validation of school-based asthma and allergy screening instruments for parents and students. Ann Allergy Asthma Immunol 90:516–528
45. Redline S, Gruchalla RS, Wolf RL, Yawn BP, Cartar L, Gan V, Nelson P, Wollan P (2004) Development and validation of school-based asthma and allergy screening questionnaires in a 4-city study. Ann Allergy Asthma Immunol 93:36–48
46. Jenkins MA, Clarke JR, Carlin JB, Robertson CF, Hopper JL, Dalton MF, Holst DP, Choi K, Giles GG (1996) Validation of questionnaire and bronchial hyperresponsiveness against respiratory physician assessment in the diagnosis of asthma. Int J Epidemiol 25:609–616

47. Mata Fernandez C, Fernandez-Benitez M, Perez Miranda M, Guillen Grima F (2005) Validation of the Spanish version of the Phase III ISAAC questionnaire on asthma. J Investig Allergol Clin Immunol 15:201–210
48. Fuso L, de Rosa M, Corbo GM, Valente S, Forastiere F, Agabiti N, Pistelli R (2000) Repeatability of the ISAAC video questionnaire and its accuracy against a clinical diagnosis of asthma. Respir Med 94:397–403
49. Kim MH, Kwon JW, Kim HB, Song Y, Yu J, Kim WK, Kim BJ, Lee SY, Kim KW, Ji HM, Kim KE, Shin YJ, Kim H, Hong SJ (2012) Parent-reported ISAAC written questionnaire may underestimate the prevalence of asthma in children aged 10–12 years. Pediatr Pulmonol 47:36–43
50. Hong SJ, Kim SW, Oh JW, Rah YH, Ahn YM, Kim KE, Koh YY, Lee SI (2003) The validity of the ISAAC written questionnaire and the ISAAC video questionnaire (AVQ 3.0) for predicting asthma associated with bronchial hyperreactivity in a group of 13–14 year old Korean schoolchildren. J Korean Med Sci 18:48–52
51. Miller CJ, Joseph J, Safa W, Flood PE, Dunn EV, Shaheen HM (2007) Accuracy of Arabic versions of three asthma symptoms questionnaires against the clinical diagnosis of asthma. J Asthma 44:29–34
52. Nwaru BI, Lumia M, Kaila M, Luukkainen P, Tapanainen H, Erkkola M, Ahonen S, Pekkanen J, Klaukka T, Veijola R, Simell O, Knip M, Virtanen SM (2011) Validation of the Finnish ISAAC questionnaire on asthma against anti-asthmatic medication reimbursement database in 5-year-old children. Clin Respir J 5:211–218
53. Sole D, Vanna AT, Yamada E, Rizzo MC, Naspitz CK (1998) International Study of Asthma and Allergies in Childhood (ISAAC) written questionnaire: validation of the asthma component among Brazilian children. J Investig Allergol Clin Immunol 8:376–382
54. Ublagger E, Schreuer M, Eder W, von Mutius E, Benz MR, Braun-Fahrlander C, Moeller A, Brunekreef B, Schram D, Wickman M, Swartz J, Pershagen G, Riedler J (2005) Validation of questions on asthma and wheeze in farming and anthroposophic children. Clin Exp Allergy 35:1033–1039
55. Santos MC, Cunha AA (2005) A brief questionnaire for screening asthma among children and adolescents in Rio de Janeiro. Brazil Allergol Immunopathol (Madr) 33:20–26
56. Galant SP, Crawford LJ, Morphew T, Jones CA, Bassin S (2004) Predictive value of a cross-cultural asthma case-detection tool in an elementary school population. Pediatrics 114:e307–e316
57. Pearce N, Sunyer J, Cheng S, Chinn S, Bjorksten B, Burr M, Keil U, Anderson HR, Burney P (2000) Comparison of asthma prevalence in the ISAAC and the ECRHS. ISAAC Steering Committee and the European Community Respiratory Health Survey. International Study of Asthma and Allergies in Childhood. Eur Respir J 16:420–426
58. Pekkanen J, Pearce N (1999) Defining asthma in epidemiological studies. Eur Respir J 14:951–957
59. Welty C, Weiss ST, Tager IB, Munoz A, Becker C, Speizer FE, Ingram RH Jr (1984) The relationship of airways responsiveness to cold air, cigarette smoking, and atopy to respiratory symptoms and pulmonary function in adults. Am Rev Respir Dis 130:198–203
60. Enarson DA, Vedal S, Schulzer M, Dybuncio A, Chan-Yeung M (1987) Asthma, asthmalike symptoms, chronic bronchitis, and the degree of bronchial hyperresponsiveness in epidemiologic surveys. Am Rev Respir Dis 136:613–617
61. Dales RE, Ernst P, Hanley JA, Battista RN, Becklake MR (1987) Prediction of airway reactivity from responses to a standardized respiratory symptom questionnaire. Am Rev Respir Dis 135:817–821
62. Rijcken B, Schouten JP, Weiss ST, Speizer FE, van der LR (1987) The relationship of nonspecific bronchial responsiveness to respiratory symptoms in a random population sample. Am Rev Respir Dis 136:62–68
63. Abramson MJ, Hensley MJ, Saunders NA, Wlodarczyk JH (1991) Evaluation of a new asthma questionnaire. J Asthma 28:129–139

64. Ponsonby AL, Couper D, Dwyer T, Carmichael A, Wood-Baker R (1996) Exercise-induced bronchial hyperresponsiveness and parental ISAAC questionnaire responses. Eur Respir J 9:1356–1362
65. Gibson PG, Henry R, Shah S, Toneguzzi R, Francis JL, Norzila MZ, Davies H (2000) Validation of the ISAAC video questionnaire (AVQ3.0) in adolescents from a mixed ethnic background. Clin Exp Allergy 30:1181–1187
66. Lai CK, Chan JK, Chan A, Wong G, Ho A, Choy D, Lau J, Leung R (1997) Comparison of the ISAAC video questionnaire (AVQ3.0) with the ISAAC written questionnaire for estimating asthma associated with bronchial hyperreactivity. Clin Exp Allergy 27:540–545
67. Leung R, Wong G, Lau J, Ho A, Chan JK, Choy D, Douglass C, Lai CK (1997) Prevalence of asthma and allergy in Hong Kong schoolchildren: an ISAAC study. Eur Respir J 10:354–360
68. Pearce N, Weiland S, Keil U, Langridge P, Anderson HR, Strachan D, Bauman A, Young L, Gluyas P, Ruffin D (1993) Self-reported prevalence of asthma symptoms in children in Australia, England, Germany and New Zealand: an international comparison using the ISAAC protocol. Eur Respir J 6:1455–1461
69. Pekkanen J, Remes ST, Husman T, Lindberg M, Kajosaari M, Koivikko A, Soininen L (1997) Prevalence of asthma symptoms in video and written questionnaires among children in four regions of Finland. Eur Respir J 10:1787–1794
70. Shaw R, Woodman K, Ayson M, Dibdin S, Winkelmann R, Crane J, Beasley R, Pearce N (1995) Measuring the prevalence of bronchial hyper-responsiveness in children. Int J Epidemiol 24:597–602
71. Crane J, Mallol J, Beasley R, Stewart A, Asher MI (2003) Agreement between written and video questions for comparing asthma symptoms in ISAAC. Eur Respir J 21:455–461
72. Yu DS, Lee DT, Woo J (2004) Issues and challenges of instrument translation. West J Nurs Res 26:307–320
73. Ellwood P, Williams H, Ait-Khaled N, Bjorksten B, Robertson C (2009) Translation of questions: the International Study of Asthma and Allergies in Childhood (ISAAC) experience. Int J Tuberc Lung Dis 13:1174–1182
74. Weiland SK, Kugler J, von Mutius E, Schmitz N, Fritzsch C, Wahn U, Keil U (1993) The language of pediatric asthma patients. A study of symptom description. Monatsschr Kinderheilkd 141:878–882
75. ISAAC Steering Committee (1993) International Study of Asthma and Allergies and Childhood manual. ISAAC, Auckland/Münster

Nomenclature

5

Hasse Melbye

5.1 Introduction

The various adventitious lung sounds are associated with certain pulmonary diseases, although the strength of the associations may vary [1]. When this diagnostic knowledge is applied in clinical practice and also when physicians communicate their observations on chest auscultation, it is important to have unambiguous terms for the lung sounds. The terminology used today dates back to Laennec's thesis from 1819 [2]. Inadequate translations from French and further elaboration in national languages have led to inconsistent use of terms [3]. Inspired by new knowledge on how lung sounds are generated, a new standardized terminology was introduced by the International Lung Sound Association (ILSA) in the 1980s [4]. The implementation of this nomenclature has varied between countries [5].

5.2 Onomatopoeia and Other Describing Terms

Onomatopoeias are words imitating natural sounds. Laennec used the word "râle" as a common term for abnormal lung sounds, a French term that imitates what we hear when air passes through secretions in the trachea and central bronchi [3]. "Rattle" is the corresponding English term. When Laennec named the different kinds of "rales," some terms were onomatopoetic, like rale "sibilant," whereas others indicated pathophysiological associations, like "rale muqueux." Since patients could connect the term "rale" with death rattling, Laennec decided to exchange

Electronic supplementary material The online version of this article (https://doi.org/10.1007/978-3-319-71824-8_5) contains supplementary material, which is available to authorized users.

H. Melbye
General Practice Research Unit, UIT the Arctic University of Norway, Tromsø, Norway
e-mail: hasse.melbye@uit.no

K. N. Priftis et al. (eds.), *Breath Sounds*, https://doi.org/10.1007/978-3-319-71824-8_5

"rale" with "rhonchus," a Latin onomatopoeia for snoring [3]. "Rale" continued to be used in English language for a rattling-like sound, but when pronounced in English, it was no longer an onomatopoeia. When the International Lung Sound Association proceeded to standardize the terminology, the most common adventitious sounds were divided into two categories, continuous and discontinuous sounds, inspired by acoustic analysis. Terms with onomatopoetic qualities were chosen: wheezes and rhonchi for the continuous sounds and crackles (instead of rales) for discontinuous sounds (Audio 1). The crackles were further divided into "fine" and "coarse" [4] and wheezes into high pitched and low pitched. An updated terminology was recently presented in a review paper by Bohadana and coworkers in *New England Journal of Medicine* in 2014 [1] and is shown in Table 5.1.

The new terminology has to some extent been implemented in English-speaking countries and scientific literature. However, "crepitation" is still much used instead of fine crackles. The term "wheezes" does not have onomatopoetic qualities to cover all continuous sounds, and "whistling" is sometimes used for high-frequency musical wheezes. Terms with onomatopoetic qualities are also preferred in other languages, and adaption of English terms is rarely chosen [6]. For instance, "rasseln" is used for "crackles" in Germany [6].

Table 5.1 Lung sound nomenclature as presented by Bohadana et al. [1]. *Modified with permission from Massachusetts Medical Society*

Respiratory sound	Clinical characteristics
Normal tracheal sound	Hollow and nonmusical, clearly heard in both phases of respiratory cycle
Normal lung sound	Soft, nonmusical, heard only on inspiration and on early expiration
Bronchial breathing	Soft, nonmusical, heard on both phases of respiratory cycle
Stridor	Musical, high pitched, may be heard over the upper airways or at a distance without a stethoscope
Wheeze	Musical, high pitched, heard on inspiration, expiration, or both
Rhonchus	Musical, low pitched, similar to snoring, lower in pitch than wheeze, may be heard on inspiration, expiration, or both
Fine crackle	Nonmusical, short, explosive; heard on mid-to-late inspiration and occasionally on expiration; unaffected by cough, gravity dependent, not transmitted to the mouth
Coarse crackle	Nonmusical, short, explosive sounds; heard on early inspiration and throughout expiration; affected by cough; transmitted to the mouth
Pleural friction rub	Nonmusical, explosive, usually biphasic sounds; typically heard over basal regions (Audio 2)
Squawk	Mixed sound with short musical component (short wheeze) accompanied or preceded by crackles

5.3 Agreement on the Use of Terms

In general, there is a considerable interobserver variation in physicians' reporting of clinical findings, and the agreement on adventitious lung sounds is no exception [7]. Physicians may perceive the sounds differently, and they may also choose different terms when describing the sounds heard. To advance the standardization of lung sound terminology, a task force was established by the European Respiratory Society in 2012. Audiovisual recordings of 20 patients were recorded by the task force members, and these constitute an initial reference collection which is available online [6]. In a separate study, interobserver variation in the classification of lung sounds in these 20 recordings was calculated among 12 observers: six task force members and six other experienced physicians [8]. The optional categories were fine and coarse crackles, high-pitched and low-pitched wheezes, as well as the category of rhonchi. Identification by inspiratory and expiratory phases thus offered ten non-exclusive choices. The study showed poor agreement on detailed descriptions of the sounds (fine and coarse crackles and high-pithed and low-pitched wheezes) and in particular for the category of rhonchi (Fig. 5.1). In contrast, acceptable agreement was found for the combined categories of crackles and wheezes, not inferior to agreement reached in other pulmonary examinations like chest radiography and CT [8].

5.4 Subclassification of Crackles

When applying computerized lung sound analysis, crackles can be subclassified into "fine" and "coarse." There is little doubt about the diagnostic relevance of this subclassification [9]. However, the low agreement on whether crackles are fine or coarse when

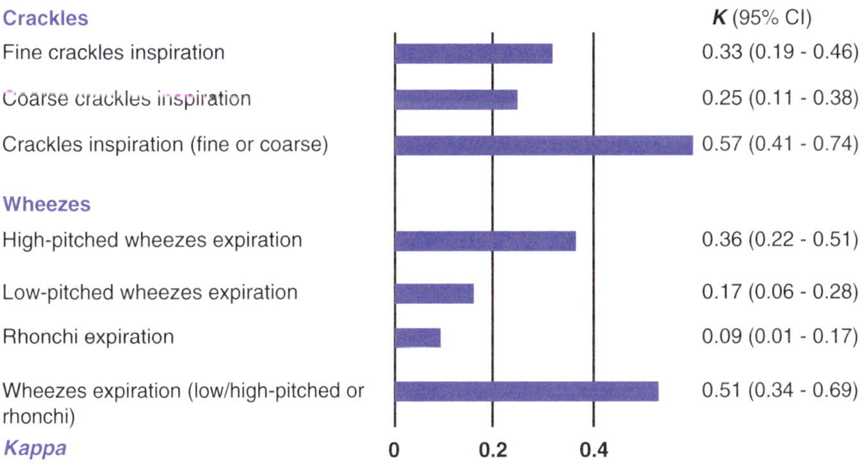

Fig. 5.1 Multirater kappa agreement among 12 observers in identifying inspiratory crackles and expiratory wheezes from audiovisual lung sound recordings [8]. *Modified with permission from BMJ Publishing Group Ltd*

listening to the sound makes the clinical application of this distinction questionable. Crackles can also be described by other characteristics, their quantity and whether they appear early or late during inspiration or expiration. Their timing has also been shown to be of diagnostic significance [9], and agreement on this characteristic may be more easily reached than the agreement on whether the crackles are fine or coarse.

5.5 Wheezes and Rhonchi

The pitch of a wheeze can be determined by computerized acoustic analysis, but it may often be difficult to say after just listening whether it is high pitched or low pitched, as shown in interobserver studies [8]. Another characteristic of wheezes that may be as useful as the pitch in the diagnosis of pulmonary diseases is the duration of each wheeze [10] or the fraction of the respiratory phases occupied by wheezes. "Rhonchi" is a puzzling term, and the listening doctors find it particularly difficult to agree on its use. This may partly be explained by its history as a common term for all adventitious sounds, as defined by Laennec, and as a term for all wheezes in countries like Poland (where sibilant rhonchi is used for high-pitched wheezes) [11] and partly by disagreement on which low-pitched continuous sounds the term should be applied. In the paper by Bohadana and coworkers, a rhonchus is defined as a variant of wheeze with a low pitch, but it is discussed whether it should be regarded as a separate category. "Rhonchi" should probably be applied when mucus is involved in the bronchial obstruction and accordingly be restricted to the nonmusical and often complex snoring-like sounds that tend to disappear after coughing [6]. However, so far, it seems difficult to reliably differentiate between rhonchi and low-pitched wheezes. This gives support to a terminology, in which the two terms may be regarded as interchangeable (Audio 3).

5.6 Clinical Application and Future Development

The terms for the lung sounds should be both reliably shared and clinically useful. When we use our stethoscopes, it will often be preferable to stick to terms reflecting broad categories of lung sounds, such as crackles and wheezes. More detailed descriptions can be used when computerized analyses has been applied. In the future, electronic stethoscopes for clinical use will probably offer computerized analysis and detailed descriptions of the sounds. With more specific terms and a broader range of lung sound categories, there will also be a potential for increased diagnostic specificity of the auscultation findings. The recommended English nomenclature is based on extensive research and is a sound basis for further development and not only for the English language.

References

1. Bohadana A, Izbicki G, Kraman SS (2014) Fundamentals of lung auscultation. N Engl J Med 370(8):744–751
2. Sakula A (1981) R T H Laennec 1781–1826 his life and work: a bicentenary appreciation. Thorax 36(2):81–90

3. Robertson AJ, Coope R (1957) Rales, rhonchi, and Laennec. Lancet 273(6992):417–423
4. Mikami R, Murao M, Cugell DW et al (1987) International Symposium on Lung Sounds. Synopsis of proceedings. Chest 92(2):342–345
5. Francis NA, Melbye H, Kelly MJ et al (2013) Variation in family physicians' recording of auscultation abnormalities in patients with acute cough is not explained by case mix. A study from 12 European networks. Eur J Gen Pract 19(2):77–84
6. Pasterkamp H, Brand PL, Everard M, Garcia-Marcos L, Melbye H, Priftis KN (2016) Towards the standardisation of lung sound nomenclature. Eur Respir J 47(3):724–732
7. Benbassat J, Baumal R (2010) Narrative review: should teaching of the respiratory physical examination be restricted only to signs with proven reliability and validity? J Gen Intern Med 25(8):865–872
8. Melbye H, Garcia-Marcos L, Brand P, Everard M, Priftis K, Pasterkamp H (2016) Wheezes, crackles and rhonchi: simplifying description of lung sounds increases the agreement on their classification: a study of 12 physicians' classification of lung sounds from video recordings. BMJ Open Respir Res 3(1):e000136
9. Piirila P, Sovijarvi AR (1995) Crackles: recording, analysis and clinical significance. Eur Respir J 8(12):2139–2148
10. Shim CS, Williams MH Jr (1983) Relationship of wheezing to the severity of obstruction in asthma. Arch Intern Med 143(5):890–892
11. Raciborski F, Tomaszewska A, Komorowski J et al (2012) The relationship between antibiotic therapy in early childhood and the symptoms of allergy in children aged 6-8 years—the questionnaire study results. Int J Occup Med Environ Health 25(4):470–480

Part II

Sound Recording, Analysis and Perception

Physics and Applications for Tracheal Sound Recordings in Sleep Disorders

6

Thomas Penzel and AbdelKebir Sabil

6.1 Introduction

Advances in technology have made it possible to reliably and not invasively record physiological parameters to diagnose sleep disorders. The most common sleep-related breathing disorder is sleep apnea. Complete cessation of airflow, apneas, or reduction of airflow, hypopneas occurs during sleep [1]. Based on the underlying pathophysiology, these respiratory events are classified as obstructive or central, with or without respiratory efforts. Accurate and reliable detection and classification of apneas and hypopneas are critical for the diagnosis and quantifying of the disease severity, morbidity, or mortality, as well as for appropriate therapy selection.

Sleep-related breathing disorders and other sleep disorders are diagnosed using polysomnography (PSG) with a recording of sleep electroencephalography, respiration, cardiac signals, and movement signals. Polysomnography is performed in general in a sleep laboratory environment attended by trained sleep technicians during the night. Because sleep apnea is so common, systems without attendance and using fewer signals, possibly for use at home, were developed. These specific systems are commonly denoted as polygraphy (PG) or home sleep testing (HST) or out-of-center (OOC) technology. Their complexity is rated according to SCOPER criteria, which stands for sleep, cardiac, oxygen, position, effort of respiration, and respiratory flow, as later explained.

The method of choice to detect respiratory events during sleep according to international recommendations is by detecting reductions in airflow or tidal volume [1].

T. Penzel (✉)
Interdisciplinary Sleep Medicine Center, Charité – Universitätsmedizin Berlin, Berlin, Germany
e-mail: thomas.penzel@charite.de

A. Sabil
Research and Development at CIDELEC, Paris, France
e-mail: kebir.sabil@hotmail.com

K. N. Priftis et al. (eds.), *Breath Sounds*, https://doi.org/10.1007/978-3-319-71824-8_6

Pneumotachography and body plethysmography have traditionally been considered the gold standards for these measurements. However, neither technique is suitable for routine sleep studies with a polysomnography (PSG), which includes sleep electroencephalography or a polygraphy (PG) without sleep electroencephalography. Alternative methods to measure airflow include thermistors and nasal cannula pressure transducers. Thermistors use the difference between the temperature of exhaled and ambient air to estimate airflow. While they may be a reliable method to detect apneas and mouth breathing, these sensors do not provide quantitative measures of airflow for detection of hypopneas. The nasal pressure transducers are an alternative that can be adapted to detect flow limitation. While all previous studies comparing different transducers show that more events are identified by nasal transducers than by thermistors, some data indicate that the nasal pressure transducer may overestimate the magnitude of airflow reduction and misclassify hypopneas as apneas. Different reasons for this are discussed. Mouth breathing, especially in pediatric patients and in the case of nasal obstruction, can have an important impact on respiratory event classification when using a nasal pressure transducer. Furthermore, while thermistors and nasal cannulas are the recommended sensors for detection of apneas and hypopneas, the validity of their signals for more than 6 h of recording is less than 60% for both children [2] and adults [3]. These two sensors are placed in the same very sensitive area for patients, between the nose and the mouth, and can cause patients much discomfort and even affect their sleep. These two sensors are therefore often displaced or even removed by the patients during recording at night, and their signals become then unusable.

For the detection of respiratory efforts and classification of events, esophageal manometry is considered as the golden standard to estimate respiratory effort [1]. However, this method is invasive and can affect sleep quality [4] and, thus, is not used for routine sleep studies.

To counter these problems, indirect ventilation measurement techniques have been developed. Respiratory inductance plethysmography (RIP) estimates volume changes through the measurement of thoracic and abdominal movements. This method uses two belts placed around the thorax and the abdomen. When the nasal pressure and the thermistor signals are of bad quality, the RIP sum signal can be used as a surrogate respiratory flow. In addition, the RIP signals are also recommended for the evaluation of respiratory efforts [1] during sleep studies. However, reliable results by these sensors are dependent on accurate placement and stability of the belts, which are challenging in patients, particularly in young children and obese patients. In addition, accuracy during recording can be diminished by displacement of the belts due to body movements during the night. Thus, there are circumstances where intrathoracic pressure changes do not correspond to proportional changes of thoracic and abdominal circumferences.

Alternative sensors have been advocated for screening OSA, including indirect identification of OSA from the analysis of signals measured using a single sensor, such as oximetry for oxygen saturation [5], ambient microphone for snoring [6], or nocturnal breathing sounds [7–9]. Breathing sound analysis provides valuable information about airway structure and respiratory disorders including

OSA. Analysis of breathing sounds recorded overnight has been used for OSA detection [7–9] with reasonable accuracy compared to PSG. Tracheal sounds, heard at the suprasternal notch, are currently the topic of significant interest. Tracheal sound signals are louder and cover a wide frequency range compared to lung sounds heard on the chest wall [10]. They are very rich in information regarding breathing, and therefore, they could play an important role in monitoring respiratory activity, as well as in the detection and characterization of respiratory events during sleep.

6.2 Historical Background

The detection of tracheal sounds for the measurement of sleep-related respiratory disorders has already been investigated in many studies. In 1980, Krumpe et al. [11] were first to show that laryngeal sound monitoring could be useful in sleep studies. They recorded laryngeal sounds using a microphone coupled to a stethoscope head firmly fixed to the patients' lateral neck or manubrium with adhesive tape. The recorded signal was conditioned using a commercially available amplifier and displayed on a time-based recorder [11]. They found that apnea could be identified by the cessation of laryngeal sounds during continuous monitoring. In a 1982 study, Cummiskey et al. used a tracheal sound sensor associated with a thermistor, a nasal pressure cannula, and pulse oximetry for the detection of apneas and hypopneas. In this study, tracheal breathing sounds were recorded over the manubrium using the same apparatus as in the study by Krumpe et al. [11]. They showed that there was no significant difference in the number of events detected with the tracheal sounds or the reference sensors [12]. In 1988, Penzel et al. developed a new technique for online snoring analysis using a combination of filtered and unfiltered output signals from one laryngeal microphone. One signal was the high-frequency component (800–2000 Hz); the second one was the output of a low-frequency filter (50–800 Hz) that allowed the distinction between snoring and physiological breathing sounds. Using the volume of the breathing sound as the third signal, this method could differentiate between obstructive apneic events characterized by low-volume snoring and hyperventilation at the termination of apneas characterized by loud snoring [13]. However, in these studies, tracheal sound recording was compared only with the conventional method of thermistors, but not with direct measurements of airflow using a pneumotachograph.

In 1989, Meslier et al. [14] simultaneously recorded the tracheal sound and pneumotachograph signals during sleep in healthy patients. In this study, the tracheal breathing sounds were detected by a microphone air-coupled to a stethoscope head as in the first studies but placed right on the sternal notch, which was not the case for the previous studies. There was no difference in the number of apneas and their duration recorded by the tracheal sound method and the pneumotachograph. However, when comparing the tracheal sound method with the thermistor method, apneas appear to be more frequent and of shorter duration using the thermistor [14]. In 1990, Soufflet et al. [15] studied the interaction between tracheal sounds and respiratory rate. In nine healthy subjects, they recorded respiratory flow by means of tracheal microphones and a pneumotachograph and showed that tracheal sounds correlated with the respiratory flow and could be used to measure the flow rate [15].

These studies mainly analyzed the tracheal sound signal in the time domain and looked at how the tracheal intensity signal changes with time, whereas later studies systematically explored frequency analysis of tracheal sound signals and examined how much of the signal lies within each given frequency band over a range of frequencies. In 2004, Nakano et al. [16] tested the automatic spectral analysis of tracheal sounds in 383 patients. They recommended the use of tracheal sound signals in ambulatory diagnostic devices especially for patients with a high probability of OSA [16]. In 2010, Yadollahi et al. [8] investigated the evaluation of tracheal sounds and pulse oximetry in 66 patients in comparison to PSG. They evaluated tracheal sounds, either as the presence of acoustic sound (breathing, snoring, noise) or as the absence of sound (silence). A high correlation was demonstrated between events defined by changes in tracheal sounds and oxygen saturation and standard PSG scoring [8]. Yadollahi et al. [17] examined the agreement between tracheal sounds measured directly at the sternal notch with those recorded 20–30 cm away from the patient. There was a clear advantage of the measurement at the sternal notch [17]. In a recently published study, Mlynczak et al. [18] used a wireless acoustic sensor placed on the tracheal notch to measure breathing sounds during sleep. The study investigated the accuracy of a new method that could differentiate between normal breathing sounds and snoring episodes, using acoustic breathing sounds and artificial neural network techniques. While the system was not validated against full PSG, it gave a good discrimination accuracy of 88.8% with a specificity of 95% [18]. This system was the first to propose a wireless tracheal sound sensor and to use a smartphone application for its interface. Thus, this new system could qualify as a good potential tool for simple OSA screening.

6.3 Tracheal Sounds

Tracheal sounds, heard at the suprasternal notch, are a measure of the body surface vibrations set into motion by pressure fluctuations. These pressure variations are transmitted through the inner surface of the trachea from turbulent airflow in the airways, including the trachea, pharynx, glottis, and subglottic regions [19]. The vibrations are determined by the magnitude and frequency content of the pressure and by the mass, elastance, and resistance of the tracheal wall and surrounding soft tissue. Thus, the surface sensor detects tracheal wall vibrations, not regular acoustic sounds. This characteristic could be used not only to detect tracheal breathing sounds (flow and snoring) but also to record suprasternal pressure, a good surrogate for respiratory efforts evaluation [20, 21].

Given the relatively short distance between the sensor and the various sound sources in the airways, the tracheal sound intensity is robust enough, even at low airflow rates, and an acceptable signal-to-noise ratio can be achieved without the use of preamplification. This makes tracheal sounds more sensitive to changes in respiratory flow in comparison to lung sounds. In addition, the response characteristics for most sensors are linear over a wide range of frequencies [22]. Furthermore, tracheal sounds are better correlated with airflow than lung sounds, and if properly processed, they could distinguish inspiration from expiration [23]. Compared to lung sounds measured through the chest wall, tracheal sounds are often considered as pure and less filtered breath sounds and therefore more useful for the study of breathing and the diagnosis of various respiratory disorders, particularly OSA. In addition, the placement of sound sensors at the trachea notch is relatively easy, and the sensors are less likely to be displaced or removed by patients compared to other sensors during a recording session, especially for sleep studies. However, the quality of the measurement is also influenced by the characteristics of the sensor as well as the quality of air tightness between the sensor and the skin. Furthermore, only signals with surface wavelength larger than the diameter of the tracheal sound sensor could be detected [24]. This makes the tracheal sensors less sensitive to ambient noise.

Compared to normal subjects, OSA patients have specific upper airway (UAW) characteristic differences, such as higher airway collapsibility and smaller cross-sectional area at several levels of the pharynx [25]. The UAW characteristics can affect the resonance produced by the UAW onto the tracheal breathing sounds. The measurements of tracheal sounds provide valuable information concerning upper airways obstruction [25]. Thus, apnea monitoring by simple recording and analysis of tracheal sounds is of interest to sleep physicians. Today, most commercial apnea monitoring devices include tracheal sound sensors in their systems. However, most of these applications use tracheal sounds only for the detection, monitoring, and analysis of snoring in general, an indication of upper airway narrowing during sleep.

To our knowledge, the only tracheal sound sensor commercially available for sleep studies, that detect apneas and not only snoring, is the PneaVoX®. The company CIDELEC, France, investigated the recording of tracheal sounds generated by breathing and developed the sensor to be used with various PG and PGS systems. In 1995, a study by Van Surell et al. [26] compared a PG system that uses tracheal sounds for detection and classification of apneas, with a routine PSG recording in 50 patients. They concluded that the PG system with tracheal sound sensor can be used to detect severe OSA [26].

6.4 Tracheal Sound Sensors

Like stethoscopes, tracheal sound sensors consist of an acoustic sensor inserted into thick protective plastic chamber with thick cuff creating a deep airtight space between the transducer and the skin of the patient (Fig. 6.1a, b). The shape and dimensions of the chamber must display certain characteristics to assure good quality of the recorded tracheal sound signal and practicability of the sensor. Usually, the cavity has a cylindrical shape, and the skin contact face of the sensor is convex so that it fits the curve just above the suprasternal notch. To ensure that the acoustic sensor never touches the skin of the patient during recording, the sensor's cavity allows an air gap of 2–3 mm, between the sensor and the contact surface of the

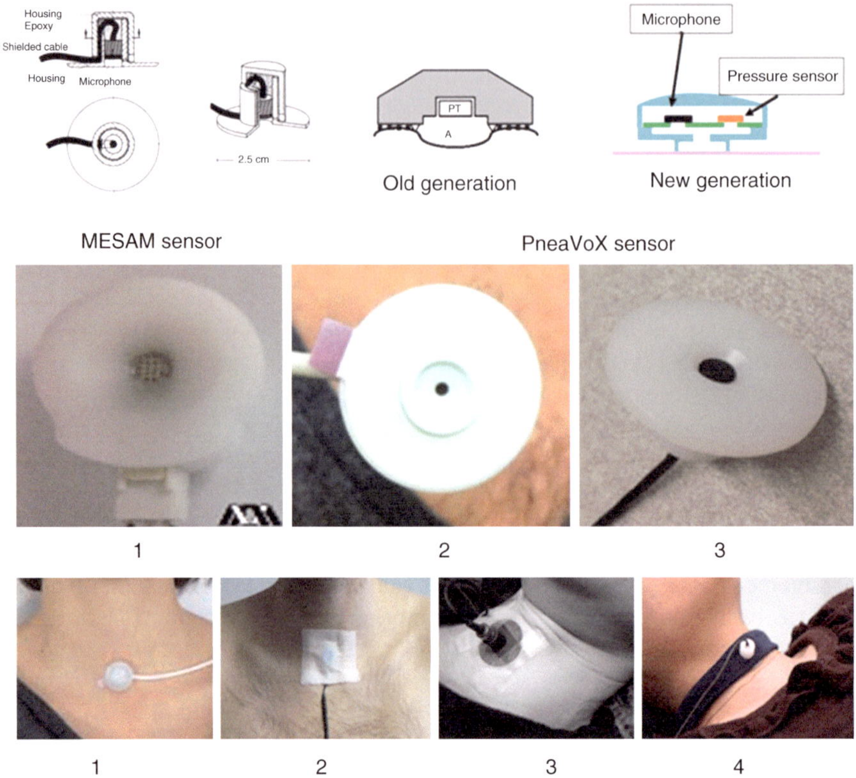

Fig. 6.1 (**a**) Diagrams of three different tracheal sound transducers. The MESAM and the old-generation PneaVoX transducers only used an acoustic sensor. The new-generation PneaVoX uses both an acoustic sensor and a suprasternal pressure sensor. The sensors are inserted in a protective plastic housing. These designs ensure an airtight acoustic chamber between the skin and the transducer. (**b**) Photographs of three different tracheal sound sensors (*1* Reyes et al. [27], *2* PneaVoX, and *3* El Wali et al. [28]) that have been used in published studies over the past 25 years. (**c**) Illustrations of different methods of attachment to the skin of tracheal sound sensors using a double-faced adhesive tape with or without adhesive bandage over the sensor (Meslier et al. [20] and Yadollahi et al. [8]) or a soft elastic band to wrap the sensor around the neck (Nakano et al. [16])

chamber. This kind of sensor had been used for the design of sleep apnea recorders [29]. Airtightness is crucial to insure insulation against ambient noise, and a double-sided ring tape is used to attach the cavity on the patient's skin. However, during recordings, signal saturation may occur since the sensor is air-coupled to the skin by a closed cavity. To solve the saturation problem, a calibrated hole at the back of the sensor is necessary to decrease the sensitivity of the sensor and increase its low-frequency cutoff. The recorded signal is usually amplified, but this amplification may not always be necessary given the high intensity of the tracheal sound signals. The signal is, however, band-pass filtered to separate high-pitch frequencies of the breathing sound from low-pitch frequencies of the snoring sound. Depending on the tracheal sound systems used, the flow sound is usually detected at frequencies between 200 Hz and 2000 Hz with an intensity no greater than a certain threshold level. On the other hand, the snoring sound is usually detected in a frequency range between 20 Hz and 200 Hz with an intensity that exceeds a predetermined threshold level. Specific settings for children for filtering ranges and threshold level may sometimes be applied. Furthermore, advanced systems, such as the PneaVoX®, use a third band-pass filter at a much lower frequency range to extract the suprasternal pressure variations that could be used for the detection of respiratory effort and help characterize the respiratory events during a sleep study. The signal is then sampled and digitized using analog-to-digital converters before analysis. To avoid erroneous sampling, a low-pass antialiasing filter is usually used. The choice of the sampling rate and the number of bits used for the A/D conversion varies from one system to another and depends on the sensitivity and the frequency range of the microphones used. However, the signal quality is affected by these choices. Incorrect application of the tracheal sound sensor, not ensuring an airtight cavity between the skin and the transducer, can also result in poor quality or absence of the signal. The sensor should be placed on the skin above the sternal notch and then secured in place using an adhesive tape. In addition, some systems use an adhesive bandage over the sensor or a soft elastic band to wrap the sensor around the neck (Fig. 6.1c). Correct positioning of the transducer right on the sternal notch is an essential element to obtain a good quality signal.

Cardiogenic oscillations can sometimes be present and may interfere with the breathing sound signal recorded over the tracheal notch. Because the frequency of the heart sounds is lower than the tracheal breath sounds, the heart sound signal can be filtered out. However, these oscillations are more likely to remain visible on the low-frequency suprasternal pressure signal, especially in the absence of effort during central respiratory events. Furthermore, the intensity of the breathing sounds might vary with the different sleep stages in the same individual and among individuals of different age and size. These variations may result in shallow breaths during regular breathing that are misclassified as hypopneas or apneas. This problem may be solved by adjusting the gain on the acoustic sensor and by filtering out background noise more effectively to optimize the signal-to-noise ratio [10].

For a reliable OSA diagnosis, the tracheal sound sensors should be able to detect the respiratory phases as well as detect the complete (apnea) or partial (hypopnea) upper airway obstruction during sleep. While few applications use time domain visual analysis to process tracheal sound signals, most studies use frequency domain automatic analysis.

6.5 Clinical Applications for Sleep Studies

6.5.1 Detection of Events

It has been established that tracheal sounds correlate well with respiratory flow and could be used to estimate airflow. Several features of respiratory sounds have been investigated to find a model that best describes flow-sound relationship [30–33]. Yadollahi et al. [34] examined the relationship between respiratory flow measured using a pneumotachograph (PNT) and four features of tracheal sound evaluated at inspiration and expiration with variable flow rates. These features were average power, logarithm of the variance, logarithm of the range, and logarithm of the envelope of tracheal sound. A linear model at each flow rate was fitted to each feature and to the reference PNT flow. The results showed that the flow-sound relationship is described best with the logarithm of the variance feature as it changes linearly with the changes of the PNT flow signal. However, in terms of the average values of different features in the time domain, the study showed that average values of variance and envelope of tracheal sounds correlate better with the PNT flow at different rates, while average power values present a nonlinear variation at higher flow rates [34]. Regardless of the proposed analysis, to provide easily interpretable signals, breathing sound flow must display a reliable respiratory cycle delimitation (Fig. 6.2). Therefore, it is important to automatically detect inspiration/expiration phases. Different envelope detection techniques, such as Hilbert transform, have been used for the detection of tracheal sound breathing cycle delimitation [32, 34], and breathing cycles could be divided into four different phases: inspiration, inspiratory pause, expiration, and expiratory pause [32]. In another study, Sierra et al. [35] developed a method that combined the sound envelope and the frequency content for an automatic estimation of respiratory cycles using tracheal sounds. Evaluated against pneumotachometer measurements and then compared with the respiratory rate manually counted by a respiratory technician, their algorithm had a high performance [35]. Respiratory cycle phases could easily be detected from lung sounds because of the significant intensity difference between inspiration and expiration [36–39]. Some studies proposed the use of lung sounds as a secondary channel to determine the subject's respiratory phases or simply assumed respiratory phases to be alternating. For instance, Chua et al. [38] used the average power spectrum of respiratory signal and the difference between average tracheal power spectrum and

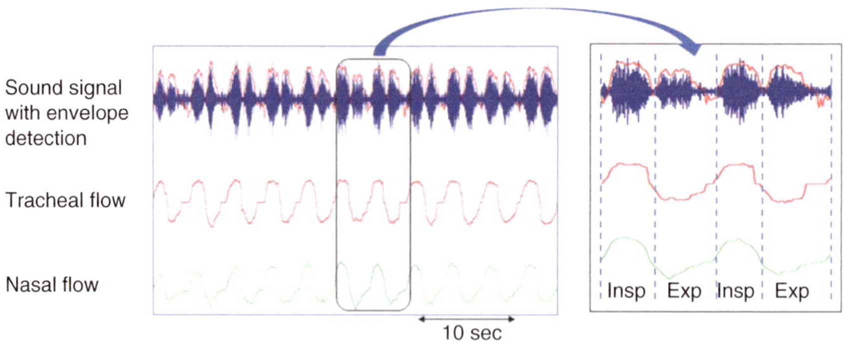

Fig. 6.2 Automatic breathing sound respiratory cycle delimitation using envelope detection techniques. The beginning and the end of inspiration and expiration are properly detected and correspond well to the respiratory cycle delimitation on the nasal pressure signal

chest wall signal to detect respiratory phases. However, for tracheal sounds, the intensity is not only related to the airflow but also to the UAW characteristics. For the same airflow, the higher the UAW resistance, the higher the intensity during either inspiration or expiration is [38]. The biggest challenge in detecting respiratory phases with tracheal sounds only is when complete obstruction, such as during apneas or swallowing, occurs within a respiratory cycle. In a recent study, Huq et al. [40] proposed a reliable method that identifies respiratory phases even when regular breathing pattern is disturbed by swallowing or apnea events. The method was tested on 93 healthy subjects and used several breathing sound parameters (duration, volume, and shape of the sound envelope) to differentiate between inspiration and expiration. Their method requires only one prior and one post breathing sound segment to identify the respiratory phases [40]. These studies showed that detection of respiratory phases using tracheal sounds is possible. Thus, the breathing sound signal could be used as any other flow signal for the analysis of respiratory events during sleep.

Apneas are defined as sleep-related events where respiratory flow is reduced by more than 90% of the reference value for at least 10 s [1]. They are easily detected using periods of tracheal sounds with the same reduction in the corresponding respiratory signal (Fig. 6.3). Hypopneas are sleep-related events where respiratory flow is reduced by more than 30% with associated oxygen desaturation of more than 3% and/or arousal [1]. The shallow breathing during hypopneas (Fig. 6.4) can be combined with snoring, which indicates partial obstruction in the upper airways. These situations are different for each subject and may change for the same patient depending on body position and sleep stage. Thus, compared to apneas, detecting hypopneas using tracheal sounds is more difficult. However, many tracheal sound automatic analysis techniques have been developed using either time domain or frequency domain exploration of the tracheal sound signals. Spectral analysis and variations of tracheal breathing sound intensity, as well as snoring sounds, correlate with respiratory events [5–8, 12, 14].

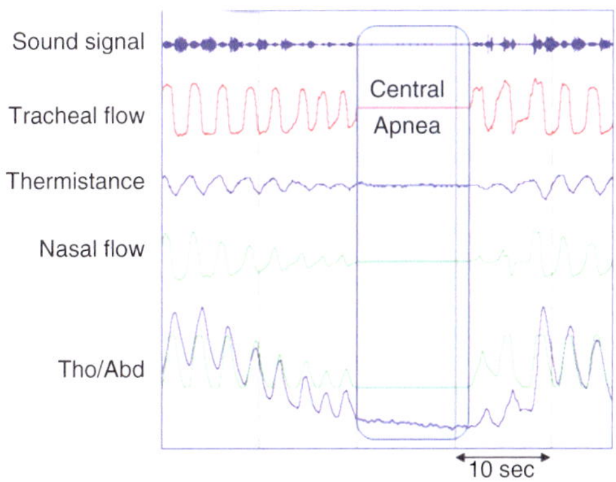

Fig. 6.3 Detection of a central apnea using tracheal sounds. Apneas are characterized by the absence of the tracheal sound signal or the reduction of its amplitude by more than 90%. However, choking sounds can be present during obstructive apneas, but no respiratory cycle is seen during these events

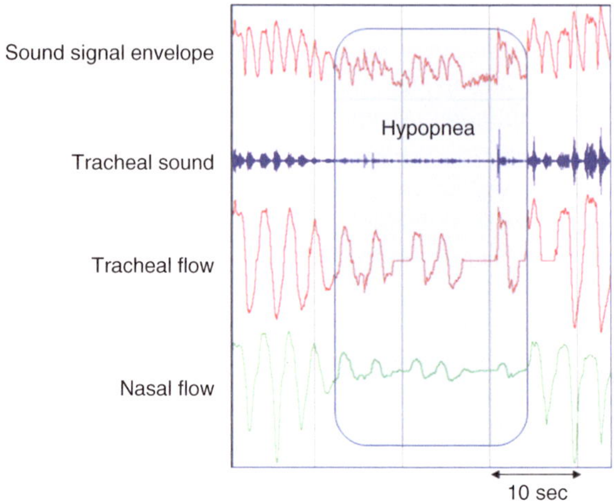

Fig. 6.4 A respiratory event with the criteria for hypopnea without snoring sounds. Persistence of respiratory cycles in the flow sound signal but reduced in amplitude both at inspiration and expiration

Penzel et al. [41] proposed one of the first ambulatory recording (MESAM) systems using a combination of heart rate and snoring analysis to detect sleep-related breathing disorders. They first used a two-channel recorder with a laryngeal microphone and ECG electrodes [41]. A four-channel recorder was developed later with an additional oximeter and a small position sensor. Using filtered breathing sounds with the low-frequency component and the total sound volume, both systems could discriminate between frequencies associated with snoring and those related to other breathing sounds. An automatic analysis algorithm was developed. Using the recorded data combined with an apnea symptoms questionnaire, the MESAM system proved to be valuable in clinical practice with more than 10,000 recordings during 6 years. The clinicians could establish the diagnosis of OSA in the recorded patients or determine if further examinations were needed for the diagnosis [29, 41]. Later the system evolved to the Poly-MESAM and the Micro-MESAM, still used under the name Apnealink. However, those systems did not analyze tracheal sounds any longer.

Kulkas et al. [42] used a temporally detailed analysis of the spectral morphology of the tracheal sound signal to develop a tracheal sound feature for separation of apneas from normal breathing or snoring sounds. For two frequency ranges from 0 to 50 Hz and 50 to 600 Hz, the sum of the amplitude spectrum was calculated and then passed through three types of smoothing filters (mean, median, and maximum) to decrease their local oscillation. The separation feature was defined as the ratio of the smoothed amplitudes of the two frequency ranges and was designed to range from 0 to 1 regardless of tracheal sound amplitudes. The tracheal sound signal amplitudes vary depending on the subjects and sometimes on the system used. Therefore, the proposed amplitude-independent method is more reliable for apnea analysis [42].

Yadollahi et al. [43] developed an automatic acoustic method to detect apnea and hypopnea events using only tracheal respiratory sounds and SpO_2. Tracheal respiratory sounds were automatically segmented to sound and silent segments. Sound segments were classified into breathing, snore, and noise segments. Their method was evaluated on 40 patients recorded simultaneously with tracheal sound monitoring and full-night PSG study. They showed high correlation (96%) of tracheal sound analysis with PSG results, and the method performed well in differentiating simple snorers from OSA patients [43].

Other techniques, such as compressed tracheal breathing sound analysis, have been used to screen for sleep-disordered breathing. Original sounds were compressed using minimum and maximum values of consecutive non-overlapping segments of the recordings. These compressed new traces were divided into plain, thin, and thick signal periods. Visual analysis, as well as automatic analysis with nonlinear filtering of compressed tracheal sounds, seemed to provide an effective tool for screening for obstructive apneas and hypopneas during sleep [44, 45].

Sanchez et al. [46] studied the characteristics of flow-standardized tracheal sounds in children and adults and the possibility of a correlation between tracheal sound spectra and body length. They found that children had significantly louder sounds and that tracheal sounds at a given flow had higher frequency components in children than in adults depending on body length. These findings suggest that sound characteristics are the result of resonance, which depends on upper airway dimensions. Thus, tracheal sounds may be used as noninvasive method to study abnormalities of the UAW [46].

In a later study, Yadullahi et al. [47] investigated the significance of different anthropometric features on the flow-sound model parameters. They compared flow-sound relationship in 93 non-OSA subjects during wakefulness and a group of 13 matched OSA patients and examined the flow-sound relationship in OSA patients during wakefulness and sleep. For non-OSA awake individuals, gender, height, and smoking were the most significant factors related to flow-sound model parameters. For OSA patients, age, gender, and height are major factors contributing to narrowing, increased resistance and collapsibility of the UAW by altering UAW length, wall thickness, and cross-sectional area [47]. These findings led to other studies using tracheal sounds analysis during wakefulness to predict OSA [48–52]. This suggests that OSA patients exhibit narrow UAW during wakefulness that modulates breathing sounds characteristics.

Using computed tomography, Heo et al. [48] have confirmed that there is a significant correlation between the AHI and the UAW minimal cross-sectional area, both during sleep and wakefulness [48]. Formant frequencies of speech, snoring, and nocturnal breathing sound allow the identification of OSA of different degrees of severity [9]. Sola-Soler et al. [53] showed that severe OSA patients could be identified during wakefulness by using information provided by formant frequencies of tracheal breathing sound. They studied several formant features, as well as their variability. Compared to severe OSA patients, mild OSA patients had distinctive formant characteristics in specific frequency bands. Used in combination with other clinical parameters such as the BMI, breathing sound intensity, and airway pressure, these formant features provided classification of OSA subjects between mild-moderate and severe groups with sensitivity, specificity, and accuracy up to 88.9%, 84.6%, and 86.4%, respectively [53].

In two separate studies, Montazeri et al. [51, 52] used tracheal sounds to screen for OSA during wakefulness. In the first study, the tracheal breathing sound was recorded in supine and upright positions with the subjects breathing exclusively through their nose or exclusively through their mouth. The power spectrum density of the tracheal breathing sound signal in each respiratory phase was calculated and averaged over the breaths. Extracted spectral features showed characteristics that could easily discriminate OSA patients from control subjects. This method provides a reliable screening tool for OSA diagnosis during wakefulness [51]. In the second study, the same posture and breathing maneuver were used on 35 apnea patients and 17 control subjects. In addition to the power spectrum analysis, Kurtosis and Katz fractal dimension of the signals were calculated. Using these advanced signal processing techniques, three features were extracted from the tracheal sound signal in different body positions and could be used as a reliable screening tool for OSA and in predicting its severity during wakefulness. The results of this study open the possibility for future clinical validation of a reliable, fast, simple, noninvasive, and inexpensive screening tool for OSA during wakefulness [52].

Sultanzada et al. [54] examined the UAW resistance variability from inspiration to expiration during wakefulness as a predictor of OSA. To estimate UAW resistance changes, tracheal breathing sounds and airflow were simultaneously recorded during PSG recordings with 15 individuals in three groups of mild, moderate, and severe OSA during wakefulness, in supine position. Due to the lack of upper airway muscles patency to dilate the airway constantly, UAW resistance during the active process of inspiration is expected to show more variability when the airways are narrower and more collapsed. UAW resistance variability within a breathing phase was shown to have a different pattern of change from inspiration to expiration in individuals with various level of OSA severity during wakefulness [54].

In a recent study, Al Wali et al. [28] used tracheal breathing sound spectra analysis for characterization of airways structure during wakefulness and daytime screening for OSA. They extracted physiologically meaningful features from the breathing sounds spectral patterns that correlated well with AHI. Based on these features, they developed a new reliable and fast algorithm that accurately separates OSA from non-OSA subjects. While this method has not been clinically validated for OSA diagnosis, this tool could be used for a quick and reliable screening of patients, prior to a surgery requiring full anesthesia, for instance [28].

6.5.2 Characterization of Events

For the snoring sound analysis, Azarbarzin et al. [55] showed in a study with 50 snorers that the ambient snoring sounds (SS) are not as characteristic as tracheal snoring sounds. The signal-to-noise ratio and the power of the signal are much higher with tracheal sounds, providing a better ability to distinguish between regular SS and SS in apneic patients [55]. Apneic SS have different acoustical properties than regular SS segments [56]. Apneic SS are characterized by the lower central tendency measure, lower skewness, and lower first formant frequency. These characteristics were not easily detected with ambient microphones, which could only detect one type of snoring and were unable to detect the acoustical property changes of SS in relation to OSA. For better analysis of snoring sounds, the placement of the sensor on the suprasternal notch is recommended [45]. Snoring sound is also useful for the characterization of hypopneas. The AASM suggests classifying hypopneas as obstructive, if snoring is detected during the event [1]. Furthermore, the presence of snoring can help to avoid misclassifying hypopneas as apneas when the magnitude of airflow reduction is overestimated due to nasal obstruction or poor positioning of the nasal cannula. However, it is possible to have another type of noise during apneas, known as "choking sound," which is induced by intense respiratory effort with a slight, transient reopening of the UAW during obstructive apneas. Scorers need to be careful not to confuse this choking sound with snoring sound.

In a recent study, Sabil et al. [57] used spectral analysis of tracheal sounds to detect choking sounds (CS) from the intermittent (during apnea) or permanent (at the end of apnea) clearing of the temporary UAW occlusion. The study aimed at establishing a link between the characteristics of CS and the nature of apneas characterized using PSG with RIP belts and suprasternal pressure signals. They characterized mixed or obstructive apneas by the presence of CS and central apneas by the absence of CS. The CS were characterized by the mid-inspiration snoring spectrum that could occur in any hyperventilation following the apnea. They showed that choking sounds (Fig. 6.5), at the end of apneas and sometimes during apneic events, correctly characterize obstructive events. During central apneas, these CS are

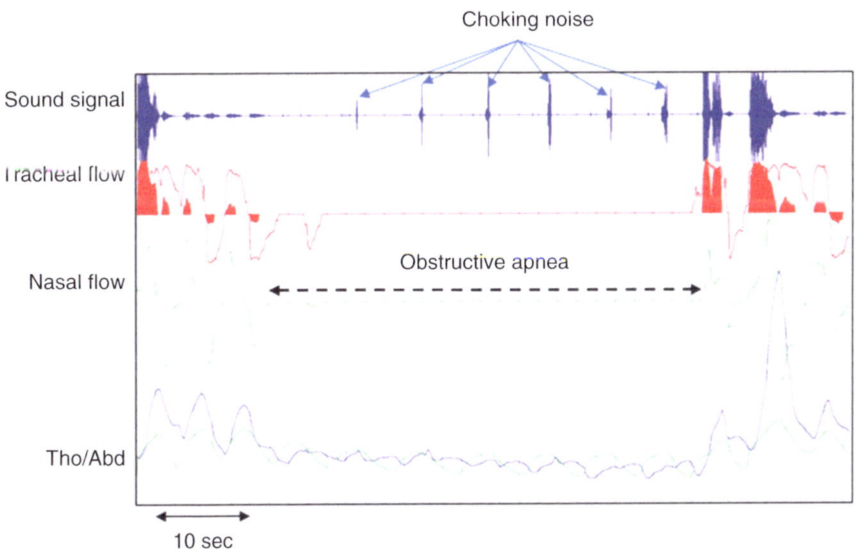

Fig. 6.5 Choking sounds during an obstructive apnea with inspiratory resumption sound and snoring amplification after the obstructive event. Note the absence of respiratory cycles during the event

absent. In addition, this study showed that the spectrum of CS is different than that of snoring, which confirms the role of efforts that generate CS during resumption of ventilation [57].

Racineux [58] examined the acoustic energy of tracheal breathing sounds in patients with increased UAW resistance. He observed a significant correlation between the acoustic energy ratio Ei/Ee (Ei, inspiratory energy, and Ee, expiratory energy) and increased UAW resistance, regardless of the presence or absence of snoring. When airflow passes through UAW without any resistance, flow sound intensity increases throughout inspiration and then throughout expiration, and the energy ratio Ei/Ee remains stable. Acoustic intensity increases with friction. With UAW resistance, friction increases and so does flow sound intensity. The energy ratio Ei/Ee increases with increased inspiratory UAW resistance (Fig. 6.6). Thus, the variation of the acoustic energy ratio Ei/Ee is a good indicator of UAW resistance evaluation [58].

The analysis of tracheal sounds may provide an easy and reliable tool for the detection of respiratory events during sleep. So far, most studies of tracheal and snoring sounds have mainly concentrated on automatic detection of apnea and hypopnea events and did not use tracheal sounds for events characterization, which is crucial for correct diagnosis. Three types of apneas are distinguished: obstructive

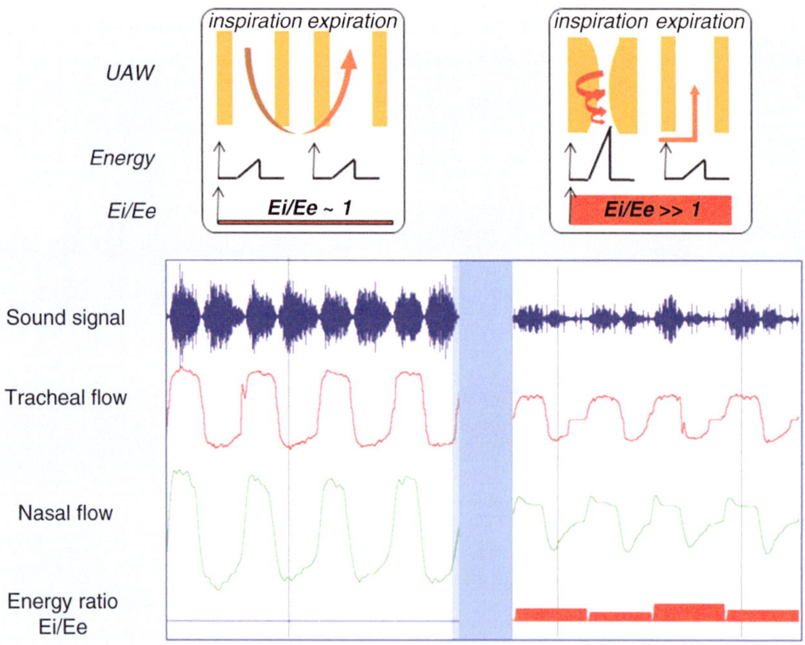

Fig. 6.6 When airflow passes through the UAW, flow sound intensity increases throughout inspiration and then throughout expiration. Acoustic intensity also increases with friction. With UAW resistance, friction increases and so does flow sound intensity. The PneaVox energy ratio Ei/Ee increases with increased inspiratory UAWR

apneas are defined as apneas with constant or increased respiratory efforts. In the absence of respiratory efforts, apneas are central, and if the event starts as central but respiratory efforts resume during the event, the apnea is mixed [1]. To distinguish between obstructive, central, and mixed apneas, in addition to flow measurement for detection of events, recording of the inspiratory effort during sleep is needed. In addition to the low-pitch snoring sound signal and the high-pitch breathing sound signal that can be extracted at different frequency bands from a raw tracheal sound signal, a non-audible much lower frequency signal corresponding to suprasternal pressure (SSP) can also be derived by means of band-pass filtering. This signal corresponds to pressure variations induced by respiratory efforts. The patient's respiratory efforts cause variations of pharyngeal pressure which induce pressure variations in the tracheal sound sensor chamber. These pressure variations are measured through movements of the skin in contact with the sensor at the sternal notch. SSP enables the characterization of an apnea as obstructive, central, or mixed [20, 21, 59]. Figure 6.7 shows an example of obstructive apnea (a) with persistence of respiratory efforts, a central apnea (b) characterized by the absence of respiratory efforts, and a mixed apnea (c) where respiratory efforts are absent at the beginning of the event and resume before the event finishes. In the absence of respiratory efforts, the RIP signals as well as the SSP signal can be reduced to a higher frequency cardiogenic oscillations (Fig. 6.8) compared to during respiratory efforts characterized by a lower frequency respiratory oscillations. The scorers must not interpret these cardiogenic oscillations as the presence of respiratory effort. In a study that used visual analysis of tracheal sound signals, Meslier et al. [20] showed a good correlation between the analysis of SSP and Pes signals in the measurement of respiratory effort for apnea classification. The PG system CID102 with an

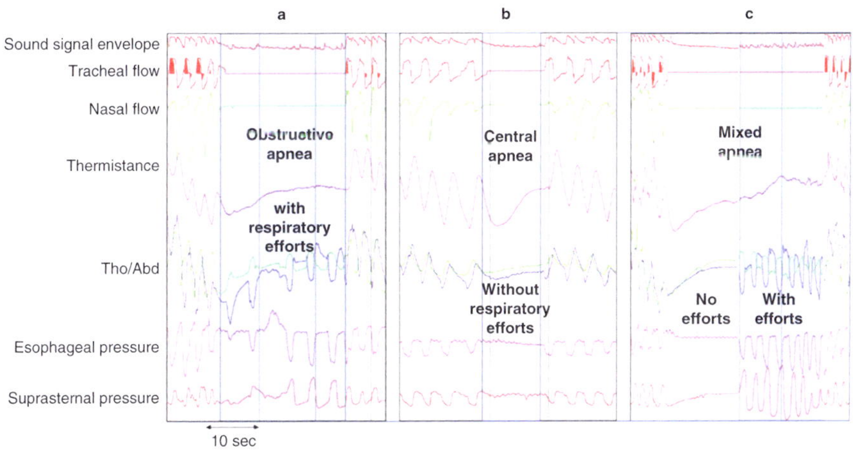

Fig. 6.7 Examples of the three types of apneas: obstructive apnea (**a**) with persistence of respiratory efforts, a central apnea (**b**) with absence of respiratory efforts, and a mixed apnea (**c**) where respiratory efforts are absent at the beginning of the event and resume before the event finishes. The respiratory efforts evaluated with the suprasternal pressure are confirmed on the RIP signals as well as on the esophageal pressure, the gold standard method for effort detection

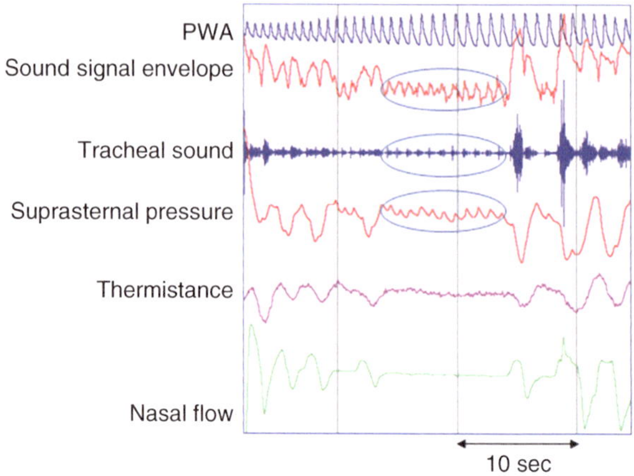

Fig. 6.8 Example of cardiogenic oscillations. In the absence of respiratory efforts, the tracheal sound signal is absent or reduced to cardiogenic oscillations. These oscillations are clearly seen on the suprasternal pressure signal because of its lower-frequency range

acoustic sensor was used in this study [20]. The acoustic sensor was placed over the trachea on the sternal notch, which enables the recording of suprasternal inspiratory pressure related to inspiratory effort, but also of tracheal sounds and snoring. The SSP has a good sensitivity (99.4%) and specificity (93.6%) for the visual evaluation of respiratory efforts in adults when compared to esophageal pressure. Measurement of SSP is recommended for the classification of apnea events with a level III of evidence in France [60]. However, due to the nonlinear nature of the microphone used in this study, there were some limitations to this approach, especially for correct intrathoracic pressure detection. The abovementioned *PneaVoX®* (Cidelec, France), a combination of a pressure transducer and a microphone in one device (Fig. 6.1a) also placed on the suprasternal notch, was developed. In a recent study, Amaddeo et al. compared the PneaVoX® sensor to the sensors recommended by the AASM, oronasal thermal sensor and RIP belts, for the characterization of sleep apneas in children in 20 patients. Compared to the usual recommended polygraph sensors, the PneaVoX sensor has a high degree of scorability in children, and it is a useful tool for characterizing apneas in children [21]. In another recent study, Penzel et al. [59] showed that the evaluation of respiratory effort in sleep apnea patients, using suprasternal pressure (SSP) recording, gives reliable differentiation between obstructive and central apneas. The study was conducted on 34 patients and compared the classification of apneas with the SSP to the RIP belts. In addition, esophageal pressure (Pes) was measured for nine patients as well. Apnea classification with SSP correlated well with the Pes and the RIP reference methods [59].

All these studies show already that tracheal sounds, recorded with appropriate sensors, being more than simple microphones, are able to pick up breathing and snoring and intrathoracic pressure variations. These three parameters are important in the diagnosis and classification of sleep disordered breathing. These parameters, even if they are not defined in the international manual for the recording and scoring of sleep studies [1], are recognized and are currently used for diagnostic studies in home sleep studies for sleep-disordered breathing. Some aspects, such as the recognition of respiratory events, are well validated. Other aspects, such as the recognition of intrathoracic pressure changes, are currently estimated and certainly need more validation studies compared to esophageal pressure recordings in order to determine their use and their limitations in distinguishing obstructive and central respiratory events. Definitely using tracheal sound recording and analysis can be a good and validated substitute for respiratory flow according to SCOPER criteria. SCOPER criteria require the recording of respiratory effort as well. Usually this is done by RIP. The PneaVoX sensor provides a substitute for respiratory effort according to SCOPER criteria. However, more studies are needed to prove the validity of this substitute.

6.5.3 Other Uses

In addition to their ability to detect respiratory efforts and characterize apnea, tracheal sound sensors can also detect oral breathing (Fig. 6.9). Oral breathing detection is important in sleep studies, and the AASM recommends their detection with thermistors. During oral breathing, the nasal pressure signal is null, and the thermistor signal detects respiratory variations. In some cases, patients inhale through their nose and exhale through their mouth or vice versa. In these situations, the use of nasal pressure alone to evaluate the respiratory flow may result in false detection of apneas. During a sleep study, tracheal sound sensors could be used as adjunct airflow sensors to reliably detect mouth breathing. Given that they are taped right on the sterna notch, in comparison to the placement of the oronasal thermistors, the tracheal sound sensors are less likely to be displaced or removed by the patient during a sleep study recording. There is however no study to date evaluating the reliability of tracheal sound analysis to detect oral breathing.

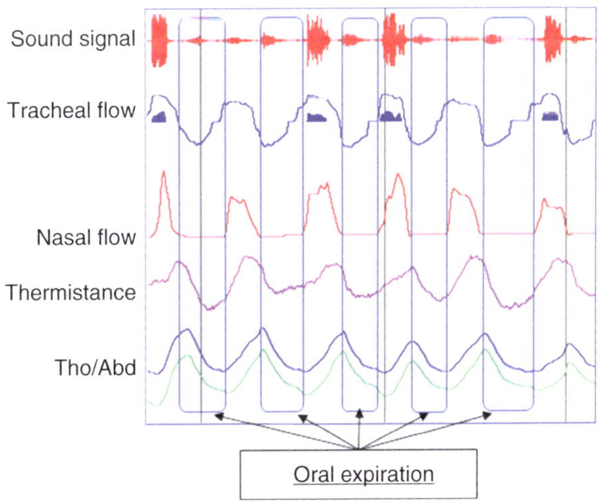

Fig. 6.9 Detection of oral breathing using tracheal sounds. During expiration, the nasal pressure signal is null, while the sound signal remains present. The oral expiration detected by the tracheal sound signal is confirmed by the thermistor signal which shows respiratory variations

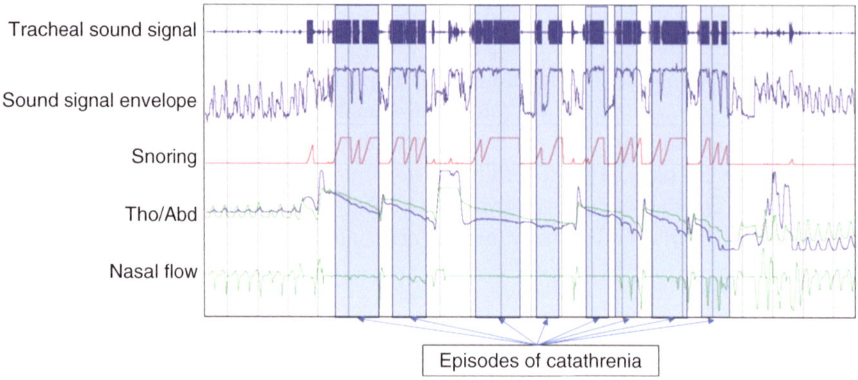

Fig. 6.10 A typical detection of catathrenia by the PneaVoX. Deep inhalation followed by a protracted exhalation. Catathrenia has a respiratory pattern that may mimic central apnea, but during which groaning sounds are produced, usually lasting much longer than regular snoring

Catathrenia is a rare condition characterized by infrequent groaning sounds and prolonged expiration that occur mainly during REM sleep [61]. Several studies have focused on the analysis of the sound and compared the results with snoring [62–65]. Iriarte et al. [65] analyzed the sound of catathrenia to characterize the origin of its sound. They compared catathrenia sounds recorded in two patients (one female) with snoring. Spectral analysis and oscillogram were used, and the sounds were classified according to the Yanagihara criteria [66]. Both sounds had formants, but catathrenia had harmonics and a very short jitter which were not found in snoring sounds. They established that catathrenia sound is laryngeal but could not be classified as expiratory snoring [65]. None of the previously published studies measured the catathrenia sounds at the tracheal notch, and this is probably the reason why the characteristics of the sounds vary among the studies. However, preliminary data from an ongoing study have shown that tracheal sound recordings provide acoustic information about catathrenia (Fig. 6.10) [67].

Conclusion

While tracheal sounds have been the subject of many research studies, we only presented in this chapter some of the original work that we thought was promising and relevant to upper airways obstruction during sleep. Tracheal sound sensors offer simple and noninvasive measurements and are more reliable compared to other breathing sensors. The development in acoustic processing techniques and the enhancement of tracheal sound signals over the past decade have led to both improved accuracy and clinical relevance of the diagnosis based on this technology. Past and current research suggest that they may have a significant role in the diagnosis of OSA.

In conclusion, associated with appropriate signal processing techniques, tracheal sound transducers could be used as threefold sensors: a snoring monitoring sensor, an oronasal respiratory flow sensor, and a respiratory effort monitoring sensor. Tracheal sound analysis is a reliable method to study the pathophysiology of the upper airway. It could be used as an adjunct tool in sleep study systems to detect breathing and snoring sound segments and estimate the respiratory cycle delimitation. It provides important physiological information about UAW narrowing and collapsibility that could be used to detect and characterize respiratory events during sleep. The tracheal sound complementarity with the routine PSG sensors makes the OSA diagnosis more reliable. In addition to their relevance during sleep, tracheal sounds could also be used as a screening tool for prediction of OSA during wakefulness. Added to the AASM-recommended sensors, the tracheal sound technology can improve detection of sleep-disordered breathing during sleep studies.

References

1. Berry RB, Brooks R, Gamaldo CE, for the American Academy of Sleep Medicine (2014) The AASM manual for the scoring of sleep and associated events: rules, terminology and technical specifications, version 2.1. American Academy of Sleep Medicine, Darien, IL
2. Goodwin JL, Enright PL, Kaemingk KL, Rosen GM et al (2001) Feasibility of using unattended polysomnography in children for research—report of the tucson children's assessment of sleep apnea study (TuCASA). Sleep 24(8):937–944
3. Redline S, Sanders MH, Lind BK, Quan SF et al (1998) Methods for obtaining and analyzing unattended polysomnography data for a multicentre study. Sleep heart health research group. Sleep 21(7):759–767
4. Chervin RD, Aldrich MS (1997) Effects of esophageal pressure monitoring on sleep architecture. Am J Respir Crit Care Med 156:881–885
5. Alvarez D, Hornero R, Marcos JV, Del Campo F et al (2008) Applying time, frequency and nonlinear features from nocturnal oximetry to OSA diagnosis. In: 30th Conf. Proc. IEEE Eng. Med. Biol. Soc., p 3872–3875
6. Solà-Soler J, Fiz JA, Morera J, Jané R (2012) Multiclass classification of subjects with Sleep Apnoea-Hypopnoea Syndrome through snoring analysis. Med Eng Phys 34(9):1213–1220
7. Azarbarzin A, Moussavi Z (2013) Snoring sounds variability as a signature of obstructive sleep apnea. Med Eng Phys 35(4):479–485
8. Yadollahi A, Giannouli E, Moussavi Z (2010) Sleep apnea monitoring and diagnosis based on pulse oximetry and tracheal sound signals. Med Biol Eng Comput 48(11):1087–1097
9. J. Solà-Soler, R. Jané, J. A. Fiz and J. Morera (2008) Formant frequencies of normal breath sounds of snorers may indicate the risk of Obstructive Sleep Apnea Syndrome. In: 30th Conf. Proc. IEEE Eng. Med. Biol. Soc., p. 3500–3503
10. Gavriely N, Cugell D (1996) Airflow effects on amplitude and spectral content of normal breath sounds. J Appl Physiol 80:5–13
11. Krumpe PE, Cummiskey JM (1980) Use of laryngeal sound recordings to monitor apnea. Am Rev Respir Dis 122(5):797–801
12. Cummiskey J, Williams TC, Krumpe PE, Guilleminault C (1982) The detection and quantification of sleep apnea by tracheal sound recordings. Am Rev Respir Dis 126:221–224
13. Penzel T, Amend G, Peter JH, Podszus T, Von Wichert P, Zahorka M (1988) Objective monitoring of therpeutical success in heavy snorers: a new technique. In: Chouard CH (ed) Chronic rhonchopathy. John Libbey Eurotext, London, pp 273–278
14. Meslier N, Racineux JL (1987) Use of tracheal sound recordings to monitor airflow during sleep. In: Peter JH, Podszus T, von Wichert P (eds) Sleep related disorders and internal diseases. Springer, Berlin, Heidelberg. https://doi.org/10.1007/978-3-642-72560-9_11
15. Soufflet G, Charbonneau G, Polit M, Attal P, Denjean A, Escourrou P, Gaultier C (1990) Interaction between tracheal sound and flow rate: a comparison of some different flow evaluations from lung sounds. IEEE Trans Biomed Eng 37(4):384–391

16. Nakano H, Hayashi M, Ohshima E, Nishikata N, Shinohara T (2004) Validation of a new system of tracheal sound analysis for the diagnosis of sleep apnea-hypopnea syndrome. Sleep 27:951–957
17. Yadollahi A, Moussavi Z (2010) Automatic breath and snore sounds classification from tracheal and ambient sounds recordings. Med Eng Phys 32:985–990
18. Mlynczak M, Migacz E, Migacz M, Kukwa W (2017) Detecting breathing and snoring episodes using a wireless tracheal sensor: a feasibility study. IEEE J Biomed Health Inform 21(6):1504–1510
19. Gavriely N (1995) Breath sounds methodology. CRC Press, Boca Raton, FL, pp 31–33
20. Meslier N, Simon I, Kouatchet A, Ouksel H, Person C, Racineux JL (2002) Validation of a suprasternal pressure transducer for apnea classification during sleep. Sleep 25(7):753
21. Amaddeo A, Fernandez-Bolanos M, Olmo Arroyo J, Khirani S, Baffet G, Fauroux B (2016) Validation of a suprasternal pressure sensor for sleep apnea classification in children. J Clin Sleep Med 12(12):1641–1647
22. Yadollahi A, Moussavi Z (2005) Measuring minimum critical flow for normal breath sounds. Conf Proc IEEE Eng Med Biol Soc 3:2726–2729
23. Beck R, Rosenhouse G, Mahagnah M, Chow RM, Cugell DW, Gavriely N (2005) Measurements and theory of normal tracheal breath sounds. Ann Biomed Eng 33(10):1344–1351
24. Sovijärvi AR, Malmberg LP, Charbonneau G, Vanderschoot J, Dalmasso F, Sacco C, Rossi M, Earis JE (2000) Characteristics of breath sounds and adventitious respiratory sounds. Eur Respir Rev 10:591–596
25. Ayappa I, Rappaport DM (2003) The upper airway in sleep: physiology of the pharynx. Sleep Med Rev 7:9–33
26. Van Surell C, Lemaigre D, Leroy M, Foucher A, Hagenmuller MP, Raffestin B (1995) Evaluation of an ambulatory device, CID 102, in the diagnosis of obstructive sleep apnoea syndrome. Eur Respir J 8:795–800
27. Reyes BA, Reljin N, Chon KH (2014) Tracheal sounds acquisition using Smartphon. Sensors 14:13830–13850
28. Elwali A, Moussavi Z (2017) Obstructive sleep apnea screening and airway structure characterization during wakefulness using tracheal breathing sounds. Ann Biomed Eng 45(3):839–850
29. Penzel T, Peter JH (1991) Design of an ambulatory sleep apnea recorder. In: Nagle HT, Tompkins WJ (eds) Case studies in medical instrument design. The Institute of Electrical and Electronics Engineers, Orlando, pp 171–179
30. Beckerman RC, Wegmann MJ, Waring WW (1982) Tracheal breath sounds for detection of apnea in infants and children. Crit Care Med 10(6):363 6
31. Que C, Kolmaga C, Durand L, Kelly S, Macklem P (2002) Phonospirometry for noninvasive measurement of ventilation: methodology and preliminary results. J Appl Phys 93:1515–1526
32. Harper V, Pasterkamp H, Kiyokawa H, Wodicka G (2003) Modeling and measurement of flow effects on tracheal sounds. IEEE TransBiomed Eng 50(1):1–10
33. Golabbakhsh M, Moussavi Z (2004) Relationship between airflow and frequency-based features of tracheal respiratory sounds. In: Proc. IEEE Canadian Conf. Elec. Comp. Eng. (CCECE), p 751–754
34. Yadollahi A, Moussavi Z (2007) Acoustical flow estimation: review and validation. IEEE Mag Biomed Eng 26(1):56–61
35. Sierra G, Telfort V, Popov B, Durand LG, Agarwal R, Lanzo V (2004) Monitoring respiratory rate based on tracheal sounds. First experiences. Conf Proc IEEE Eng Med Biol Soc, 1:317–320
36. Yadollahi A, Moussavi Z (2008) Comparison of flow-sound relationship for different features of tracheal sound. Conf Proc IEEE Eng Med Biol Soc, 2008:805–808
37. Kulkas A, Huupponen E, Virkkala J, Tenhunen M, Saastamoinen A, Rauhala E, Himanen S-L (2009) Intelligent methods for identifying respiratory cycle phases from tracheal sound signal during sleep. Comput Biol Med 39:1000–1005
38. Chuah JS, Moussavi Z (2000) Automated respiratory phase detection by acoustical means. In: Proceedings of system cyber information conference, p 228–231

39. S. Le Cam, C. Collet, F. Salzenstein (2008) Acoustical respiratory signal analysis and phase detection. In: Proceedings of IEEE international conference on acoustics, speech, and signal processing (ICASSP), p 3629–3632
40. Huq S, Moussavi Z (2012) Acoustic breath-phase detection using tracheal breath sounds. Med Biol Eng Comput 50:297–308
41. Penzel T, Amend G, Meinzer K, Peter JH, Von Wichert P (1990) MESAM: a heart rate and snoring recorder for detection of obstructive sleep apnea. Sleep 13(2):175–182
42. Kulkas A, Huupponen E, Virkkala J, Tenhunen M, Saastamoinen A, Rauhala E, Himanen S-L (2009) New tracheal sound feature for apnoea analysis. Med Biol Eng Comput 47:405–412
43. Yadollahi A, Moussavi Z (2009) Acoustic obstructive sleep apnea detection. Conf Proc IEEE Eng Med Biol Soc 2009:7110–7113
44. Kulkas A, Rauhala E, Huupponen E, Virkkala J, Tenhunen M, Saastamoinen A, Himanen S-L (2008) Detection of compressed tracheal sound patterns with large amplitude variation during sleep. Med Biol Eng Comput 46:315–321
45. Rauhala E, Hasan J, Kulkas A, Saastamoinen A, Huupponen E, Cameron F, Himanen SL (2008) Compressed tracheal sound analysis in screening of sleep-disordered breathing. Clin Neurophysiol 119:2037–2043
46. Sanchez I, Pasterkamp H (1993) Tracheal sound spectra depend on body height. Am Rev Respir Dis 148:1083–1087
47. Yadollahi A, Moussavi Z (2011) Detailed analysis of the relationship between tracheal breath sounds and airflow in relation to OSA during wake and sleep. Conf Proc IEEE Eng Med Biol Soc 2011:6797–6800
48. Heo JY, Kim JS (2011) Correlation between severity of sleep apnea and upper airway morphology: cephalometry and MD-CT study during awake and sleep states. Acta Otolaringol 131:84–90
49. Yadollahi A, Montazeri A, Azarbarzin A, Moussavi Z (2013) Respiratory flow–sound relationship during both wakefulness and sleep and its variation in relation to sleep apnea. Ann Biomed Eng 41(3):537–546
50. Montazeri A, Moussavi Z (2010) Acoustical screening for obstructive sleep apnea during wakefulness. Conf Proc IEEE Eng Med Biol Soc 2010:3662–3665
51. Montazeri A, Moussavi Z (2011) Obstructive sleep apnea prediction during wakefulness. Conf Proc IEEE Eng Med Biol Soc 2011:773–776
52. Montazeri A, Moussavi Z (2012) Assessment of obstructive sleep apnea and its severity during wakefulness. Ann Biomed Eng 40(4):916–924
53. Solà-Soler J, Fiz JA, Torres A, Jané R (2014) Identification of obstructive sleep apnea patients from tracheal breath sound analysis during wakefulness in polysomnographic studies. Conf Proc IEEE Eng Med Biol Soc 2014:4232–4235
54. Sultanzada R, Moussavi Z (2015) Upper airway resistance changes from inspiration to expiration during wakefulness is a predictor of sleep apnea: a pilot study. Conf Proc IEEE Eng Med Biol Soc 2015:2231–2234
55. Azarbarzin A, Moussavi Z (2012) A comparison between recording sites of snoring sounds in relation to upper airway obstruction. Conf Proc IEEE Eng Med Biol Soc 2012:4246–4249
56. Perez-Padilla J, Slawinski E, Difrancesco L, Feige R, Remmers J, Whitelaw W (1993) Characteristics of the snoring noise in patients with and without occlusive sleep apnea. Am Rev Respir Dis 147(3):635–644
57. Sabil A, Baffet G, Freycenon C, Pinguet J (2017) Apnea charcterization using tracheal sound spectral analysis. Sleep and Breathing conference, Marseille
58. Racineux JL (2006) Bruit trachéal et résistance des voies aériennes supérieures. Rev Mal Respir 23:7S48–7S50
59. Glos M, Sabil A, Jelavic KS, Schöbel C, Fietze I, Penzel T (2018) Characterization of respiratory events in obstructive sleep apnea using suprasternal pressure monitoring. J Clin Sleep Med. Accepted 17 Nov. 2017 (in press)
60. "Recommandations pour la pratique clinique (RPC)", for the classification of apneas with a level of evidence of III recommended

61. De Roek J, Van Hoof E, Cluydts R (1983) Sleep related expiratory groaning. A case report. Sleep Res 12:237
62. Guilleminault C, Hagen CC, Khaja AM (2008) Catathrenia is not expiratory snoring. Sleep 31(6):774–775
63. Siddiqui F, Walters AS, Chokroverty S (2008) Catathrenia: a rare parasomnia which may mimic central sleep apnea on polysomnogram. Sleep Med 9(4):460–461
64. Vetrugno R, Lugaresi E, Ferini-Strambi L, Montagna P (2008) Catathrenia (nocturnal groaning): what is it? Sleep 31(3):308–309
65. Iriarte J, Fernández S, Fernandez-Arrechea N, Urrestarazu E, Pagola I, Alegre M, Artieda J (2011) Sound analysis of catathrenia: a vocal expiratory sound. Sleep Breath 15:229–235
66. Yanagihara N (1967) Significance of harmonic changes and noise components in hoarseness. J Speech Hear Res 10:531–541
67. Baffet G, Montaron C, Sabil A (2016) A new sensor for various respiratory events detection during sleep. ESRS Conference, Bologna, 2016

Check for updates

Sound Transmission Through the Human Body

7

Steve S. Kraman

7.1 Introduction

Many parts of the human body have been probed by acoustic techniques. Ultrasound has been used to image the heart, blood, blood vessels, abdominal and pelvic organs, and the developing fetus, and it has been developed into a mature technology used in nearly every hospital and many clinics. There has also been some interest in analyzing the sounds made by the gastrointestinal system and various joints. Nevertheless, this is a chapter in a book on breath sounds, so I will focus narrowly on the acoustics of the respiratory system.

The acoustic terrain of the respiratory system is a complicated and messy place. Different lung sounds are produced in different locations within the tracheobronchial tree or lung parenchyma and take a variety of routes to get to the chest wall where they can be detected. In doing so, they traverse a variety of biological tissues of diverse thickness, density, and compressibility that all influence sound speed and may favor passage of certain acoustic wavelengths while impeding others. Of course none of this was known when Laennec invented the stethoscope and came up with the first comprehensive description of lung sounds and their association with specific diseases [1]. Had he known in advance how acoustically complicated the respiratory system is, he may have thought better of his plans and found an easier way to pass the time. However, despite his ignorance about what lay beneath his stethoscope, he was nevertheless able to use audible pattern recognition together with his long experience in personally performing autopsies on his own patients to produce a schema that provided valuable diagnostic information and continues to be used effectively today, nearly 200 years later by most clinical practitioners around the world. In fact, the only substantial changes that have been made to Laennec's diagnostic descriptions are in nomenclature, a remarkable legacy. This is even more

S. S. Kraman, M.D.
University of Kentucky, Lexington, KY, USA
e-mail: sskram01@uky.edu

K. N. Priftis et al. (eds.), *Breath Sounds*, https://doi.org/10.1007/978-3-319-71824-8_7

amazing as it could be stated that few twenty-first century practitioners understand the acoustics of the respiratory system any better than did Laennec. Rather, they, like he, just associate certain sounds with certain diseases, as they have been taught in their medical training.

Several of these sounds have been long associated with significant changes in acoustic transmission through parts of the respiratory system and are still in use today although much less commonly than in past decades. There are different percussion notes (flat, dull, resonant, hyperresonant), changes in the character of the transmitted voice (pectoriloquy, egophony), the rarely used coin test, and sternal percussion. All are more or less poorly defined and lack much scientific scrutiny. Nevertheless, in skilled hands, some of these signs effectively identify pathology that can later be proven by subjecting the patient to modern imaging techniques.

Over approximately the last 50 years, new acoustic analysis techniques and instrumentation have been used to better describe lung sounds and to try to determine how they are made and how they reach the chest wall. Although some may not agree, I would argue that the most important conclusion that has emerged from this half-century of research was the revelation of the enormous acoustic complexity of the respiratory system. Researchers have worked out parts of the puzzle regarding both generation and transmission of sound through the respiratory system, but few would argue that most of the mysteries remain unsolved. This is true because of the complexity of the problem and in significant part because other medical technological advances have attracted the majority of government and industry interest as well as the limited financial resources needed for research. The effort to improve the understanding of the physiology underlying a 200-year-old technology is not on an equal footing with the development of new and often amazing developments such as computed tomography, ultrasonography, and magnetic resonance imaging. Nevertheless, a substantial amount of research has been carried out over the past 50 years and has given us new insights into the respiratory system and what can be understood through the investigation of its acoustic properties. This should not be ignored as the technology that Laennec first invented remains useful, available, cheap, and readily at hand at a moment's notice.

Other chapters of this textbook will deal with what is known about the production of lung sounds, both normal and abnormal. However, since transmission of lung sounds is critically dependent on the location of the structure producing the sound and of the position of the sound detector, something should be said about which structures produce the sounds that we are interested in. Our knowledge about this is incomplete. Normal lung sounds are thought to be produced in the medium-sized airways, probably centered at the lobar and segmental airways. Sounds heard high-up on the anterior chest wall are probably produced at least in part, in the trachea or perhaps even the larynx. Wheezes and rhonchi are likely produced in smaller airways although this could be variable and, to my knowledge, has not been firmly established. Fine crackles appear to be produced in the most peripheral airways of the lung, usually immediately underlying the pleura, whereas coarse crackles are probably produced more proximally although exactly where is uncertain. These different locations of sound producers determine how much of the lung is traversed by the sound. Transmission paths may involve primarily airway or parenchyma or combinations that are poorly defined and difficult to investigate. Multipath transmission and reverberation occur in many acoustic environments and can complicate analysis as well. In addition, for all usual clinical situations, sound must also penetrate and traverse the chest wall which is made up of varying substances with different acoustic characteristics. The thickness of the chest wall varies from location to location and varies even more among different persons.

This chapter will deal exclusively with transmission of sound through the respiratory system. By this I mean both sounds that are produced within the respiratory system and those that are introduced, as a probing device, from outside of it but not including ultrasound which, by its nature, is of no value in penetrating air-containing tissue.

7.2 Transmission of Artificial Sound Introduced into the Airway

One of the earliest studies of sound transmission from mouth-to-chest wall was carried out by Ploy-Song-Sang et al. [2]. They placed microphones on the chest of the subjects at four anterior locations, apex to base on each side of the sternum in the midclavicular line. They recorded lung sounds as well as transmitted band-limited white noise (150–350 Hz) in the subjects in supine and upright positions. ^{133}Xe ventilation scans were also performed. Then, the transmitted sound data was used to adjust for lung sound amplitude, and the resulting compensated breath sound distribution pattern was compared with the ^{133}Xe ventilation scans. They found their compensated breath sound index to better match the ventilation scan pattern than did the raw lung sounds in both postures suggesting that this acoustic technique could perhaps supplant ventilation scans that use radioactive gases.

Kraman and Austrheim [3] examined the relationship between naturally occurring lung sounds and transmitted sound of similar frequency composition introduced at the mouth. Unlike the study of Ploy-Song-Sang et al. [2], they mapped the sounds apex to base bilaterally, front and back in 2-cm increments. Their sound amplitude maps revealed maximal lung sound amplitude at the anterior apices bilaterally in a pattern similar to the transmitted sound. Posteriorly, the transmitted sounds were also at a maximum near the apices, whereas the lung sounds were loudest at the bases. In all cases, the transmitted sounds were of greater amplitude on the right side, whereas the lung sounds were roughly symmetrical. In a secondary examination of one upright subject, the investigators mapped lung sounds and transmitted sounds in a band encircling the upper chest. They found that the two sound patterns were quite distinct with the loudest lung sounds on the left and transmitted sounds on the right side (Fig. 7.1). As all sounds were recorded at the same horizontal level, no gravitational gradient could have caused these discrepancies. The authors surmised that much of the sound introduced at the mouth exits the trachea at the right side of the mediastinum where the tracheal wall directly abuts the pleura and thereby directly couples to the parenchyma, bypassing the airways and making

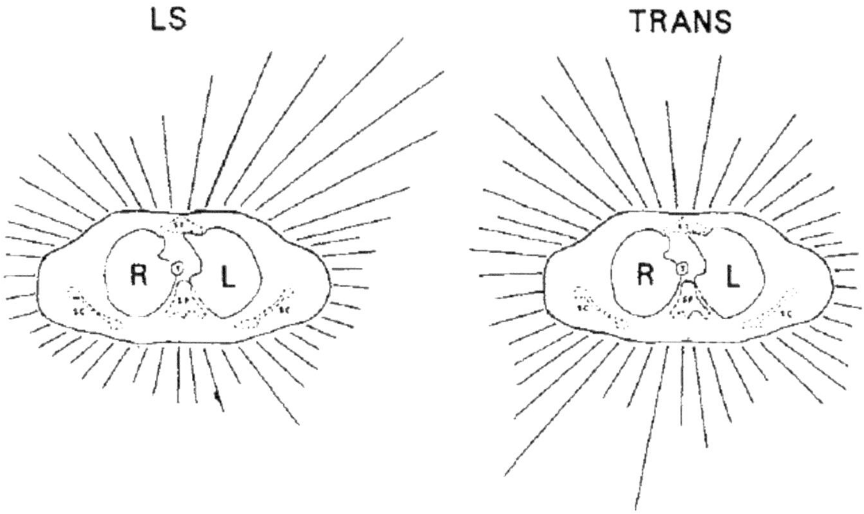

Fig. 7.1 Lung sound (LS) and transmitted sound (TRANS) maps recorded at a horizontal line encircling the chest at the level of the third thoracic vertebra in a standing subject. The length of the straight lines radiating from the chest is proportional to sound pressure measured at that point. Note the position of the trachea in direct contact with the medial aspect of the right lung. *R* right, *L* left, *T* trachea, *ST* sternum, *SC* scapula, *SP* spine [3]. Reprinted with permission of the American Thoracic Society. Copyright 2016 American Thoracic Society. The American Journal of Respiratory and Critical Care Medicine is an official journal of the American Thoracic Society

mouth-to-chest wall transmitted sound unlikely to correct for distribution of ventilation.

In a subsequent study [4], Fiz et al. confirmed similar asymmetry of naturally produced lung sounds (left > right) in subjects studied in sitting, supine, prone, and lateral decubitus positions with little change among them.

Wodicka and colleagues [5] studied the pattern of transmitted sounds through the lungs of healthy men over six posterior chest wall sites within three different frequency bands (100–600 Hz [low], 600–1100 Hz [mid], and 1100–1600 Hz [high]). They found a right-to-left dominance of transmission as Kraman and Austrheim had previously reported [3] but only in the low-frequency range. For the mid- and high-range sounds, there was no lateral dominance at all. This suggested more airway-borne transmission and less coupling of the sound to the airway wall at these higher frequencies.

Rice and colleagues have investigated transmission of sound through animal lungs, both airways and parenchyma. In a pivotal study [6], Rice measured the speed of audible, high-frequency sounds (>10 kHz) produced by a spark gap placed within a catheter in the trachea. The sound was limited at the receiving end to a band between 10 kHz and 20 kHz. This is a frequency range much higher than that of any naturally occurring lung sounds or that had been studied by others using transmitted sounds [2, 3, 5]. Rice measured the acoustic velocity of transmission (spark to lung surface) to be 349 m/s and found it to be dependent on lumen gas composition, temperature, and mean flow speed. This is virtually the same as the speed of sound through air. It was insensitive to cross-sectional area and shape, flow profile, transpulmonary pressure, and lung volume. Rice theorized that the composition of the airway walls was apparently unimportant as the airway tissue is acoustically rigid at these high sound frequencies. At frequencies at and below 1000 Hz where virtually all lung sounds (normal and abnormal) reside, airway walls appear to interact strongly with the vibrating air column resulting in a much slower sound speed.

Rice [7] also examined acoustic transmission through lung parenchyma alone by measuring sound speed through individual lobes of excised horse lungs. He used a spark gap as a broadband sound source and detected the sound with a microphone on the opposite side of the lobe. He further examined the effect on sound speed of using gasses of different densities (air, helium, and sulfur hexafluoride) and at ambient pressures of 0.1–7 atm. He found that despite the input frequency range of 5–30,000 Hz, the lung passed only frequencies between 100 and 1000 Hz. The measured trans-lobar speed was much slower than sound in air (30–60 m/s, ~20% sound speed in air), was minimally affected by gas composition, and varied with ambient pressure in a manner suggesting that the factor most responsible for sound speed limitation was volumetric stiffness of the lung tissue.

Rice and Rice [8], having demonstrated the wide differences in sound speed between airway sound and parenchymal sound, measured sound speed from the trachea to pleura in five excised horse (and one dog) lungs. The sound source was a square wave pulse delivered by a wide frequency driver delivering an acoustic frequency range of 200–8000 Hz. They found that the frequency of peak transmission averaged 252 Hz and that the dominant mode of transmission was through the airways as gas density (helium, air, carbon dioxide, and sulfur hexafluoride) affected the speed although not as much as expected in total air transmission. They found no evidence of surface or longitudinal waves. The exact point at which sound passed from the airway to the parenchyma was uncertain, but measurements of the first waves to reach the pleura suggested that about 90% of the transit was within the airways.

Kraman [9] attempted to measure the speed of band-limited sound in the frequency range of normal lung sounds (125–500 Hz) through the respiratory system from the upper trachea-to-chest wall in five healthy human subjects. This was done after breathing both air and a mixture of 80% helium in 20% oxygen (heliox). Transit times varied from 2 ms in the upper chest to 5 ms at the lower chest, giving an approximate sound speed of 30 m/s. When heliox was breathed, the sound speed increased by only 10% suggesting that gas transmission through airways was a minor component of the transmission route. The findings were also consistent with Rice's previous conclusions regarding sound speed limitation by the volumetric stiffness of the gas-filled lung tissue.

Mahagnah and Gavrieli [10] attempted to clarify the discrepancy between Rice [8] who found clear-cut dependence of transpulmonary transit time on gas density and previous studies that found minimal dependence [3, 7]. Mahagnah and Gavrieli measured mouth to upper and lower chest wall transmission time of sound with the subjects breathing air or heliox. They reported average transit times of 1.5 ms at the apex and 5.2 ms at the base that was similar to what has been previously reported [3, 7, 9] for low-frequency sound (<~500 Hz). They also found no effect of gas density on the transit time. They were unable to explain the marked density-dependent transit time found by Rice [8]. However, it must be recognized that measuring sound transmission from mouth-to-chest wall in an intact human as these studies have been usually done is fundamentally different than transmission from trachea to lung surface in an excised horse lung. In the excised lung, there is no direct contact between the trachea and lung parenchyma as exists in an intact human. As previously mentioned, the likely coupling of low-frequency sound energy from the tracheal wall to the parenchyma probably shortens the path of the transmission through the airway lumen. Regarding their findings in the excised lung, Rice and Rice state in their discussion "this result applies only to the fastest mode(s) of transpulmonary sound. There may be found in the larger airways more energetically favorable points of sound transfer from the airway to the parenchyma" [8]. There is also the matter of interaction with the chest wall that will be discussed in the following section of this chapter. Its effect on mouth-to-chest wall sound transmission is not at all defined.

Bergstresser and colleagues carried out a study of trachea-to-chest wall sound transmission [11] in 12 intact human subjects using the stethographic multichannel lung sound analyzer that permits simultaneous acquisition of sound at 14 posterior chest wall locations as well as the trachea. They used the cross-correlation technique to measure transit times at lung volumes ranging from total lung capacity to residual volume. To decrease ambiguity and improve identification and measurement of the received signals, they encoded the input sound as a train of 11-cycle polyphonic pulses of frequencies ranging from 130 to 150 Hz. They found transit times of between 1 and 5 ms for central and peripheral locations. From the transit times and estimated path length, they calculated a trachea-to-chest wall sound speed of 37 m/s, a value similar to that found by other investigators [7, 9, 12]. In addition, they found that the transit times consistently decreased as lung volume increased. To explain this behavior, they modeled the acoustic behavior of the respiratory system as a two-phase system with sound introduced at the mouth traveling through the tracheal lumen at near free-field speeds until "jumping" to the parenchyma and proceeding at much slower speed determined by the parenchymal stiffness due mainly to the bulk modulus of air.

One attempt has been made to model, mathematically, the acoustic behavior of nearly the entire respiratory system including the vocal tract, trachea, and first five bronchial generations. Although the model, described by Wodicka et al. [13], necessarily contained numerous assumptions and estimations derived from experimental data up to that time, the predictions of their model are instructive and could lead to improved models that incorporate more experimental data. The authors modeled the respiratory system as a series of acoustic circuits for frequencies between 100 and 600 Hz (that encompass nearly all normal and abnormal lung sounds audible through a stethoscope). The large airways were modeled as a single-tube radiating acoustic energy into the lung parenchyma that was itself modeled as a mixture of air bubbles in water. The thermal effects of the massive boundary of the chest wall were also included. The total system was analyzed as a complex electronic circuit and the output compared with experimental results. Although this model was necessarily simplified, not taking into consideration the repetitively bifurcating bronchial tree, the results did qualitatively model the actual respiratory system behavior including the enhanced transmission of low-frequency sound compared with higher-frequency sound within the experimental range of 100–600 Hz and suggest that this results from thermal losses within the lung parenchyma. While a necessarily simplified model of a very complex biological system, Wodicka and colleagues' model shows promise for a possibly finer grained computational surrogate of the acoustical behavior of the respiratory system in health and disease.

The following year, Wodicka and Shannon [14] measured the trachea-to-chest wall acoustic transfer function in eight healthy adults using input sound at the mouth limited to 75–1400 Hz. The sound was picked up by accelerometers over the trachea at the neck and over the right posterior upper and lower lung zones. As the signal/noise was poor above ~650 Hz, the authors limited their analyses to the range of 100–600 Hz. The transfer function spectra revealed the peak transmission of 143 Hz ± 13 (SD) over the apex and 129 Hz ± 6 (SD) over the base with Q values of 2.0 and 2.2, respectively. Roll-off of energy above 300 Hz of 10 ± 4 (SD) dB/octave at the upper site and 17 ± 2 (SD) dB/octave at the lower site was in general agreement with predictions generated by their previously described acoustic circuit model [13]. They concluded that the interaction between the lung and chest wall is important in enhancing the transmission of lower-frequency sounds.

Cohen and Bernstein [15] carried out a similar experiment but using vocal input rather than an externally introduced sound. They studied 19 healthy subjects and 5 subjects with a variety of lung diseases including one with interstitial fibrosis, measuring both the autoregressive (AR) spectral analysis and the more computationally demanding autoregressive moving average (ARMA) transfer function with input vocal sounds low-pass filtered at 1000 Hz. For the normal subjects, they found the peak transmitted frequency to be 130–250 Hz with decreased transmission at higher frequencies similar to previous findings by Wodicka et al. [13]. In the single patient with pulmonary fibrosis (a disease in which the lung parenchyma progressive stiffens), there was a first peak at about the same frequency as the normal subjects but unusually enhanced transmission as well at about 700 Hz. Suggesting that the acoustic transmission properties of the lung are significantly modified in that disease.

In an attempt to define the acoustic transpulmonary transmission characteristics during acute lung injury, Rasanen and colleagues have carried out several studies using an oleic acid-induced lung injury model in pigs. Acute lung injury is a common and devastating lung condition that may complicate a variety of clinical situations such as major trauma, drowning, burns, poisoning, toxic gas exposure, and shock, among others. The common underlying defect in this condition is capillary leak with fluid filling the alveoli leading to collapse of dependent lung zones and consequent oxygen desaturation. Besides treating the underlying cause, supportive treatment, using positive pressure ventilation, is commonly employed to maintain the patient until gradual recovery which may take days to weeks. Positive end-expiratory pressure (PEEP), used to stent open collapsed lung zones and improve oxygenation, has been the standard treatment for decades. The safe use of PEEP requires knowledge of how much is enough due to the risk of serious adverse effects such as barotrauma and cardiac dysfunction that increase as the intrathoracic pressure is increased. Commonly used techniques to achieve the right amount of PEEP are measurements of oxygen saturation, lung compliance, cardiac output, the radiographic appearance of the lungs on plain radiographs, and CT scans. A simple and rapid technique to determine when the dependent lung zones have been adequately expanded would be welcomed.

Rasanen and Gavrieli [16] studied six healthy pigs that were anesthetized and placed on mechanical ventilation. They injected broadband noise (70–20,000 Hz) through the endotracheal tube and detected the sound at the trachea and at six locations over the dependent and nondependent lung areas. After baseline recording, acute lung injury was produced in the pig's lungs by the administration of oleic acid through a pulmonary artery catheter until a predefined difference in the ratio of arterial oxygen partial pressure-to-inspired oxygen fraction of <250 was achieved. During the development of lung injury, sound transfer function, amplitude, and coherence were measured at 20-min intervals. The investigators found a consistent increase in sound transfer function in the range of 1500–2500 Hz (where sound transmission was most efficient) of >fivefold in the dependent lung zones, two- to threefold in the lateral zones, and no increase at the nondependent lung zones. This probably results from enhanced impedance matching of the fluid-filled (and relatively airless)-dependent lung tissue to the chest wall reducing acoustic reflections from the interface. Radiographs and postmortem examinations of the lungs confirmed the distribution of the pulmonary edema to the dependent lung zones. This well-done study established the potential utility of using transpulmonary sound transmission to detect the distribution of lung injury in situations similar to what is encountered in patients with acute lung injury.

These same authors followed this study with a similar one in which the effects of PEEP were assessed [17]. As explained above, PEEP is used to reinflate the atelectatic (airless) lung to improve ventilation and oxygenation. Rasanen and Gavriely predicted that this would also reverse the enhancement of acoustic transmission that they had previously found in the dependent areas of lungs affected by acute lung injury. They used their previously described oleic acid-treated lung model to produce acute lung injury in six healthy pigs. Sound signals limited to 350–4000 Hz were introduced through the endotracheal tube and detected at the same six chest wall sites used in their previous study. Transfer function magnitude, coherence, and phase were measured at baseline airway pressure and after 15 min of PEEP at 5, 10, and 15 cmH_2O pressure followed by two 15-min recordings at ambient airway pressure. The animals were subsequently killed and the lungs examined. The results clearly showed the reversal in enhanced transmission in the dependent regions of the pig lungs with the effect at 10 cmH_2O greater than 5 cmH_2O and similar to that of 15 cmH_2O. Removal of PEEP resulted in a rapid reversal of the PEEP effect (Fig. 7.2). Radiographs confirmed the regional atelectasis of the dependent lung, and postmortem examination showed hemorrhagic edema in the dependent zones with well-aerated nondependent lung tissue.

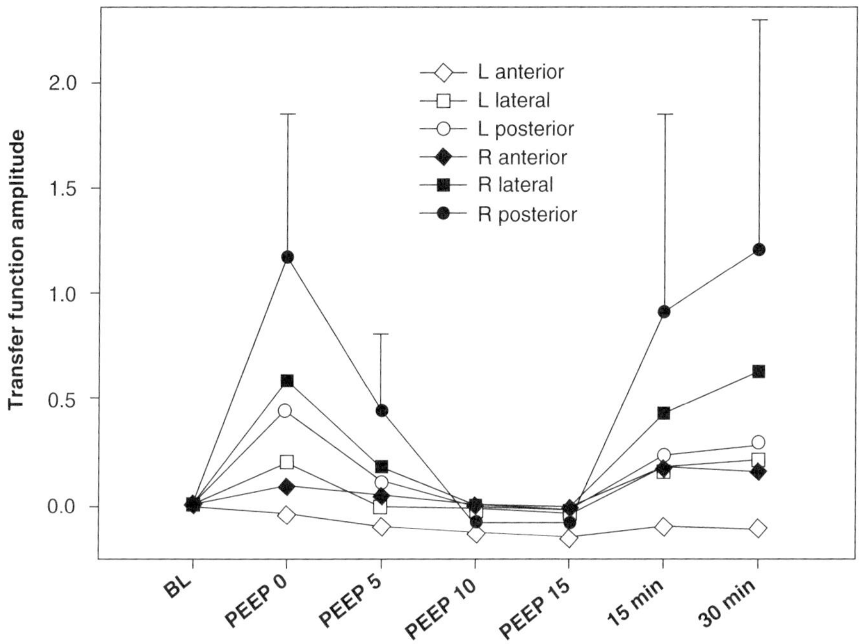

Fig. 7.2 Peak amplitude of the lung sound transfer function relative to baseline level over a frequency band from 1200 to 3500 Hz, recorded with six sensors overlying three lung regions bilaterally, during development of oleic acid-induced lung injury and subsequent application and withdrawal of PEEP. Data points are average values for all six animals. *BL* baseline [17]. Reprinted with permission from Springer

These studies establish the potential viability of monitoring the progression of acute lung injury and controlling the level of PEEP by using regional transpulmonary sound analysis. Currently, the only techniques used to asses this are radiography and CT scanning, which are techniques unsuited to frequent use. There has not been, to my knowledge, any widespread usage of transpulmonary sound transmission to manage PEEP levels in mechanically ventilated patients. Lev et al. [18] have studied the distribution of lung sounds in such patients with the absence or presence of lung sounds serving as surrogates for the introduced sounds previously used by Rasanen and Gavrieli. In Lev and colleagues' study, 34 patients with a wide variety of lung diseases or injuries resulting in respiratory failure were studied using a commercial device produced by Deep Breeze Ltd., Or Akiva, Israel. This consisted of a bilateral, posterior chest microphone array with sound analysis and display. The posterior lung sound distribution was displayed and measured at PEEP levels of 0, 5, and 10 cmH_2O and, in 15 of the patients, additional measurements at 15 cmH_2O. Repeated measurements were made in most of the patients. The authors found that the application of PEEP was accompanied by an increase the lung sound amplitude at the bases and a decrease at the apex with no significant change in the mid-lung region. This shift also corresponded with an increase in dynamic compliance. The study carried out in real-world ventilated patients suggests that atelectasis at the bases of the lungs of these patients opened with PEEP resulting in the appearance or increase in corresponding lung sound amplitude. It seems logical that similar technology could be employed to detect the transmission of sound introduced into the airway as done by Rasanen and Gavrieli [17]. Unfortunately, the study by Lev et al. suffers from multiple methodologic shortcomings, some of which they acknowledge. The patients are a heterogeneous group with apparently only a minority having acute lung injury that would be expected to benefit from ventilation with PEEP. Some had unilateral lung disease, others no lung disease. Many were breathing spontaneously. The ventilation modes varied and no patients were deeply sedated. There is no indication that most of the patients required PEEP to treat hypoxemia. Although these shortcomings weaken the findings, the lung sound recording technology appears attractive as a simple means to examine transpulmonary sound introduced into the airway in an appropriately selected group of patients with acute lung injury or acute respiratory distress syndrome where PEEP would be required for adequately oxygenation.

7.3 Transpulmonary (Auscultatory) Percussion

The technique of direct percussion has been around since the eighteenth century [19] and remains a useful technique today. In direct percussion, the body part of interest is sharply tapped, usually with an intervening finger helping create a sharp note, and the resulting tone and feel are interpreted to gain information about the condition of the underlying tissue (hollow, air-filled, solid). Auscultatory percussion is a variation of this technique in which one side of the body part is percussed and the sound is accessed at a distance or even on the opposite side of the body using a stethoscope, the theory being that a greater thickness of tissue can be probed that way. Guarino published several papers describing the use of this technique in different parts of the body [20–23]. He also reported a controlled study of 28 patients purporting to reveal a surprising ability of auscultatory percussion to detect intrapulmonary masses as small as 2 cm diameter [24]. This was intriguing and, six years later, Bohadana and colleagues attempted to replicate Guarino's findings [25]. Bohadana et al. studied 98 patients who were found to have abnormal chest films as part of a group of 281 subjects referred for chest radiography. The authors used two independent examiners who employed both auscultatory percussion and direct percussion. A third blinded examiner evaluated the chest films of the subjects to characterize the radiological findings. They found that both auscultatory percussion and direct percussion were about equally effective at detecting pleural effusions but that neither technique was able to detect any other abnormalities including intrapulmonary masses of any size below 6 cm diameter.

Two years later, Bohadana came to my lab to spend a research year. The first study we carried out [26] was an investigation of percussion sound paths through the chest to attempt to discover the reason behind the finding in the previous study [25]. We studied five healthy subjects by percussing repeatedly over the sternum and recording the sounds over the upper and lower parts of both posterior lungs at total lung capacity (TLC), functional residual capacity (FRC), and residual volume (RV). Percussion was first practiced to assure consistency, and 40 percussion notes were recorded at each location and at each studied lung volume. For each series, we calculated the average peak-to-peak pulse amplitude, and the average frequency was calculated from Fourier waveform analysis. After the series was completed while the subjects breathed air, we repeated the entire series with the patients breathing 80% helium in 20% oxygen (heliox). We found that the peak-to-peak amplitude was higher at TLC and RV then at FRC. The results on air and heliox were nearly identical. Our findings were best interpreted as indicating that the sounds of sternal percussion were transferred primarily through the skeleton rather than through the lungs and that the stiffening of the chest wall at high and low lung volumes enhanced transmission.

We followed the above study with another in which we performed three-dimensional mapping of sternal percussion sounds on the posterior chest wall in three healthy subjects and four patients with large intrapulmonary masses [27], ranging from 6 to 10 cm in largest diameter. We performed sequential recordings at each of 63 locations covering the back in a 7 × 9 point matrix with 2-cm point separation and created sound amplitude maps of the resultant sound distribution (Fig. 7.3). We found that the only anatomic structures that altered the sound pattern were chest wall structures, most notably the scapulae. Neither the lung masses in the patients nor mediastinal structures in any of the patients or subjects were revealed in the percussion maps. From this, along with our previous studies, we concluded that the sounds of sternal percussion travel to the back of the chest primarily via chest wall structures with intrathoracic structures having little effect. Whereas direct percussion and auscultatory percussion may help detect the presence of large masses or fluid in contact with the chest wall, the evidence suggests that auscultatory percussion plays no role in the detection of intrapulmonary lesions.

There are theoretical issues that should be mentioned regarding the question of whether it is possible for a solid mass within the lung to affect a sound wave traversing the lung. This is related to the size of the mass and wave length of the sound, which can be estimated using knowledge of the frequency of the sound and its speed through the lung. As the frequency of percussion sounds are limited to 100 Hz or less [26] and the speed of low-frequency sound has been measured at about 30 m/s [9], the percussion pulse wavelength within the lung is calculated at approximately 30 cm, comparable to the anterior-posterior diameter of the chest. To be detectable by a passing wave, the object must be of substantial size with respect to the wavelength, generally stated as at least ½ the wavelength [28]. That suggests that to be detectable by sternal percussion, the mass would have to be about 15 cm in diameter assuming that the percussion wave did pass through the lung parenchyma rather than the skeleton.

Since my own investigations into auscultatory percussion were carried out, the Internet was established and with it, the ability to discover writings that had been obscured by time but were now easily accessible as they were put online by various libraries. Among these was a short letter related to auscultatory percussion that was published in 1896 in which the author states the following about the technique in

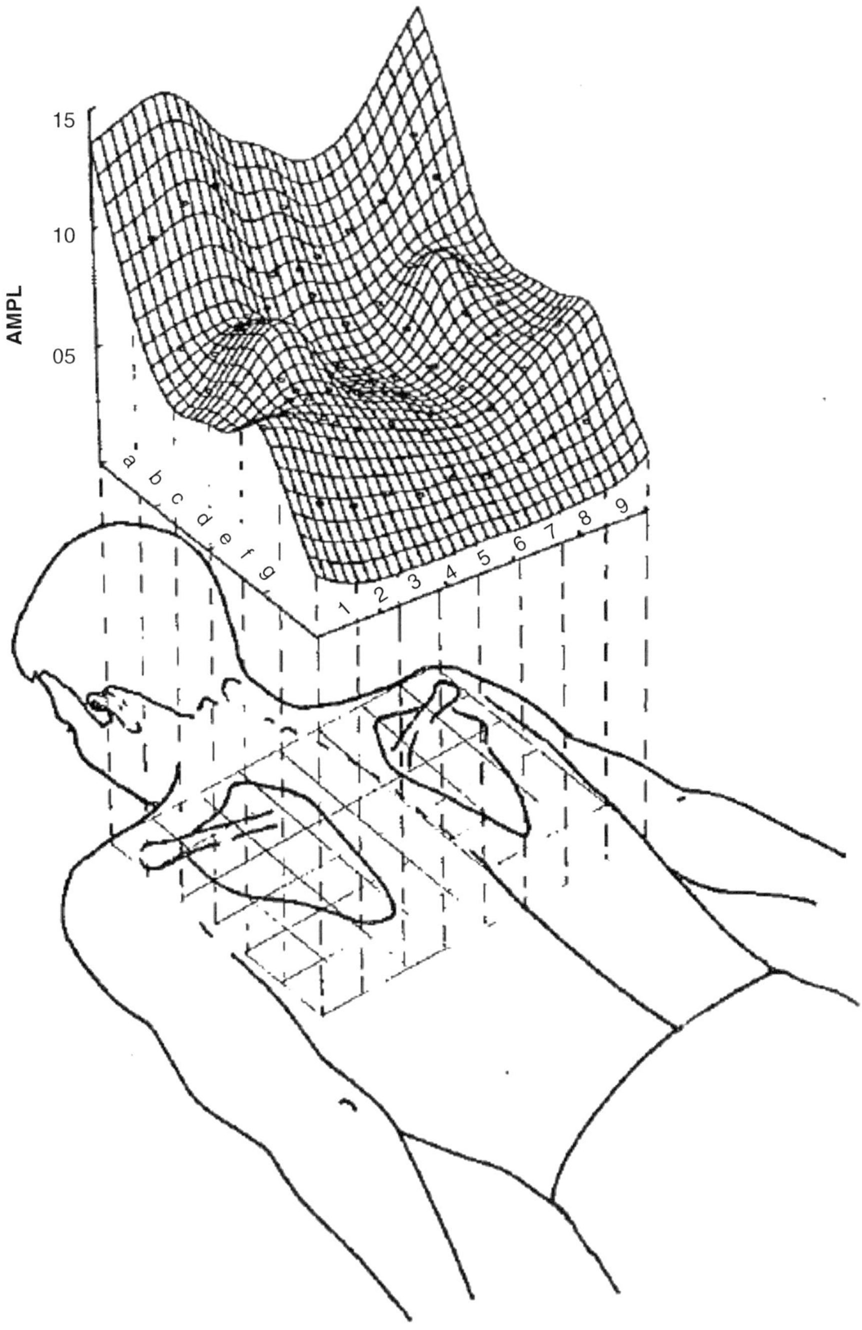

Fig. 7.3 Correspondence between the osseous structures of the posterior chest and the three-dimensional contour maps of percussion amplitude in one subject [27]. Reprinted with permission from Springer

question: "My own observations would lead me to believe that the waves of sound are, as regards the thorax, mainly conducted by the walls" [29]. Had we known of this note at the time of our study, we would have been sure to credit his insight.

Conclusion

Much of the utility of auscultation that has made the practice so useful for 200 years is due to the changes in lung sounds and percussion notes that result from alterations in the density of the underlying thoracic contents mainly consisting of the lung and material, mainly liquid, that can intrude between it and the chest wall. Although the abnormal sounds are generally interpreted as changes in intensity and character, the underlying mechanism is transmission through a modified medium. We generally only recognize this overtly when listening to the transmitted voice and the practitioner still mostly relies on pattern recognition as did Laennec. However, technology has arrived at the point that, in appropriate clinical situations, sound transmission through the lung can now be readily and inexpensively measured with sufficient resolution to clearly detect regional differences and time-to-time changes in lung density. There is opportunity for investigators to develop and prove this technology. I hope that we will see this in the near future.

References

1. Laennec RTH (1819) De l'Auscultation Médiate ou Traité du Diagnostic des Maladies des Poumons et du Coeur (On mediate auscultation or treatise on the diagnosis of the diseases of the lungs and heart). Brosson and Chaudé, Paris
2. Ploy-Song-Sang Y, Martin RR, Ross WR, Loudon RG, Macklem PT (1977) Breath sounds and regional ventilation. Am Rev Respir Dis 116(2):187–199. https://doi.org/10.1164/arrd.1977.116.2.187
3. Kraman SS, Austrheim O (1983) Comparison of lung sound and transmitted sound amplitude in normal men. Am Rev Respir Dis 128(3):451–454
4. Fiz JA, Gnitecki J, Kraman SS, Wodicka GR, Pasterkamp H (2008) Effect of body position on lung sounds in healthy young men. Chest 133(3):729–736. https://doi.org/10.1378/chest.07-1102
5. Wodicka GR, DeFrain PD, Kraman SS (1994) Bilateral asymmetry of respiratory acoustic transmission. Med Biol Eng Comput 32(5):489–494
6. Rice DA (1980) Sound speed in the upper airways. J Appl Physiol Respir Environ Exerc Physiol 49(2):326–336
7. Rice DA (1983) Sound speed in pulmonary parenchyma. J Appl Physiol Respir Environ Exerc Physiol 54(1):304–308
8. Rice DA, Rice JC (1987) Central to peripheral sound propagation in excised lung. J Acoust Soc Am 82(4):1139–1144
9. Kraman SS (1983) Speed of low-frequency sound through lungs of normal men. J Appl Physiol Respir Environ Exerc Physiol 55(6):1862–1867
10. Mahagnah M, Gavriely N (1995) Gas density does not affect pulmonary acoustic transmission in normal men. J Appl Physiol 78(3):928–937
11. Bergstresser T, Ofengeim D, Vyshedskiy A, Shane J, Murphy R (2002) Sound transmission in the lung as a function of lung volume. J Appl Physiol 93(2):667–674. https://doi.org/10.1152/japplphysiol.00050.2002

12. Wodicka GR, Stevens KN, Golub HL, Shannon DC (1990) Spectral characteristics of sound transmission in the human respiratory system. IEEE Trans Biomed Eng 37(12):1130–1135. https://doi.org/10.1109/10.64455
13. Wodicka GR, Stevens KN, Golub HL, Cravalho EG, Shannon DC (1989) A model of acoustic transmission in the respiratory system. IEEE Trans Biomed Eng 36(9):925–934. https://doi.org/10.1109/10.35301
14. Wodicka GR, Shannon DC (1990) Transfer function of sound transmission in subglottal human respiratory system at low frequencies. J Appl Physiol 69(6):2126–2130
15. Cohen A, Berstein AD (1991) Acoustic transmission of the respiratory system using speech stimulation. IEEE Trans Biomed Eng 38(2):126–132. https://doi.org/10.1109/10.76377
16. Rasanen J, Gavriely N (2002) Detection of porcine oleic acid-induced acute lung injury using pulmonary acoustics. J Appl Physiol 93(1):51–57. https://doi.org/10.1152/japplphysiol.01238.2001
17. Rasanen J, Gavriely N (2005) Response of acoustic transmission to positive airway pressure therapy in experimental lung injury. Intensive Care Med 31(10):1434–1441. https://doi.org/10.1007/s00134-005-2745-7
18. Lev S, Glickman YA, Kagan I, Dahan D, Cohen J, Grinev M, Shapiro M, Singer P (2009) Changes in regional distribution of lung sounds as a function of positive end-expiratory pressure. Crit Care 13(3):R66. https://doi.org/10.1186/cc7871
19. https://en.wikipedia.org/wiki/Leopold_Auenbrugger
20. Guarino JR (1986) Auscultatory percussion to detect ascites. N Engl J Med 315(24):1555–1556
21. Guarino JR (1981) Auscultatory percussion of the bladder to detect urinary retention. N Engl J Med 305(12):701
22. Guarino JR (1974) Auscultatory percussion. A new aid in the examination of the chest. J Kans Med Soc 75(6):193–194
23. Guarino JR (1982) Auscultatory percussion of the head. Br Med J (Clin Res Ed) 284(6322):1075–1077
24. Guarino JR (1980) Auscultatory percussion of the chest. Lancet 1(8182):1332–1334
25. Bohadana AB, Coimbra FT, Santiago JR (1986) Detection of lung abnormalities by auscultatory percussion: a comparative study with conventional percussion. Respiration 50(3):218–225
26. Bohadana AB, Kraman SS (1989) Transmission of sound generated by sternal percussion. J Appl Physiol 66(1):273–277
27. Bohadana AB, Patel R, Kraman SS (1989) Contour maps of auscultatory percussion in healthy subjects and patients with large intrapulmonary lesions. Lung 167(6):359–372
28. Anon. https://en.wikipedia.org/wiki/Nyquist-Shannon_sampling_theorem. Wikipedia. Accessed 9 July 2016
29. Thorne WB (1896) Auscultatory percussion: a reply. Br Med J 1(1845):1140–1141

Breath Sound Recording

8

Yasemin P. Kahya

8.1 Introduction

Auscultation of the lung dates back more than 2000 years, but it has become a diagnostic tool since Laennec introduced the first form of the stethoscope [1]. The stethoscope is a widely used instrument to the extent that it has become the symbol of medical profession. Nevertheless, auscultation with a traditional stethoscope, which amplifies frequencies lower than 112 Hz and attenuates those higher than 112 Hz [2], is regarded to have low diagnostic value due to the attenuation of higher frequencies, which contain valuable diagnostic information regarding respiratory sounds, and due to the subjectivity involved in the evaluation of these sounds by medical doctors. With the advances in computer technology and signal processing algorithms, computerized analysis of respiratory sounds has provided new understanding in correlating lung sounds with diseases and disease states [3] and, also, in relating pulmonary acoustics with lung mechanics. Computational methods for the analysis of breath sounds offer additional advantages, such as digital storage, monitoring in critical settings, computer-supported analysis, comparison among different recordings, and provision of objective parameters in their evaluation. Despite this aroused research activity in breath sound processing and analysis, the main concern is in the standardization of the recording of breath sounds. Different approaches to record breath sounds have been reported in various publications, such as in [4–7]. Moreover, there have been efforts to offer guidelines for data acquisition equipment, such as the Computerized Respiratory Sound Analysis (CORSA) project financed by the European Community [8]; such efforts will eventually culminate in the commercial development of respiratory sound acquisition equipment, which will be accepted with general consensus by the medical community.

Y. P. Kahya
Electrical and Electronic Engineering Department, Bogazici University, Istanbul, Turkey
e-mail: kahya@boun.edu.tr

K. N. Priftis et al. (eds.), *Breath Sounds*, https://doi.org/10.1007/978-3-319-71824-8_8

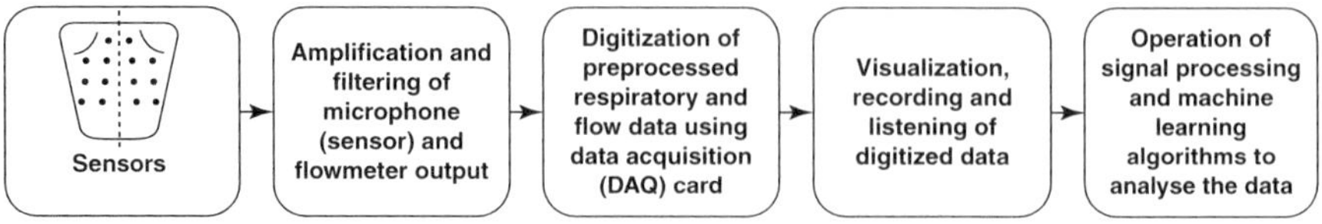

Fig. 8.1 Overview of lung sound data acquisition, recording, and computerized analysis system

8.2 Breath Sound

The term "breath sound" is used to include normal and adventitious sounds recorded over the chest wall, the trachea, or at the mouth [9]. The characteristics of breath sounds are closely correlated with the airflow in the respiratory tract; therefore, when breath sounds are recorded, some form of airflow measurement is also made, either directly using a flowmeter or indirectly estimating from tracheal or chest sounds [10]. Lung sounds are all respiratory sounds heard over the chest wall. The most commonly used bandwidth in the measurement of lung sounds is from 60–100 Hz to 2 kHz when recorded over the chest. Tracheal sounds are recorded from the extrathoracic part of the trachea with a bandwidth from 60–100 Hz to 4 kHz. Cough sounds are also measured with a bandwidth from 50 Hz to 3 kHz. Snoring sounds, which are induced by abnormal vibrations in the walls of the oropharynx, are low-frequency noisy sounds with periodic components of 30–250 Hz fundamental frequencies and are usually detected during sleep. The acquisition system of the breath sound is designed according to the location and type of breath sound to be recorded. A block diagram of a lung sound acquisition, recording, and analysis system is depicted in Fig. 8.1.

8.3 Sensors Used in Breath Sound Recording

8.3.1 Specifications and Definitions

In discussions relating to sensors, certain specifications have been given as guidelines in building data acquisition instruments for breath sound recording. In this section these specifications and their definitions are presented [11].

Decibel scale: The basis for most microphone specifications is the decibel (dB) scale. The dB scale is logarithmic and is used because it is analogous to the way the human ear perceives changes in sound pressure. Furthermore, the changes in dB are more comprehensible than the large numbers that might occur in pressure scales (e.g., Pascal, Newton, or Bar). The dB scale expresses a given pressure in proportion to a reference pressure, mostly 20 μPa (i.e., Pa, a measurement of pressure). The reference pressure 20 μPa is chosen to be equal to 0 dB. It is important to note that 0 dB does not mean that there is no sound; it is considered to be the lower limit in the sound pressure level which can be detected by the average human ear.

The frequency response: The frequency response of a microphone is usually represented with the frequency response curve, which illustrates the microphone's ability to transform acoustic energy into electric signals. A flat response curve, which would indicate that the microphone does no coloring, is required in the frequency range of the respiratory sounds. The frequency response is different from the microphone's frequency range, which indicates which frequency range the microphone reproduces sound within a given tolerance. The frequency range is sometimes also referred to as "bandwidth" where the tolerance is usually −3 dB. In [12], it is recommended that the maximum deviation within the frequency range of respiratory sounds be 6 dB in breath sound recording systems.

Sensitivity: The sensitivity of a microphone is the electrical response at its output to a given standard acoustic input. The standard reference input signal for microphone sensitivity measurements is a 1 kHz sine wave at 94 dB sound pressure level (SPL) or 1 Pascal (Pa). According to the IEC 268-4 norm, the sensitivity is measured in mV per Pascal at 1 kHz whereas at 250 Hz for measuring microphones. Alternatively, the sensitivity can be stated in dB relatively to 1 V/Pa, resulting in a negative value. Tolerances in sensitivity, according to production differences, are also stated and would normally be in the region of 2 dB. Sensitivity represents the microphone's ability to convert acoustic pressure to electric voltage. The sensitivity indicates the voltage a microphone produces at a certain sound pressure level. A microphone with high sensitivity gives a high-voltage output and therefore does not need as much amplification as a model with lower sensitivity. In applications with low sound pressure levels, a microphone with a high sensitivity is required in order to keep the amplification noise low. In [12], it is recommended that the sensitivity of breath sound recording systems be stable and steady and be independent of variations in static pressure and sound direction.

The equivalent noise level: The equivalent noise level of a microphone, or microphone's self-noise, indicates the sound pressure level that will create the same voltage, as the self-noise from the microphone will produce. A low noise level is required when working with low sound pressure levels, and self-noise determines the lower limit in the microphone's dynamic range.There are two typical standards:

1. The dB(A) scale will weigh the SPL according to the ear's sensitivity, especially filtering out low-frequency noise. Good results (very low noise) in this scale are usually below 15 dB(A).
2. The CCIR 468-1 scale uses a different weighing, so in this scale, good results are below 25–30 dB.

Signal-to-noise ratio (SNR): The signal-to-noise ratio (SNR) is the ratio of a reference signal to the noise level of the microphone output. This noise level includes noise contributed both by the microphone element and the electronic circuit included in the microphone package. The SNR is the difference in decibels between the noise level and a standard 1 kHz, 94 dB SPL reference signal. SNR is calculated by measuring the noise output of the microphone in a quiet, echoless environment. A weighed value, dB(A), which means that it includes a correction factor that corresponds to the human ear's sensitivity to sound at different frequencies, is used to specify SNR over a 20 kHz bandwidth. When comparing SNR measurements of different microphones, it is important to make sure that the specifications are presented using the same weighing and bandwidth; a reduced bandwidth measurement makes the SNR specification better than it is with a full 20 kHz bandwidth measurement. The CORSA recommendation [12] is to have a minimum SNR of 60 dB, with a sensitivity of 1 mV/Pa on a load of 200 Ω in breath sound recording systems.

The dynamic range: The dynamic range of a microphone is a measure of the difference between the loudest and quietest SPLs to which the microphone responds linearly. The SNR of the microphone measures the difference between the noise floor and a 94 dB SPL reference, but the microphone still has a great deal of useful signal response above this reference level. Druzgalski [13] recommended that microphones used for respiratory sounds have dynamic ranges greater than or equal to 40–50 dB; however, the minimum dynamic range acceptable for sound sensors is 60 dB as recommended by CORSA [12].

Total harmonic distortion: Total harmonic distortion (THD) is a measurement of the level of distortion on the output signal for a given single-frequency input signal. This measurement is presented as a percentage. It is the ratio of the sum of the powers of all harmonic frequencies above the fundamental frequency to the power of the input at the fundamental frequency. This parameter is expressed in percentage. The input signal for this test is typically at 105 dB SPL, which is 11 dB above the reference SPL of 94 dB. THD is measured at a higher SPL than other specifications because, as the level of the acoustic input signal increases, the THD measurement typically increases as well. A rule of thumb is that the THD triples with every 10 dB increase in input level. Therefore, THD less than 3% at 105 dB SPL means that the THD will be less than 1% at 95 dB SPL.

Polar pattern: Polar pattern is also called directional pickup pattern or directionality. The polar pattern of a microphone is the sensitivity to sound relative to the direction or angle from which the sound arrives. The most common types of directionality are omnidirectional, cardioid, and supercardioid. The recommendation by CORSA [12] is the use of omnidirectional microphones. The omnidirectional microphone has equal output or sensitivity at all angles; therefore, it picks up sound from all directions.

8.3.2 Sensor Types and Recording Approaches

The basic principle in auscultation with a stethoscope is the transfer of vibrations of the chest wall to the air pressure variations that travel to the diaphragm of the ear using the medium of the stethoscope. These air pressure variations cause sound waves and are recorded using microphones that are transducers that convert sound signals to electrical signals. There are different types of microphones that employ diverse methods to convert the air pressure variations of a sound wave to an electrical signal. The most common microphones available in the market are the dynamic microphone, which uses a coil of wire suspended in a magnetic field; the condenser microphone, which uses the vibrating diaphragm as a capacitor plate; and the piezoelectric microphone, which uses a crystal of piezoelectric material.

The principle of the dynamic microphone is electromagnetic induction. A small movable induction coil is placed in the magnetic field of a permanent magnet and is attached to the diaphragm of the microphone. When sound reaches the microphone, it moves the diaphragm whose vibration causes the coil to move in the magnetic field, producing a varying current in the coil through electromagnetic induction. The dynamic microphone's main disadvantage is its narrow bandwidth, since a single dynamic membrane does not linearly respond to all audio frequencies and may introduce distortions in different regions of the frequency spectrum.

The condenser microphone, also called the capacitor microphone or electrostatic microphone, has a diaphragm which acts as one plate of a capacitor and the vibrations produce changes in the distance between the plates, causing changes in the capacitance value. A nearly constant charge is maintained externally on the capacitor with a DC bias. The fluctuations in the capacitance value due to vibrations caused by sound waves induce fluctuations in the voltage across the capacitor plates. It is to be noted that the capacitance of the parallel plate capacitor is inversely proportional to the distance between the plates. There is a specific type of condenser microphone that is called the electret microphone where the externally applied charge is replaced by a permanent charge in an electret material, which is a ferroelectric material that has been permanently electrically charged. Due to their good performance, ease of manufacture, and relatively lower cost, electret microphones are widely used in instrumentation. They have almost flat frequency response over the audio frequency range and are quite stable. They do not require an external polarizing voltage but are produced with an integrated preamplifier that requires power. When used in pulmonary sound recording, the diaphragm and the chest wall need to be coupled acoustically through a closed air cavity since the movements involved are very small.

Piezoelectricity is the ability of some materials to produce a voltage under the application of pressure. Piezoelectric microphone uses piezoelectricity to convert vibrations into an electric signal. The piezoelectric materials are used to form a piezoelectric accelerometer that senses the acceleration of the mass of the whole sensor caused by the movement of the surface it is in contact with. They are used as contact sensors directly on the skin to amplify sound signals from the body. Due to low output signal and very high output impedance, they are susceptible to noise. The earlier versions, which had high sensitivity and signal-to-noise ratio, were massive; however, the contemporary models are manufactured in much smaller dimensions.

In recording breath sounds, there are basically two major approaches:

1. "Contact sensor" for direct recording of the movement of the chest wall (e.g., piezoelectric accelerometer)
2. "Air-coupled sensor" for acoustic recording of the movement of a diaphragm exposed to the air pressure generated by the chest-wall movement (e.g., condenser, in particular, electret microphone)

These two types of sensors have been compared by Druzgalski [13] with the conclusion that the piezoelectric contact sensors have a higher sensitivity and immunity to ambient noise. However, later studies by Pasterkamp et al. [14] have found that both sensors have similar frequency response and signal-to-noise ratio in the frequency range of respiratory signals. A detailed discussion on the electro-acoustic and electromechanical analogies to illustrate the working principles of various microphone transduction techniques may be found in [11], a classic review of microphone types in [15] and more contemporary ones in [16].

8.3.3 Sensor Attachment

The type of sensor used determines the type of coupling in a breath sound recording system.

Contact sensors: If a piezoelectric accelerometer is used, then coupling is directly on the skin, since it is a contact sensor. There is no need for an air coupler, but the pressure exerted on the skin through the sensor should be kept constant. Maintaining constant pressure is difficult to achieve manually. The use of elastic bands is not suitable, since the pressure between the sensor and the skin varies as thorax moves with breathing. Adhesive rings are suggested to be used for contact sensor attachments.

Condenser microphones: There is a need of an air coupler that is used with the condenser microphone since free-field measurement is not possible for such small movements of the chest wall involved in respiratory sounds. The air that is captured in the air cavity of the coupler exerts enough force on the diaphragm to cause a displacement that produces measurable sound pressure. The geometry of the air coupler is effective in the overall performance of the sensor. Wodicka et al. [17] studied the effects of microphone air cavity depth on the frequency response of the transduction with measurements performed both using an artificial chest wall and lung sounds from a healthy subject. They concluded that the high-frequency response of the transduction diminished with increasing cavity depth and that smaller cavity depths were more appropriate for detection of lung sounds over a wide bandwidth. Kraman et al. [18] studied the effects of coupler air chamber width, shape, and venting on lung sounds. They used cylindrical chambers of 5, 10, and 15 mm in diameter at the skin and conical chambers of 8, 10, and 15 mm in diameter and 2.5, 5, and 10 mm in depth and compared the inspiratory lung sound spectra obtained using each of the couplers. They also studied the effect of various needle vents in transmitting ambient noise into the microphone chamber. The shape and diameter had insignificant effect on the lung sound spectrum below 500 Hz. From approximately 500 to 1500 Hz, the 5 mm diameter couplers showed slightly less sensitivity than the 10 and 15 mm diameter couplers. Also 2.5 mm and 5 mm depth couplers had higher sensitivity. All conical couplers provided approximately 5–10 dB more sensitivity than the cylindrical couplers. All vents allowed some ambient noise to enter the chamber, but the amount was very small using the narrowest, longest vent. They concluded that the optimal air coupler for the electret microphone was conical in shape, between 10 and 15 mm in diameter at the skin, with 2.5–5 mm in depth, and either not vented or vented with a tube no wider than 0.35 mm or shorter than 20 mm.

For all sensors used, shielded twisted pair of coaxial cables is recommended for protection from electromagnetic interference. They should also be protected from mechanical vibrations against acoustic noise.

Although many laboratories that are conducting studies on the analysis of lung sounds and CORSA guidelines [12] have attempted to set a standard for breath sound acquisition, it is still a challenge to compare data acquired with different systems. Contrary to previous studies, a later study by Kraman et al. [19] compared different lung sound transducers using a bioacoustics transducer testing system. They used two different brand accelerometers, one electret condenser microphone with different shape and size air couplers, one classic stethoscope head connected to an electret condenser microphone, and one electronic stethoscope. They found that the size and shape of the air coupler chamber they used had no important effect on the detected sound; that one accelerometer had the broadest frequency response with useful sensitivity extending to 4 kHz; that the other accelerometer, the electret condenser microphone, and the classic stethoscope head connected to an electret condenser microphone had similar flat frequency responses from 200 Hz to 1200 Hz; and that worse performance was obtained from the electronic stethoscope. Their conclusion was that there are important differences among commonly used lung sound sensors that have to be defined to allow comparison of data from different laboratories.

8.3.4 Attachment Locations

The earlier recording instruments used one or two sensors in the recording of lung sounds [20–23] from the chest. Similarly, the minimal locations recommended by CORSA task force are trachea (for tracheal sounds) and left and right posterior base of the lungs usually 5 cm laterally from the paravertebral line and 7 cm below the scapular angle for adults [24]. Later multichannel recording systems were developed in various laboratories, and multichannel analysis of respiratory sounds became popular [25–28], since the simultaneous recording and analysis of sounds from multiple sites over the chest facilitated and accelerated an otherwise slow and tedious process. In Fig. 8.2, the depiction of examples of locations used in multichannel recording of lung sounds in various studies is presented. These studies used 14–25 microphone locations on the chest wall for simultaneous recording of lung sounds. The optional locations recommended by CORSA for adults are right and left anterior area of the chest at the second intercostal space at the mid-clavicular line and right and left lateral area of the chest at the fourth or fifth intercostal space on the mid-axillary line [24].

In tracheal breath measurements, the sensor is usually attached to the neck at the anterior cervical triangle [29]. The recommendation by CORSA is also at the sternal notch [24].

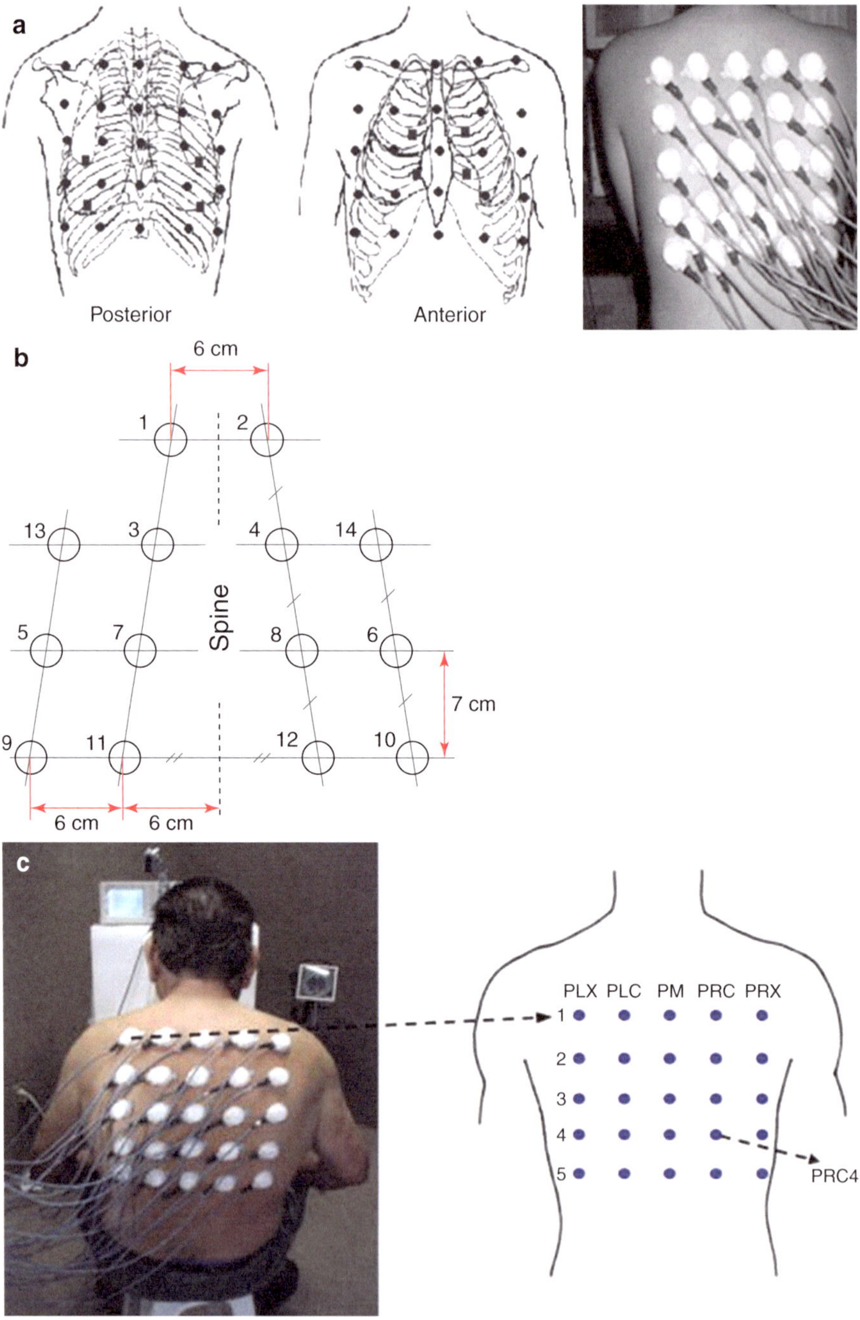

Fig. 8.2 Examples of locations used in multichannel recording of lung sounds in various studies [25–28]. (**a**) Microphone locations used in [25]. (**b**) Microphone locations used in [26]. (**c**) Microphone locations used in [27]. (**d**) Microphone locations used in [28]

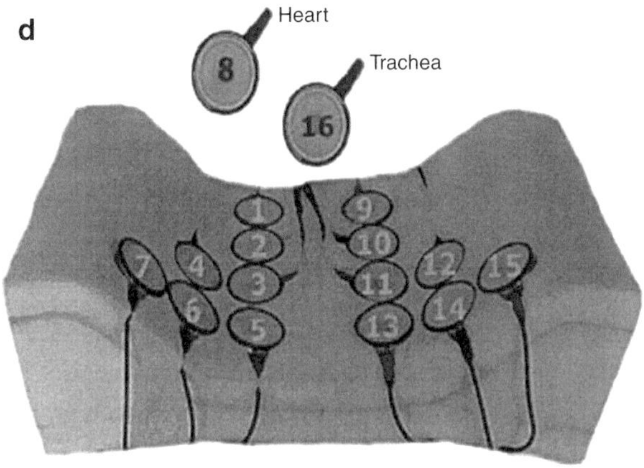

Fig. 8.2 (continued)

8.3.5 Environmental and Subject Conditions for Breath Sound Recording

There are a number of recommendations by the CORSA Task Force applicable to the environmental and subject conditions during breath sound recording [24]:

- The background noise level should preferably be less than 45 dB (A) and 60 dB (linear) with minimum ambient noise from the environment including voiced sounds. The sounds induced by airflow through the flow transducer should be taken into account.
- The recording is to be performed at comfortable room temperature, humidity, lighting, and ventilation.
- The sitting position is preferable for the subject for short-term recording, whereas supine position is preferable for long-term recording.
- For adults, tidal breathing of 7–10 respiratory cycles, with a peak expiratory and inspiratory flow of 1–1.5 l/s or 10–15% of the predicted maximum peak flow, and tidal volume of 1 L or 15–20% of predicted vital capacity are recommended for short-term recording, whereas tidal breathing without any voluntary effort is recommended for long-term recording.
- The airflow, volume, and flow/volume display should be in front of the subject.
- For babies and young children, chest movement monitoring by strain gauge bands, pneumatic belts, or chest straps should be used.

8.4 Analog Processing

8.4.1 Amplification

The electric signal coming from the sound transducer is amplified so that it is prepared for analog-to-digital conversion. The signal amplitude should be at an optimum level for the analog to digital converter input. The earlier instruments employed operational or discrete transistor amplifiers, but the more recent designs use instrumentation amplifiers available as integrated circuits in a single package. An instrumentation amplifier is a difference amplifier with an extremely high common-mode and differential mode input impedance (>100 MΩ), very low output impedance, accurate and stable gain which can usually be adjusted with a single external resistor, and an extremely high common-mode rejection ratio (CMRR). High-input impedances are needed for minimum loading of the signal input, and low-output impedance minimizes signal loss at the output stage of the amplifier. The instrumentation amplifier with its high CMRR is able to amplify a small signal from a transducer in the presence of a large common-mode component such as noise from the power lines; hence, it is widely applied in biomedical measurement and test instrumentation. The minimum required CMRR for amplifiers used in some of the other biomedical measurement instruments have been already established. For example, the minimum CMRRs for Electrocardiography (ECG or EKG) and for Electroencephalography (EEG) amplifiers are 107 dB and 140 dB, respectively [30]. No standard has been set for the breath sound recording system but in [31], a minimum CMRR of 100 dB is suggested.

Another requirement of the amplifier is low internal noise since the noise of the amplifier should be smaller than that of the sound sensor. In ECG and EEG amplifiers, the maximum internal noise voltage requirements are 2 mV and 1 mV, respectively [30]. However, no standard requirement on the noise level has been established for breath sound recording amplifiers since the requirement would depend on the type of the sound sensor used. A related parameter is the signal-to-noise ratio (SNR) of the measurement, which is usually around 40 dB in breath sound recording instrument although it is suggested that the SNR of the amplified signal should be approximately 60 dB in the frequency range of interest [12].

The frequency bandwidth of the amplifier should be adequate for the signal of interest. The gain-bandwidth product of the instrumentation amplifier is taken into consideration in the design of the recording system. The requirements relating to gain-bandwidth product are not very demanding for the signal of interest since the useful frequency range of lung sounds and tracheal sounds extends up to 2 kHz and 4 kHz, respectively [12].

Additional features, which are preferred in the amplifier, are low-power and programmable gain. Low-power is critical both for safety reasons and for portable instrument design. Programmable gain gives the user flexibility to the instrument if used to record sounds from different regions of the pulmonary system since, for example, the amplitude of tracheal sounds is much higher than the amplitude of lung sounds recorded from the posterior chest.

8.4.2 Filtering

Passband filtering is applied in breath sound recording systems. This is usually achieved by a cascade of high-pass and low-pass filters. The reason for high-pass filtering is to reduce low-frequency distortions due to heart, muscle, and friction noise and other external low-frequency noise. For the high-pass filter, the cutoff frequency is chosen somewhere in the range from 30 to 150 Hz by most researchers, but the most frequently preferred range is between 50 and 60 Hz [31]. Passband ripples are not allowed; moreover, it is recommended that linear phase or delay equalized frequency responses be used as incorrect high-pass filtering can particularly distort waveforms of signals containing crackles and other transient-type signals with a wide bandwidth and short duration [32]. This is due to the fact that filters introduce a frequency-dependent phase shift. If this shift varies linearly with frequency, its effect is simply to delay the signal by a constant amount. However, if phase varies nonlinearly, different input frequencies will experience different delays, so non-sinusoidal signals containing multiple frequencies may experience significant phase distortion in propagating through the filter. Usually, Bessel filters are used in high-pass filtering since they maximize the passband delay, resulting in nearly linear phase characteristics within the passband. The slope of the frequency response is generally chosen to be greater than 18 db/oct corresponding to a minimum filter order of three.

Low-pass filtering is needed to prevent aliasing of the digitized signal. The digitization process of the analog to digital converter creates additional spectral components, called images, at locations symmetric about half the sampling frequency, f_s, which is called the Nyquist frequency, $\frac{f_s}{2}$. Aliasing occurs when the signal contains frequencies above the Nyquist frequency because the spectral components of the signal will be distorted with the overlapping spectral components of the image, making it impossible to fully recover the original signal. So to reconstruct the signal of a given bandwidth, f_B, from its digitized version, the sampling rate, f_s, must be such that $f_s \geq 2\, f_B$. This requirement is met by band-limiting the signal below the Nyquist frequency and is achieved by using a low-pass filter which has a flat response up to f_B and which must roll off rapidly enough to provide the desired amount of suppression at $\frac{f_s}{2}$ and beyond. Usually Butterworth filters with maximally flat response in the passband are used. The order of the filter, therefore the slope of the response, depends on f_s: the higher the f_s, the smaller the order can be. However, it is recommended that there should be at least 24 dB attenuation at the aliasing frequency and that the −3 dB cutoff frequency of the filter must be at the upper frequency of the signal [32].

8.4.3 Safety Standards

The acquisition instrument is made up of the sensor, the amplifier, the filters, the analog to digital converter, and the computer. A very important concern in the design of the preprocessing circuitry and the instrument as a whole is compliance with the basic safety and performance requirements of medical equipment which are defined in IEC 60601-1 standards. The European (EN 60601-1) and Canadian

(CSA 60601-1) versions of the standard are identical to the IEC standard. The original standard has evolved to the fourth edition, and the adoption of the various revisions of IEC 60601-1 depends on the particular country. However, it should be noted that no specific standard for safety in biomedical sound recording exists.

The sensors are in direct contact with the patient and are critical components for safety concerns. Their biasing voltages should be low, and their preprocessing circuitry, i.e., the amplifier and the filters, must conform to the above-mentioned standards.

8.5 Digitization

In earlier recordings of breath sounds, analog systems, such as tape records, were used to store data for further analysis [4]. However, with the advent of digital computers and advanced digital signal processors, the format of data has become digital. The main advantage of digital form of data is its ready usability with digital signal processing algorithms for further analysis. Actually, a new research area where studies involving topics like detection of adventitious lung sounds, classification of lung sounds, evaluation of the diagnostic value of lung sounds, respiratory system modeling, etc. has evolved in the last 30 years [5, 6, 33].

Other evident advantages of digital form may be listed as ease of documentation and communication, immunity to distortion due to noise in transmission, and ease of storage and access.

The digitization process is carried out by analog-to-digital converters (ADC). Two important specifications in choosing the optimum ADC are the sampling frequency and the resolution, which corresponds to the number of bits in conversion. Different research groups have used diverse combinations of sampling rate and resolution. The CORSA task force has come up with a list of recommendations for digitization [34]. Their recommendations, however, specifically address recording systems which use sound facilities already available in the market, in particular the CD format of 44.1 kHz sampling rate. This sampling rate has been adopted for audible sound bandwidth of 20 kHz but is too high for breath sounds. So, they have suggested that submultiples of 44.1 kHz be used for different types of breath sounds. For example, for lung sounds recorded from the chest area, band-limiting the signal with a fourth order Butterworth low-pass filter with 3-dB cutoff frequency at 2 kHz is suggested with a sampling rate of 5.5125 kHz. The cutoff frequencies of recording tracheal sounds and snoring/cough sounds could be set at 4 and 8 kHz, with 11.025 and 22.05 kHz sampling rates, respectively. If the flow signal is also recorded simultaneously, then these sampling rates are very high, and digitally low-pass filtering of the signal to 20 Hz is recommended.

There are good quality ADC cards commercially available, which can be used as auxiliary units with the computer and are multichannel with programmable sampling rates. If such an ADC card is used in the recording system, then the recommendation is that the sampling rate should be chosen such that after low-pass filtering the signal, there should be at least 24 dB attenuation at the sampling frequency.

Most of the researchers have used at least an ADC resolution of 12 bits in their breath sound recording systems [4]. However, because of internal noise generated in the ADC, the actual resolution corresponds to smaller number of bits. So, in [6], it is recommended that 16-bit resolution is used so that even in mediocre ADC cards, an actual resolution of about 12 bits is achieved. However, if a good quality, professional ADC card is used with 12-bit resolution, it is recommended that the least significant 4 bits be padded with zeroes and a 16-bit word in two's complement format be used for data representation.

Also, the CORSA task force has come up with some recommendations [34], regarding the input signal level for the ADC, assuming Gaussian-like input signals. For an ADC with a voltage range of –V to +V, the maximum allowed signal power should be around $V^2/16$, resulting in a maximum signal-to-quantization noise ratio (SQNR) of around 65 dB for 16 bits. Thus, the minimum power of 35 dB less than this figure should be used assuming a minimum SNR of 30 dB.

They have also recommended that a calibration procedure to determine the gain and phase responses of the amplifier and filter unit be available for the breath sound recording system along with a verification procedure to check that no clipping, overload, and excessive noise level exist.

8.6 Upper Airway Sounds

Measurement and computerized analysis of upper airway sounds have aroused scientific research interest with a view to correlate pathologies with these sounds. Of particular interest are the cough sounds and snoring sounds.

8.6.1 Cough Measurement

Cough is one of the most common complaints for which people seek medical consultation [35] and consume vast number of drugs. It is a challenge for a physician to evaluate the significance of cough clinically and its response to treatment. It is possible to measure cough by assessing different aspects and effects of cough, and these approaches involve the assessment of such attributes like severity, frequency, intensity, and impact on quality of life. There are basically two approaches to assessment of coughs: subjective tools and objective tools. A systematic review of these tools is given in [36] and in [37]. The most commonly used subjective measurement tools of cough severity, frequency, impact, or their combination are cough diaries, visual analog scale (VAS) scores, the Leicester cough questionnaire (LCQ), and cough-specific quality of life questionnaire (CQLQ) in clinical environment although other subjective questionnaires are also available.

Subjective tools of cough assessment: A widely used subjective assessment tool, VAS, is brief and easy to use, where the subject is asked to evaluate the severity of cough on a 100 mm scale from "no cough" to "the worst cough severity." The other advantages of VAS can be listed as free availability, familiarity to clinicians, and clinical meaningfulness. Its drawback is the lack of published data reporting its validity and the minimal important difference [37]. Different effects of cough such as chest pain, vomiting, headache, sleep disorder, and similar disturbances may be more widely acquired using health-related quality of life questionnaires (HRQOL). Of these, LCQ and CQLQ are the most common, especially for adult patients with chronic cough. The LCQ has 19 items addressing physical, psychological, and social aspects of the effects of cough [38]. It was originally developed for patients with chronic cough but later was also validated for patients with chronic obstructive pulmonary disease (COPD), bronchiectasis, and acute cough [39–41]. LCQ is validated with good reliability, repeatability, and responsiveness to change. The other popular subjective tool, CQLQ, has 28 items and was developed in the USA. It is well validated in patients with chronic and acute cough [42]. Some other subjective questionnaires which are less commonly used in clinical assessment of cough are cough severity score (CSS) which refers to symptoms during the day time and night time separately and acquires data relating to cough frequency, intensity, and impact and cough severity diary (CSD) which has seven items to evaluate the severity and impact of the cough and was developed using patient feedback [43]. The latter two assessment tools have not been accepted in clinical use as extensively and have not been validated.

Objective tools of cough assessment: Cough frequency measurement is considered the gold standard for objective assessment of cough [44]. Electronic recording devices have been used in cough detection monitoring, and the earlier approaches were based either on sound measurement alone [45] or on simultaneous recording of sound and electromyography (EMG) [46, 47]. The earlier versions of these devices were mostly used in research applications rather than in clinical trials. The technical developments like MP3 recorders and longer-lasting batteries led to the design of systems that could be used in clinical environments or in ambulatory, 24-h monitoring of cough frequency [48]. Moreover, the advances in signal processing techniques made the fast handling and processing of large data possible [49]. There are several instruments that have been validated and are being widely used in clinical settings. One commonly used device uses a free-field miniature condenser lapel microphone with a flat frequency response between 20 Hz and 20 kHz and an MP3 recorder with a recording duration of more than 24 h [50]. It has an especially custom-developed software, based on the Hidden Markov model, for automated detection of cough sound. Another popular device has two sensors, one chest wall air-coupled electret condenser microphone and one free-field lapel condenser microphone, both microphones being omnidirectional. The frequency range for the microphones is between 100 Hz and 4 kHz. Recordings are made at a sampling rate of 8 kHz with 16 bits per sample bit rate, stored on a compact flash memory card [49, 51]. The algorithm for cough detection involves data reduction before manual counting by a trained technician. Both monitors have been validated and utilized in patients with chronic cough, acute cough, and COPD and have been used to evaluate antitussive therapy in clinical trials [52, 53]. The two main challenges in the design of cough measuring instruments are the discrimination of cough sounds from other sounds like throat clearing, speech, sneezing, laughing, and other ambient sounds and the variability of the cough sound characteristics between subjects, which requires the development of a general model that is applicable to different patients [48].

Cough reflex sensitivity challenge tests: The most common tussive agents to evaluate the sensitivity of the cough reflex are capsaicin and citric acid although other agents such as fog, low-chloride solution, bradykinin-prostaglandin E2, mannitol, and cinnamaldehyde are also used [54]. The most extensively employed procedure is the inhalation of nebulized tussive agents, and the test result is expressed as the concentration of tussive agent that causes two or five coughs (C2 or C5). Although cough reflex sensitivity assessment is reproducible, its major drawback in clinical practice is that it cannot discriminate healthy subjects from patients with cough.

Among the numerous available validated tools to assess cough, a combination of subjective and objective measures is preferable in clinical settings [54]. By combining these methods, the severity and the effect of cough can be assessed more completely. However, there is still a need for very large-scale studies which include different patterns of cough to cross validate evaluations of cough-specific quality of life questionnaires and cough monitoring devices before they can be recommended for extensive use [55].

8.6.2 Snoring Sound Measurements

Snoring sound, which is commonly heard during sleep, is measured especially in the diagnosis of obstructive sleep apnea (OSA). According to the International Classification of Sleep Disorders, "primary snoring is characterized by loud upper-airway of breathing sounds in sleep, without episodes of apneas or hyperventilation" [56]. The snore is an inspiratory sound but can occur during expiration in OSA instances. It contains periodic components with a fundamental frequency between 30 and 250 Hz and is loud with an intensity higher than 50 dB(A) [57]. To understand the clinical importance of snoring sounds, it is essential to record these sounds using standardized techniques so that studies from different sleep laboratories may be compared. No European standards are available for the measurement of snoring, but there are three methods, which are considered equivalent by the American Academy of Sleep Medicine (AASM) [58, 59]. These methods use an acoustic sensor such as a microphone, a nasal pressure sensor such as a cannula or a piezoelectric vibration sensor. However, in a study which was conducted to compare these three methods, it was concluded that there was a lack of consistency among these three methods in detecting snore events, and it was recommended that audio-based measurement was the most accurate [60].

8.7 Future Perspectives for Breath Sound Recording

Breath sound recording is a stimulating area of scientific research; however, even with more than 30 years of research activity, it has not yet established itself as a clinical investigation tool for diagnosis. Although many intelligent signal processing algorithms have been developed, the real bottleneck in the widespread application of breath sound recording as a routine clinical procedure is the lack of standardization in the sound signal acquisition from the surface of the body.

Consequently, objective comparisons and correlations of data from different recording systems cannot be made for an established diagnostic practice. The two main sensors used in the breath recording instruments, namely, the air-coupled electret microphone and the piezoelectric contact accelerometer, have their own shortcomings. An ideal sensor should be small and lightweight with a broad and reproducible frequency response. It should be immune to ambient noise and be enhanced with noise cancellation abilities so that it can record breath sounds in clinical settings where silent recording conditions may be difficult to achieve. There are new developments in microelectromechanical systems (MEMS) which have resulted in sensors with high-quality detection of breath and heart sounds [7]. With the progress of sensor research, an unanimously accepted transducer for breath sound recording is expected to be attained.

With the development of more efficient methods of recording breath sounds, multi-sensor arrays are being designed for acoustic mapping of the lung [25, 28, 61, 62]. The use of acoustic data for visual representation of the lung may be a promising alternative due to its practical, inexpensive, noninvasive, and harmless nature.

Wireless recording is another promising area for breath sound recording development. There have been several studies, such as [63], where wireless microphones are utilized to transmit breath sound to a receiver for further processing. A similarly active and expanding area in medicine is remote monitoring. Telemetry is of two types, namely, asynchronous and synchronous telemedicine. In asynchronous medicine, data are collected and sent electronically to a medical professional for further analysis and diagnosis. Synchronous telemedicine is real time and even interactive. Moreover, in synchronous telemedicine, distant examination may be enabled through audiovisual technology. There have been reports of self-monitoring of asthma [64, 65] and COPD [66] patients at home using telemedicine tools, and the results were accurate and satisfactory, without affecting the quality of care received by these patients. A study using telemedicine with intelligent algorithms is presented in [67]. Similarly, with the advances in smartphone and Bluetooth technology, wireless stethoscopes working with mobile phones have been developed [68]. Furthermore, with the miniaturization of sensors and widespread use of Internet communication, wearable monitoring systems are being cultivated [69, 70].

References

1. Laënnec RTH (1819) De l'auscultation médiate ou traité du diagnostic de maladies des poumons et du coeur, fondé principalement sur ce nouveau moyen d'exploration. Brosson et Chaudé, Paris
2. Abella M, Formolo J, Penney DG (1992) Comparison of the acoustic properties of six popular stethoscopes. J Acoust Soc Am 91:2224–2228
3. Murphy RLH (2008) In defense of the stethoscope. Respir Care 53(3):355–369
4. Gavriely N (1995) Breath sounds methodology. CRC Press, Boca Raton, FL
5. Pasterkamp H, Kraman SS, Wodicka GR (1997) Respiratory sounds: advances beyond the stethoscope. Am J Respir Crit Care Med 156:974–987
6. Reichert S, Gass R, Brandt C, Andres E (2008) Analysis of respiratory sounds: state of the art. Clin Med Circ Respirat Pulm Med 2:45–58

7. Zhdanov DS, Bureev AS, Khokhlova LA, Seleznev AI, Zemlyakov IY (2014) Short review of devices for detection of human breath sounds and heart tones. Biol Med 6(3):1–7
8. Sovijarvi ARA, Vanderschoot J, Earis JE (2000) Standardization of computerized respiratory sound analysis. Eur Respir Rev 10:77. 585
9. Sovijarvi ARA, Dalmasso F, Vanderschoot J, Malmberg LP, Righini G, Stoneman SAT (2000) Definitions of terms for applications of respiratory sounds. Eur Respir Rev 10:77. 597–610
10. Yadollahi A, Moussavi ZMK (2007) Acoustical respiratory flow: a review of reliable methods for measuring air flow. IEEE Eng Med Biol Mag 26(1):56–61
11. Kleiner M (2013) Electroacoustics. CRC Press, Boca Raton, FL
12. Vannuccini L, Earis JE, Helistö P, Cheetham BMG, Rossi M, Sovijärvi ARA, Vanderschoot J (2000) Capturing and preprocessing of respiratory sounds. Eur Respir Rev 10(77):616–620
13. Druzgalski CK, Donnerberg RL, Campbell RM (1980) Techniques of recording respiratory sounds. J Clin Eng 5(4):321–330
14. Pasterkamp H, Kraman SS, DeFrain PD, Wodicka GR (1993) Measurement of respiratory acoustical signals. Comparison of sensors. Chest 104:1518–1525
15. Bauer BB (1962) A century of microphones. Proc IRE 50:719–729
16. Rayburn RA, Eargle J (2004) Eargle's the microphone book: from mono to stereo to surround—a guide to microphone design and application, 2nd edn. Focal Press, London
17. Wodicka GR, Kraman SS, Zenk GM, Pasterkamp H (1994) Measurement of respiratory acoustic signals. Effect of microphone air cavity depth. Chest 106:1140–1144
18. Kraman SS, Wodicka GR, Oh Y, Pasterkamp H (1995) Measurement of respiratory acoustic signals. Effect of microphone air cavity width, shape, and venting. Chest 108:1004–1008
19. Kraman SS, Wodicka GR, Pressler GA, Pasterkamp H (2006) Comparison of lung sound transducers using a bioacoustics transducer testing system. J Appl Physiol 101:469–476
20. Jin F, Krishnan S, Sattar F (2011) Adventitious sounds identification and extraction using tempora-spectral dominance-based features. IEEE Trans Biomed Eng 58(11):3078–3087
21. Sankur B, Kahya YP, Güler ÇE, Engin T (1994) Comparison of AR-based algorithms for respiratory sounds classification. Comput Biol Med 21(4):67–76
22. Waitman LR, Clarkson KP, Barwise JA, King PH (2000) Representation and classification of breath sounds recorded in an intensive care setting using neural networks. J Clin Monit Comp 16(2):95–105
23. Alsmadi S, Kahya YP (2008) Design of a DSP-based instrument for real-time classification of pulmonary sounds. Comput Biol Med 38(1):53–61
24. Rossi M, Sovijärvi ARA, Piirila P, Vannuccini L, Dalmasso F, Vanderschoot J (2000) Environmental and subject conditions and breathing manoeuvres for respiratory sound recordings. Eur Respir Rev 10(77):611–615
25. Charleston-Villalobos S, Cortés-Rubiano S, González-Camarena R, Chi-Lem G, Aljama-Corrales T (2004) Respiratory acoustic thoracic imaging (RATHI): assessing deterministic interpolation techniques. Med Biol Eng Comput 42(5):618–626
26. Sen I, Kahya YP (2005) A multi-channel device for respiratory sound data acquisition and transient detection. In: Proc 27th IEEE Eng Med Biol Soc (EMBS), p 6658–6661
27. Charleston-Villalobos S, Martinez-Hernandez G, Gonzalez-Camarena R, Chi-Lem G, Carrillo JG, Aljama-Corrales T (2011) Assessment of multichannel lung sounds parameterization for two-class classification in interstitial lung disease patients. Comput Biol Med 41(7):473–482
28. Murphy R (2007) Computerized multichannel lung sound analysis: development of acoustic instruments for diagnosis and management of medical conditions. IEEE Eng Med Biol Mag 26(1):16–19
29. Beck R, Rosenhouse G, Mahagnah M, Chow RM, Cugell DW, Gavriely N (2005) Measurement and theory of normal tracheal breath sounds. Ann Biomed Eng 33(10):1344–1351
30. Webster JG (2006) Encyclopedia of medical devices and instrumentation. Volume I. Wiley-Interscience, Hoboken, NJ
31. Earis JE, Cheetham BMG (2000) Current methods used for computerized respiratory sound analysis. Eur Respir Rev 10(77):586–590

32. Katila T, Piirila P, Kallio K, Paajanen E, Rosqvist T, Sovijarvi AR (1991) Original waveform of lung sound crackles: a case study of the effect of high-pass filtration. J Appl Physiol 71:2173–2177
33. Hadjileontiadis LJ (2009) Lung sounds: an advanced signal processing perspective. Morgan & Claypool Publishers, San Rafael, CA
34. Cheetham BMG, Charbonneau G, Giardano A, Helistö P, Vanderschoot J (2000) Digitization of data for respiratory sound recordings. Eur Respir Rev 10(77):621–624
35. National Ambulatory Medical Care Survey: 2008 summary tables. Centers for Disease Control and Prevention website. http://www.cdc.gov/nchs/ahcd.htm
36. Schmit KM, Coeytaux RR, Goode AP, McCrory DC, Yancy WS Jr, Kemper AR, Hasselblad V, Heidenfelder BL, Sanders GD (2013) Evaluating cough assessment tools: a systematic review. Chest 144(6):1819–1826
37. Spinou A, Birring SS (2014) An update on measurement and monitoring of cough: what are the important study endpoints? J Thorac Dis 6(S7):S728–S734
38. Birring SS, Prudon B, Carr AJ et al (2003) Development of a symptom specific health status measure for patients with chronic cough: Leicester Cough Questionnaire (LCQ). Thorax 58:339–343
39. Berkhof FF, Boom LN, ten Hertog NE et al (2012) The validity and precision of the Leicester Cough Questionnaire in COPD patients with chronic cough. Health Qual Life Outcomes 10:4
40. Murray MP, Turnbull K, MacQuarrie S et al (2009) Validation of the Leicester Cough Questionnaire in non-cystic fibrosis bronchiectasis. Eur Respir J 34:125–131
41. Yousaf N, Lee KK, Jayaraman B et al (2011) The assessment of quality of life in acute cough with the Leicester Cough Questionnaire (LCQ-acute). Cough 7:4
42. French CT, Irwin RS, Fletcher KE et al (2002) Evaluation of a cough-specific quality-of-life questionnaire. Chest 121:1123–1131
43. Vernon M, Kline Leidy N, Nacson A et al (2010) Measuring cough severity: development and pilot testing of a new seven-item cough severity patient-reported outcome measure. Ther Adv Respir Dis 4:199–208
44. Morice AH, Fontana GA, Belvisi MG et al (2007) ERS guidelines on the assessment of cough. Eur Respir J 29:1256–1276
45. Subburaj S, Parvez L, Rajagopalan TG (1996) Methods of recording and analysing cough sounds. Pulm Pharmacol 9:269–279
46. Munyard P, Busst C, Logan-Sinclair R, Bush A (1994) A new device for ambulatory cough recording. Pediatr Pulmonol 18(3):178–186
47. Chang AB, Newman RG, Phelan PD, Robertson CF (1997) A new use for an old holter monitor: an ambulatory cough meter. Eur Respir J 10:1637–1639
48. Matos S, Birring SS, Pavord ID, Evans DH (2007) An automated system for 24-h monitoring of cough frequency: the Leicester Cough Monitor. IEEE Trans Biomed Eng 54(8):1472–1479
49. Barton A, Gaydecki P, Holt K et al (2012) Data reduction for cough studies using distribution of audio frequency content. Cough 8:12
50. Birring SS, Fleming T, Matos S et al (2008) The Leicester Cough Monitor: preliminary validation of an automated cough detection system in chronic cough. Eur Respir J 31:1013–1018
51. JAK V (2015) Model 7100, user training manual. Vitalograph, Maids Moreton, Buckingham
52. Smith J et al (2006) Effect of codeine on objective measurement of cough in chronic obstructive pulmonary disease. J Allergy Clin Immunol 117:831–835
53. Woodcock A et al (2010) The efficacy of a NOP1 agonist (SCH486757) in subacute cough. Lung 188(Suppl 1):S47–S52
54. Birring SS, Spinou A (2015) How best to measure cough clinically. Curr Opin Pharmacol 22:37–40
55. Leconte S, Ferrant D, Dory V, Degryse J (2011) Validated methods of cough assessment: a systematic review of the literature. Respiration 81:161–174
56. American Academy of Sleep Medicine (2001) International classification of sleep disorders, revised: diagnosis and coding manual. American Academy of Sleep Medicine, Chicago, IL
57. Gavriely N, Jensen O (1993) Theory and measurement of snores. J Appl Physiol 74:2828–2837

58. Berry RB, Brooks R, Garnaldo CE et al (2015) The AASM manual for the scoring of sleep and associated events: rules, terminology and technical specifications, version 2.2. American Academy of Sleep Medicine, Darlen, IL
59. Iber C, Ancoli-Israel S, Chesson AL, Quan SF (2007) The AASM manual for the scoring of sleep and associated events: rules, terminology and technical specifications, version 1. American Academy of Sleep Medicine, Westchester, IL
60. Arnardottir ES, Isleifsson B, Agustsson JS et al (2016) How to measure snoring? A comparison of the microphone, cannula and piezoelectric sensor. J Sleep Res 25:158–168
61. Sen I, Saraclar M, Kahya YP (2010) Acoustic mapping of the lung based on source localization of respiratory sound components. In: Proc 32rd IEEE Eng Med Biol Soc (EMBS), p 3670–3673
62. Kompis M, Pasterkamp H, Wodicka G (2001) Acoustic imaging of the human chest. Chest 120(4):1309–1321
63. Lu BY (2016) Unidirectional microphone based wireless recorder for the respiration sound. J Bioeng Biomed Sci 6(3):195. 1–8
64. Finkelstein J, Cabrera MR, Hripcsak C (2000) Internet-based home asthma telemonitoring: can patients handle the technology? Chest 117:148–155
65. Chan D, Callahan C, Sheets S, Moreno C, Malone F (2003) An internet-based store-and-forward video home telehealth system for improving asthma outcomes in children. Am J Health Syst Pharm 60:1976–1981
66. Casas A, Troosters T, Garcia-Aymerich J et al (2006) Integrated care prevents hospitalisations for exacerbations in COPD patients. Eur Respir J 28:123–130
67. Palaniappan R, Sundaraj K, Sundaraj S, Huliraj N, Revadi SS (2015) Appl Soft Comput 37:952–959
68. Reyes BA, Reljin N, Chon KH (2014) Tracheal sounds acquisition using smartphones. Sensors 14:13830–13850
69. Corbishley P, Rodriguez-Villegas E (2008) Breathing detection: towards a miniaturized, wearable, battery-operated monitoring system. IEEE Trans Biomed Eng 55(1):196–204
70. Li SH, Lin BS, Tsai CH, Yang CT, Lin BS (2017) Design of wearable breathing sound monitoring system for real-time wheeze detection. Sensors 17:171. 1–15

9 Current Techniques for Breath Sound Analysis

Leontios J. Hadjileontiadis and Zahra M. K. Moussavi

9.1 Introduction

This chapter aims to provide some insight in the current techniques used for breath sound analysis, in order to reveal, as accurately as possible, their underlying diagnostic value. This process leads to the construction of feasible models and tools that assist the physician during lung-related disease assessment and treatment. The main problems that drive the development of such techniques are (1) overcoming subjective interpretation of the breath sounds performed during auscultation by the doctor and (2) the elimination, as much as possible, of the contamination noise imposed during the breath sound acquisition by various noise sources (internal and/or external).

Breath sounds were the locus of interest even from the ancient Greeks, who followed vast medical experimentation to better understand the anatomy and functionality of the human body. Breath sounds are mentioned and described in the writings of the Hippocratic school (circa 400 BC) as *splashing*, *crackling*, *wheezing*, and *bubbling* sounds emanating from the chest [1]. All these different sound impressions reveal the variation in the breath sound perception that makes their interpretation a quite hard task to accomplish.

L. J. Hadjileontiadis (✉)
Department of Electrical and Computer Engineering, Aristotle University of Thessaloniki, Thessaloniki, Greece

Department of Electrical and Computer Engineering, Khalifa University of Science and Technology, Abu Dhabi, UAE
e-mail: leontios@auth.gr; leontios.h@kustar.ae.ac

Z. M. K. Moussavi
Department of Electrical and Computer Engineering, University of Manitoba, Winnipeg, MB, Canada
e-mail: Zahra.Moussavi@umanitoba.ca

K. N. Priftis et al. (eds.), *Breath Sounds*, https://doi.org/10.1007/978-3-319-71824-8_9

A profound idea, yet with great impact on the qualitative appreciation of breath sounds, was proposed by René Theophil Hyacinthe Laënnec in 1816, who invented the *stethoscope*. This simple gadget, which was originally made of wood, replaced the "ear-upon-chest" detection procedure enhancing the emitted breath sounds [2]. Nevertheless, this invention has changed a lot the way medicine was performed. Actually, medicine was one of the first sites where the conceptual tools of rationality and empiricism were combined with techniques of investigation to make the human body a source of knowledge [3]. The stethoscope significantly contributed to the combination of conceptual tools of rationality and empiricism with techniques of investigation, transforming the human body to "an object of knowledge" (ibid). It was not so much about the actual artifact as the technique that it crystallized, i.e., mediated auscultation [4]. In this way, listening became important to the construction of medical knowledge and its application through the development of a technique and a technology to go with it, to such extent that doctor's hearing tool became the symbol of a profession, even from the 1820s [5]. Clearly, *a 'good doctor' is the one that has the technology and possesses the technique to effectively use it.*

The development of the stethoscope and mediated auscultation coincided with the development of new theories of sense perception based on a "separation of the senses." To this end, seeing and hearing are to be understood as fundamentally and absolutely different modes of knowing the world, though neither form of knowledge is guaranteed as truth [6]. This was the moment when empiricism collided with subjectivism [7]. If the sensorium was, before this moment, a kind of complex whole, it then became an accumulation of parts. Thus, not only vision but hearing became its own, specific object of knowledge over the course of the nineteenth century, supplemented through technique and technology. From then, audition became a key modality in perceiving states of patients' bodies.

Attempts of quantitative analysis of breath sounds date to 1930, but the first systematic, quantitative measurement of their characteristics (i.e., amplitude, pitch, duration, and timing in controls and in patients) is attributed to McKusick in 1958 [1]; with his work, a new window toward the exploration of acoustics in medicine was widely opened.

Before embarking on the description of the advanced signal processing approaches in the area of breath sound analysis, their characteristics are epitomized in the succeeding section, facilitating the understanding of the nature of the examined breath sound signals.

9.2 Breath Sound Characteristics

The whole book serves as a valuable source of information regarding the breath sound characteristics according to their categorization. Here, some issues that relate with the essence of breath sound analysis approaches are presented, mainly focused on lung sounds (LSs).

From a general perspective, a LS is nothing but an audible sound; the latter consists of audible vibrations transmitted through an elastic solid or a liquid or gas, created by alternating regions of compression and rarefaction of the elastic medium. The density of the medium determines the ease, distance, and speed of sound transmission. The higher the density of the medium, the slower sound travels through it. Sound waves are characterized by the generic properties of waves, which are frequency, wavelength, period, amplitude, intensity, speed, direction, and polarization (for shear waves only). Due to the variety of LSs, a commonly accepted categorization is needed. In the latter, the principal characteristics, i.e., frequency, intensity, duration, and quality (timbre/texture), are mainly considered.

9.2.1 Categorization

In fact, LSs are divided into two main categories, i.e., *normal* and *abnormal* ones. The normal are certain sounds heard over specific locations of the chest during breathing in healthy subjects. The character of the normal LSs and the location at which they are heard define them. Hence, the category of the normal LSs includes [8]:

Tracheal (heard over the trachea having a high loudness)

Vesicular (heard over dependent portions of the chest, not in immediate proximity to the central airways)

Bronchial (heard in the immediate vicinity of central airways but principally over the trachea and larynx)

Bronchovesicular, which refers to normal breath sounds with a character in between vesicular and bronchial (heard at intermediate locations between the lung and the large airways)

Normal crackles, inspiratory breath sounds (heard over the anterior or the posterior lung bases) [9, 10]

The abnormal LSs consist of LSs of a bronchial or bronchovesicular nature that appear at typical locations (where vesicular LS is the norm). The abnormal LSs are categorized between *continuous adventitious sounds* (CAS) and *discontinuous adventitious sounds* (DAS) [11] and include [12–16]:

Wheezes: musical CAS that occur mainly in expiration and are invariably associated with airway obstruction, either focal or general

Rhonchi: low-pitched sometimes musical CAS that occur predominantly in expiration, associated more with chronic bronchitis and bronchiectasis than with asthma

Stridors: musical CAS that are caused by a partial obstruction in a central airway, usually at or near the larynx

Crackles: discrete, explosive, non-musical DAS, further categorized between:

Fine crackles are high-pitched exclusively inspiratory events that tend to occur in mid-to-late inspiration, repeat in similar patterns over subsequent breaths, and have a quality similar to the sound made by strips of Velcro™ being slowly pulled apart; they result from the explosive reopening of small airways that had been closed during the previous expiration

Coarse crackles are low-pitched sound events found in early inspiration and occasionally in expiration as well, develop from fluid in small airways, are of a "popping" quality, and tend to be less reproducible than the fine crackles from breath to breath

Squawks (SQ): short, inspiratory wheezes that usually appear in allergic alveolitis and interstitial fibrosis [17] and predominantly initiated with a crackle, caused by the explosive opening and fluttering of the unstable airway that causes the short wheeze

Friction rub: DAS localized to the area overlying the involved pleura which occur in inspiration and expiration when roughened pleural surfaces rub together, instead of gliding smoothly and silently.

Analytical description can be found in Part III of the current book.

9.2.2 Intrinsic Characteristics

The variety in the categorization of LSs implies changes in the acoustic characteristics, either of the source or the transmission path of the LSs inside the lungs, because of the effect of a certain pulmonary pathology. It is likely that the time- and frequency-domain characteristics of the LS signals reflect these anatomical changes [18].

In particular, the time-domain pattern of the normal LSs resembles a noise pattern bound by an envelope, which is a function of the flow rate (ibid). Tracheal sounds have higher intensity and a wider frequency band (0–2 kHz) than the chest wall sounds (0–600 Hz) and contain more acoustic energy at higher frequencies [19]. The CAS time-domain pattern is a periodic wave that may be either sinusoidal or a set of more complex, repetitive sound structures [18]. In the case of wheezes, the power spectrum contains several dissonant-like peaks ("polyphonic" wheezes) or a single peak ("monophonic" wheeze), usually in the frequency band of 200–800 Hz, indicating bronchial obstruction (ibid). Crackles have an explosive time-domain pattern, with a rapid onset and short duration (ibid). It should be noted that this waveform may be an artifact of high-pass filtering [20]. Their time-domain structural characteristics (i.e., a sharp, sudden deflection usually followed by a wave) provide a means for their categorization between fine and coarse crackles [21].

For an extensive description and a variety of examples regarding LS structure and intrinsic characteristics, the reader should refer to [12, 16, 18] and Chaps. 2, 5, and 6 of the current book.

9.3 Analysis Mainstream Pathways

LSs analysis has long lived between two main representations, i.e., in time and frequency domain, following a variety of directions; the most popular include:

Respiratory flow estimation [22–29]

Heart sound cancellation [30–45]

DAS detection and denoising [46–68]
Nonlinear analysis of LS [69–79]
Feature extraction and classification [6, 18, 46, 52, 60, 80–108]

Although LS time and spectral characteristics proved to be so far quite efficient in the interpretation of LSs, they cannot always provide the full image of the diagnostic power of LSs. In this vein, some new analysis domains have been proposed, approaching some LSs properties from different angles, capturing, perhaps, in a more pragmatic way their behavior. The latter could drive more efficiently machine learning algorithms applied in the diagnosis of lung sound [109]. The presentation of such methodologies aims at not only revealing the importance of LSs as indicators of respiratory health and disease but also shedding light upon the inherent characteristics of the advanced signal processing techniques that manage to adapt to the specific properties of LSs, providing a new viewpoint in the evaluation of respiratory acoustics. These interesting representations and features of LSs are gleaned in the subsequent sections, based on the relevant literature, where more detailed (mathematical) description is provided, accordingly.

9.4 Beyond Spectrum: Higher-Order Spectrum (HOS)

9.4.1 Rationale

Many real-world signals, such as almost all the biomedical ones, are non-Gaussian random processes. As a result, distinguishing features, such as non-Gaussianity, non-minimum phase, colored noise, and nonlinearity, are important and must be accounted for in a signal processing context. To this end, a class of tools has been developed to the point of practical application, known as higher-order statistics (spectra) (HOS), which have proven to be of potential value when dealing with non-Gaussian random processes [110, 111].

Higher-order statistics, also known as cumulants, are related to and may be expressed in terms of the moments of a random process. In general, the k th-order cumulant of a random process is defined in terms of the process's joint moments of orders up to k (ibid). Just as the power spectrum (PS) (the Fourier transform of the autocorrelation) is a useful tool in the signal analysis, so too are the higher-order spectra, also known as polyspectra, which are the associated Fourier transforms of the cumulants. In PS estimation, the process under consideration is treated as a superposition of statistically uncorrelated harmonic components, and the distribution of power among them is the estimation outcome. As such, only linear mechanisms governing the process are investigated due to the suppression of the phase relations among the frequency components [112]. Consequently, the information contained in the PS suffices for the complete statistical description of a Gaussian process of known mean. Looking beyond the PS to obtain information regarding deviations from Gaussianity and presence of nonlinearities, the polyspectra should be employed. The most often used ones are the third- and fourth-order spectra, also called bispectrum and trispectrum, respectively. From this perspective, the PS should be considered, in fact, as a member of the class of higher-order spectra, i.e., as a second-order spectrum.

Cumulants not only reveal amplitude information about a process but also reveal phase information. This is of great importance, since, as is well known, second-order statistics, i.e., correlation, are phase-blind. A key characteristic, which differentiates cumulants from correlation, is that cumulants are blind to all kinds of Gaussian processes, whereas correlation is not. From a practical point of view, this means that when cumulant-based methods are applied to non-Gaussian (or, possibly, nonlinear) processes contaminated by additive Gaussian noise (even colored Gaussian one), they provide an analysis field of automatically improved signal-to-noise ratio (SNR).

Practically speaking, many biomedical signal processes are non-Gaussian yet corrupted by measurement noise, which can often be realistically described as colored Gaussian process; hence, in these practical applications, the value of the HOS is apparent. Another very attractive property of cumulants refers to the ability to work with them as operators. On a practical level, this means that the cumulants of the sum of two statistically independent random processes equals the sum of the cumulants of the individual processes. Higher-order moments, by contrast, do not have that property; hence, they are much less convenient [111].

Based on the aforementioned HOS characteristics, placing LSs in the HOS-based domain could reveal their true character and, hence, could disclose further their underlined diagnostic value, as exemplified next.

9.4.2 Epitomized Definitions and Examples of HOS-Based Analysis of LSs

9.4.2.1 LS Quadratic Phase Coupling (QPC) Detection

Quadratic phase coupling (QPC) refers to peaks at harmonically related positions in the power spectrum. As the existence of phase coupling denotes existence of nonlinearity, which, in turn, in many cases, is related to the existence of pathology, detection of QPC in LS signals could possibly provide an indicator of the anatomical changes of lungs due to the pathology. The detection of the QPC is facilitated via the HOS-defined bicoherency index (BI). The latter is the magnitude of the bicoherence, i.e., ($|P_3^x(\omega_1, \omega_2)|$), defined as

$$P_3^x(\omega_1,\omega_2) = \frac{C_3^x(\omega_1,\omega_2)}{\left[C_2^x(\omega_1)C_2^x(\omega_2)C_2^x(\omega_1+\omega_2)\right]^{\frac{1}{2}}}, \tag{9.1}$$

where $C_2^x(\omega)$ and $C_3^x(\omega_1,\omega_2)$ correspond to the power spectrum and the bispectrum of a stationary stochastic process $\{X(k)\}$, given, accordingly, by

$$C_2^x(\omega) = \sum_{\tau=-\infty}^{+\infty} c_2^x(\tau)e^{-j(\omega\tau)}, |\omega| \le \pi, \tag{9.2}$$

$$C_3^x(\omega_1,\omega_2)=\sum_{\tau_1=-\infty}^{+\infty}\sum_{\tau_2=-\infty}^{+\infty}c_3^x(\tau_1,\tau_2)\mathrm{e}^{-j(\omega_1\tau_1+\omega_2\tau_2)}$$
$$|\omega_1|\le\pi,|\omega_2|\le\pi,|\omega_1+\omega_2|\le\pi, \tag{9.3}$$

and $c_2^x(\tau)$ denotes the autocorrelation function, whereas $c_3^x(\tau_1,\tau_2)$ are the third-order cumulants of $\{X(k)\}$, defined (for a zero-mean $\{X(k)\}$) as

$$c_3^x(\tau_1,\tau_2)=E\{X(k)X(k+\tau_1)X(k+\tau_2)\}. \tag{9.4}$$

Due to the even symmetry of $c_2^x(-\tau)=c_2^x(\tau)$, $C_2^x(\omega)=C_2^x(-\omega)$ and $C_2^x(\omega)\ge 0$; thus $C_2^x(\omega)$ is a real nonnegative function. This observation is quite vital for the use of the power spectrum when phase carries the important information, where, unlike $C_3^x(\omega_1,\omega_2)$, it becomes useless, as $C_2^x(\omega)$, being real, cannot express any phase information.

A nonlinear analysis of musical LSs based on BI was first presented in [76]. In the latter, the third-order statistics and spectra were used both for the detection of QPC between distinct frequency components of musical lung sounds and as a measure of their nonlinear interaction. This harmonic analysis was conducted on pre-classified signals (wheezes, rhonchi, stridors) selected from international teaching tapes. The derived results have shown a high degree of deviation from Gaussianity along with quadratic self-coupling within the distinct frequencies of the corresponding power spectrum of musical lung sounds. This is depicted in Fig. 9.1, where the estimated $C_2^x(\omega)$ and $C_3^x(\omega_1,\omega_2)$ of an inspiratory stridor recorded from an infant with croup [76] are depicted in Fig. 9.1a, b, respectively. From the three distinct peaks seen in the $C_2^x(\omega)$ in Fig. 9.1a, i.e., (410.2, 820.4, 1230.6) Hz, a self-coupling is revealed in the bispectrum domain, $C_3^x(\omega_1,\omega_2)$ in Fig. 9.1b, denoted by the clear peak at the (410.2, 410.2) Hz.

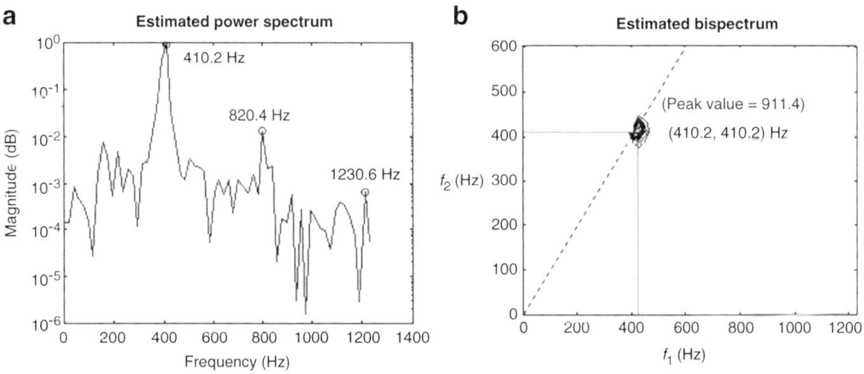

Fig. 9.1 An example of QPC seen in the case of a recorded inspiratory stridor: (**a**) the corresponding power spectrum and (**b**) the corresponding bispectrum estimated within the principal region in the bi-frequency domain [76]. The distinct peak in the bispectrum denotes existence of the QPC and strong deviation from the Gaussian assumption

As reported in [76], in case of monophonic wheezes, the frequency pair of QPC belongs into the low-frequency band. The fundamental frequency is revealed in inspiratory phase of breath cycle, while its first harmonic dominates in the expiratory phase. This fact leads to the conclusion that the monophonic wheeze consists of a single note or a single tonality, established by the octaves of the fundamental frequency, due to a nonlinear mechanism. In case of polyphonic wheezes, the frequency pair of QPC belongs into a higher frequency band than that of monophonic wheezes. In the inspiratory phase, pairs of high frequencies perform QPC, while in the expiratory phase, submultiple frequencies of those in the inspiratory phase perform QPC. The harmonics which are involved result in a polyphonic chord, since apart from the fundamental frequency (f_0), the octave ($2f_0$) and the fifth of the chord ($3f_0$) perform QPC. This result is consistent with the accepted theory that polyphonic wheezes are made up of several dissonant notes starting and ending simultaneously, like a chord [14].

In the same works, in case of random wheezes, the nonlinearity and non-Gaussianity of the process were found to be evident both in inspiratory and expiratory cases. In cases of sibilant (SBR) and sonorous (SNR) rhonchi, high- and low-frequency pairs perform QPC, since they correspond to high and low wheezes, respectively. From $(f_1,f_2)\Big|_{(\text{expiratory SNR})}=\left(\frac{1}{3}\right)\times(f_1,f_2)\Big|_{(\text{inspiratory SBR})}$ it can be concluded that sibilant and sonorous rhonchi have similar nonlinear production mechanism but different transmission, since high frequencies are only amplified in case of sibilant rhonchi. Moreover, in case of stridors, high-frequency pairs, both in inspiration and expiration, perform QPC. The frequencies with QPC corresponding to inspiratory stridors from an infant with croup are higher than those corresponding to inspiratory stridors from a 9-year old child with croup. As it is well known, stridor (ST) intensity is the only thing that distinguishes a stridor from a monophonic wheeze (MW) [14]. From the nonlinear analysis, it can be seen that $(f_1,f_2)\Big|_{(\text{inspiratory MW})}=\left(\frac{1}{5}\right)\times(f_1,f_2)\Big|_{(\text{inspiratory ST})}$ justifying their relationship, but the degree of nonlinearity is much larger in stridor than in monophonic wheeze. This difference can introduce another field of separating these associated abnormal musical LSs categories.

From the examples presented above, clearly, differences in the degree of QPC, the nonlinearity, and the non-Gaussianity of the processed LS signals could establish a new field in characterization and feature extraction of the pulmonary pathologies associated with musical lung sounds, such as asthma and chronic obstructive pulmonary dysfunction [52, 75, 76].

9.4.2.2 AR-HOS Modeling of LSs Source and Transmission

Analysis and modeling of the system that produces the LSs and their transmission channel inside the lungs contribute to the understanding of both the way LSs are produced and, even more, the way the pathology affects these production and transmission mechanisms. Such modeling could offer more sparse representation of the lung functionality via the model parameters, which, with efficient modeling, could lead to an objective description of the changes a disease imposes to the production or transmission path of the LSs.

LSs originated inside the airways of the lung are modeled as the input to an all-pole filter, which describes the transmission of LSs through the parenchyma and chest wall structure [113]. The output of this filter is considered to be the LSs recorded at the chest wall. The recorded LSs also contain heart sound interference. Muscle and skin noise, along with instrumentation noise, are modeled as an additive Gaussian noise. With this model, given a signal sequence of LSs at the chest wall, an autoregressive (AR) analysis based on third-order statistics (TOS), namely, AR-TOS, can be applied to compute the model parameters. Therefore, the source and transmission filter characteristics can be separately estimated, as it is thoroughly described in [52, 75].

The AR-TOS is described from the following equation:

$$y_n + \sum_{i=1}^{p} a_i y_{n-i} = w_n, a_0 = 1, \tag{9.5}$$

where y_n represents a pth order AR process of N samples ($n = 0, \ldots, N - 1$), a_i are the coefficients of the AR model, and w_n are independent and identically distributed (i.i.d.), third-order stationary, zero-mean, random variables, with $E\left\{w_n^3\right\} = \beta \neq 0$ and y_n independent of w_l for $n < l$. Since w_n is third-order stationary, y_n is also third-order stationary, assuming it is a stable AR model. For the model of (9.5), we can write the cumulant-based "normal" equations [114]:

$$\sum_{i=0}^{p} a_i c_3^y \left(\tau_1 - i, \tau_2\right) = 0, \tau_1 = 1, \ldots, p;\ \tau_2 = -p, \ldots, 0, \tag{9.6}$$

where $c_3^y\left(\tau_1, \tau_2\right)$ are the third-order cumulant sequence of the AR process. In practice, sample estimates of the cumulants are used. The (9.6) yields consistent estimates of the AR parameters maintaining the orthogonality of the prediction error sequence to an instrumental process derived from the data [115].

The profound motivations behind the use of the AR-TOS model is the suppression of Gaussian noise, because TOS of Gaussian signals are identically zero. Hence, when the analyzed waveform consists of a non-Gaussian signal in additive symmetric noise (e.g., Gaussian), the parameter estimation of the original signal with TOS takes place in a high-SNR domain, and the whole parametric presentation of the process is more accurate and reliable [111].

The model used for the LSs originated inside the airways considers the LSs source as the output from an additive combination of three kinds of noise sequences [116]. The first sequence (periodic impulse) describes the CAS sources, because they have characteristic distinct pitches, and they are produced by periodic oscillations of the air and airway walls [14, 18]. The second sequence (random intermittent impulses) describes the crackle sources, because they are produced by sudden opening/closing of airways or bubbling of air through extraneous liquids in the airways, both phenomena associated with sudden intermittent bursts of sounds energy (ibid).

Finally, the third sequence (white non-Gaussian noise) describes the breath sound sources, because they are produced by turbulent flow in a large range of airway dimensions (ibid). The estimation of the AR-TOS model input (LSs source) can be derived from the prediction error by means of inverse filtering [52, 117]. An example of AR-TOS ($p = 2$) modeling for the case of fine crackles corresponding to pulmonary fibrosis [117] is shown in Fig. 9.2.

For the acquired fine crackles (Fig. 9.2a), the estimated source waveform based on (9.5) and (9.6) (Fig. 9.2b) contains impulsive bursts, corresponding to the fine crackles of Fig. 9.2a. This could be explained by the associated with fine crackles phenomenon of explosive reopening of small airways that had closed during the previous expiration. The abnormal airway closure that precedes the "crackling" reopening is due to increased lung stiffness [18]. Moreover, the transmission filter response (Fig. 9.2c) is centered at high frequencies (≈530 Hz); hence, pulmonary fibrosis converts the transmission path to a band-pass filter (350–700 Hz). From the magnitude of parametric bispectrum (Fig. 9.2d), it can be noticed that a self-QPC exists at (530, 530) Hz, denoting that nonlinear mechanisms are involved in the transmission path of fine crackles through the lungs.

In the same vein, in the work of Li and Liu [118], QPC peaks of bispectrum, normalized bispectral entropy and parameters of slice spectrum are selected to form the feature vector for lung sounds classification for the classes of controls, patients with pneumonia and patients with asthma. Their results, although qualitative, have

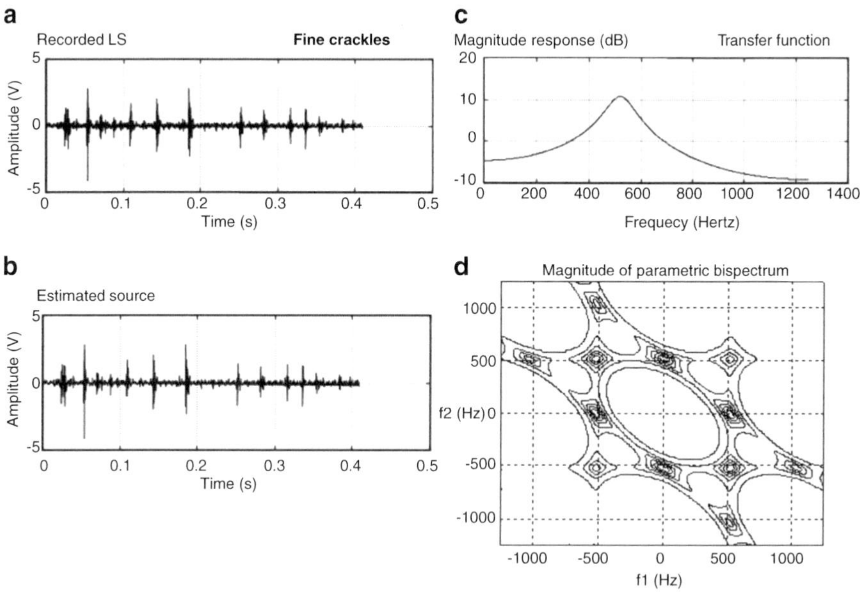

Fig. 9.2 An example of AR-TOS modeling of LS source and transmission for the case of fine crackles [75, 117]. (**a**–**d**) Correspond to the recorded LSs signal, the AR-TOS-based estimated source, the AR-TOS-based estimated transfer function, and the corresponding magnitude of the parametric bispectrum, respectively

shown that bispectrum analysis of lung sounds is applicable and effective and could provide a field to yield more reliable classification features than the conventional power spectrum.

9.5 Beyond Fourier Transform: Wavelet Transform (WT)

9.5.1 Rationale

The notion of a wavelet (i.e., a small wave) has evolved rapidly from its introduction by Grossmann and Morlet in the middle of the 1980s as applied to the analysis of properties of seismic and acoustic signals [119]. Nowadays, the family of analyzing functions dubbed wavelets is being increasingly used in problems of pattern recognition, in processing and synthesizing various signals (like speech), in analysis of images of any kind (e.g., iris images, X-rays, satellite images, an image of mineral, etc.), for study of turbulent fields, for contraction (compression) of large volumes of information, and in many other cases.

The wavelet transform (WT) of a one-dimensional signal involves its decomposition over a basis obtained from a soliton-like function (wavelet), possessing some specific properties, by dilations and translations. Each of the functions of this basis emphasizes both a specific spatial (temporal) frequency and its localization in physical space (time). Thus, unlike the Fourier transform traditionally used in signal analysis, the WT offers a two-dimensional expansion of a given one-dimensional signal, with the frequency and the coordinate treated as independent variables. Consequently, the signal could be analyzed simultaneously in physical (time, coordinate) and frequency spaces. This ability has spawned a number of sophisticated wavelet-based methods for signal manipulation and interrogation. WT has been found to be particularly useful for analyzing signals which can best be described as aperiodic, noisy, intermittent, and transient [120].

One faces known difficulties when processing short high-frequency signals or signals with localized frequencies. The WT proves to be an extremely efficient tool in adequately decoding such signals, since elements of its basis are well localized and possess a moving time-frequency window. It is not a coincidence that many researchers refer to wavelet analysis as a "mathematical microscope," as this term accurately conveys the remarkable capability of the method to offer a good resolution at different scales. This so-called microscope reveals the internal structure of an essentially inhomogeneous process (or field) and exposes its local scaling behavior [121]. In this vein, WT picks out "coherent structures" in a time signal at various scales by shifting the wavelet along the signal, so coherent structures related to a specific dilation in the signal to be identified.

The decomposition of the input signal into approximation and detail space is called *multiresolution approximation* [122], which can be realized using a pair of finite impulse response (FIR) filters (and their adjoints), which are low pass and high pass, respectively, defining a multiresolution decomposition–multiresolution reconstruction scheme (MRD–MRR).

Wavelets can be successfully applied to solve various problems, as the vast relevant literature justifies. An analytical description and details regarding the implementation of wavelet analysis can be found in [120, 123–127] and in their references.

9.5.2 Epitomized Definitions and Examples of WT-Based Analysis of LSs

Wavelet transform analysis uses wavelets to convolve them with the signal under investigation [120]. The continuous wavelet transform (CWT) of a continuous signal $x(t)$ with respect to the wavelet function is defined as [120]

$$W_x(a,b) = \int_{-\infty}^{\infty} x(t)\psi^*_{a,b}(t)\,\mathrm{d}t, \tag{9.7}$$

where $\psi^*_{a,b}(t)$ is the conjugate of the mother wavelet scaled by a factor a ($a > 0$) and dilated by a factor b, i.e.,

$$\psi_{a,b}(t) = \frac{1}{\sqrt{a}}\psi\left(\frac{t-b}{a}\right). \tag{9.8}$$

Assuming $x(t)$ to be a sine wave (e.g., like a musical LS signal, i.e., wheeze), then $x(t) = A \sin(\omega_x t + \varphi)$, with ω_x and φ being its angular frequency and phase, respectively; it holds that $\omega_x = \lambda\omega_c/a$, where ω_c/a is the angular frequency of the analyzing mother wavelet of (9.8), and ω_c is the central angular frequency that corresponds to $a = 1$; $\lambda = \omega_x / \left(\frac{\omega_c}{a}\right)$ and for a real mother wavelet and $b = 0$, (9.7) could be written in the form of

$$W_x(a) = A\sqrt{a}\int_{-\infty}^{\infty} \sin(\lambda\omega_c t + \varphi)\psi_\alpha(t)\,\mathrm{d}t. \tag{9.9}$$

The inverse CWT (ICWT) is defined as [120]

$$x(t) = \frac{1}{C_g}\int_{-\infty}^{\infty}\int_{0}^{\infty} W_x(a,b)\psi_{a,b}(t)\frac{\mathrm{d}a\mathrm{d}b}{a^2}, \tag{9.10}$$

where C_g is an admissibility constant [120], and its value depends on the chosen wavelet.

By selecting discrete values for a, b parameters, a discrete form of the wavelet of (9.8) is produced. When a power-of-two logarithmic scaling of both the dilation and translation steps is adopted (known as the "dyadic grid arrangement"), then a dyadic grid wavelet is formed. Discrete dyadic grid wavelets are commonly chosen to be orthonormal; they are both orthogonal to each other and normalized to have unit energy.

Considering the characteristics of various LS signals, a series of research efforts were developed toward the application of WT to LS analysis. In the work of Gross et al. [128], parameters based on multiresolution approximation were able to detect typical pneumonia LS at an early stage of the disease in all 16 examined patients. In particular, using Daubechies 8 coefficient quadratic mirror filters [123], a multiresolution approximation was performed, and the bronchial breathing sound pattern was detected by using WT-based ratio R between inspiration and expiration of the frequency band 345–690 Hz (scale 3) described in [129]. WT coefficients in the pneumonia site exhibited reduced amplitude compared to the ones from the healthy site, following a reversed pattern (healthy site, higher amplitude in inspiration and lower in expiration; pneumonia site, lower amplitude in inspiration and higher in expiration). The successful WT-based detection of bronchial breathing can be considered as a first step in developing a monitoring system for pneumonia-risk patients.

Ayari et al. [130] applied the WT transform to normal LS, crackles, and wheezes. In their work, they used wavelets formed by the first derivative of a Gaussian. Derivatives of Gaussian are most often used to guarantee that all maxima lines propagate up to the finest scale. They used the WT modulus maxima method [131] to characterize the local regularity of LS. The localized singularities correspond to the sharp and slow variations. WT of LS across scales presents local maxima when using a wavelet that is a first derivative of a smoothing function. Consequently, the sharp and slow variations are indicated by the location of the local modulus maxima obtained by one vanishing moment wavelet. The analysis of the behavior of WT modulus maxima across scales permits detection of singularities and estimation of Lipschitz exponents for the sharp and slow variation [132]. Numerical results for the crackle sound showed that singularity at sharp variation was Lipschitz 1. For wheezes the singularity at sharp variations was Lipschitz 1. This is quite expected, as wheezing sound seems more like a sinusoidal signal, so it looks to be more regular than the normal lung sound.

WT has also been used in combination with artificial neural networks (ANNs) to form a LS classification scheme. In the work of Kandaswamy et al. [94], LS signals were decomposed into the frequency sub-bands using multiresolution approximation, and a set of statistical features was extracted from the sub-bands to represent the distribution of wavelet coefficients. An ANN-based system, trained using the resilient back-propagation algorithm (RPROP) [133], was implemented to classify LS to one of the six categories: normal, wheeze, crackle, squawk, stridor, or rhonchus. RPROP is a local adaptive learning scheme, performing supervised batch learning in feed-forward neural networks. The basic principle of RPROP is to eliminate the harmful influence of the size of the partial derivative on the weight step. As a consequence, only the sign of the derivative is considered to indicate the direction of the weight update. The authors used some statistics from the WT coefficients as features for the ANN-based classification. In particular, they used (1) the mean of the absolute values of the coefficients in each sub-band, (2) the average power of the wavelet coefficients in each sub-band, (3) the standard deviation of the coefficients in each sub-band, and (4) the ratio of the absolute mean values of adjacent sub-bands. The first two features represent the frequency distribution of the signal whereas the next two the amount of changes in frequency distribution. These feature vectors, calculated for the frequency scales of 3–7, were used for classification of the LS signals by the ANN. The authors achieved classification accuracy >90%, when using Daubechies wavelet of order 8 [123].

Various combinations of WT-based approaches in DAS detection and extraction from the background vesicular sound were also proposed. As already mentioned, WT provides a new perspective in analysis of LS, since it can decompose them into multi-scale details, describing their power at each scale and position (ibid). Applying a threshold-based criterion at each scale, a filtering scheme which weights WT coefficients according to signal structure can be composed. Separation of signal from "noise" can be achieved through an iterative reconstruction–decomposition process, based on the derived weighted WT coefficients at each iteration. The aforementioned concept was introduced in [49], where the implementation of a wavelet transform-based stationary–nonstationary (WTST–NST) filter for the separation of DAS (nonstationary waves) from vesicular ones (stationary waves) is described. WTST–NST is a wavelet domain filtering technique, based on the fact that explosive peaks (DAS) have large components over many wavelet scales, while "noisy" background (VS) dies out swiftly with increasing scale. This fact allows characterization of the wavelet transform coefficients with respect to their amplitude; the most significant coefficients at each scale, with amplitude above some threshold, correspond to DAS, while the rest correspond to VS. Consequently, a wavelet domain separation of WT coefficients corresponding to DAS and vesicular sound, respectively, can offer a time-domain separation of DAS from vesicular sound using an iterative MRD–MRR scheme. Figure 9.3 illustrates an example of the application of the WTST–NST filter to recorded LS that contains coarse crackles.

In Fig. 9.3, the top subplot illustrates the original recorded LS sounds; the nonstationary character of CC is clearly evident. The result of the application of the WTST–NST filter to the recorded LS is depicted in the middle subplot of Fig. 9.3, whereas the estimated VS signal (serving as background noise) is shown in the bottom subplot of Fig. 9.3. When comparing the output of the WTST–NST filter with the original signal, the ability of the WTST–NST filter to efficiently identify and extract DAS from VS is realized. Extended implementation details and further experimental results can be found in [49].

In the work of Ulukaya et al. [104], a rational-dilation WT (RADWT) [134] was used, in which the *Q*-factor of the analysis and synthesis filters can be adjusted according to the properties of signal of interest. When high *Q*-factor filters are used, oscillatory wavelets similar to wheeze signals in the time domain and better frequency resolution for low and middle frequency bands in frequency domain can be achieved. From the decomposed sub-band coefficients with the RADWT, various feature subsets, namely, energy, Shannon entropy, standard deviation, minimum/maximum, and kurtosis values of each sub-band, were derived. These new feature subsets were fed into *k*-nearest neighbor (*k*-NN) and support vector machine (SVM) classifiers, in order to discriminate the classes of crackle, wheeze, and normal signals. Their results show that by using high *Q*-factor wavelet analysis, higher individual crackle, wheeze, normal signal detection rates, and average accuracy (mean of individual rates) could be achieved (>95% with SVM), when compared to the low *Q*-factor wavelet analysis.

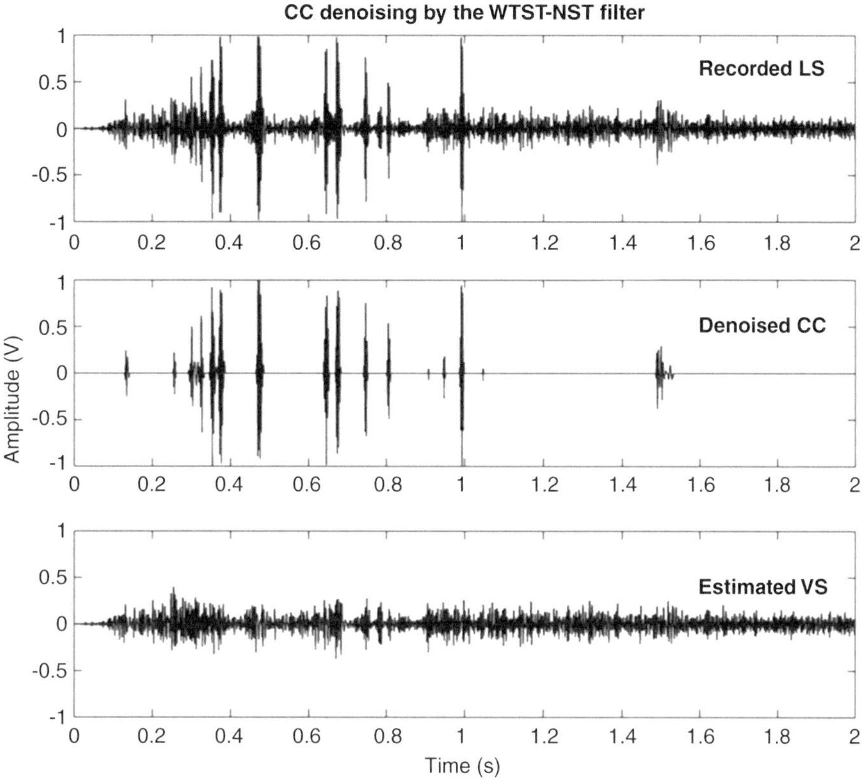

Fig. 9.3 An example of the application of the WTST–NST filter [49] to recorded LS that contain coarse crackles (CC), illustrating the efficient performance of the WTST–NST filter to identify and extract DAS from vesicular sound (VS). (top) The original recorded LS, (middle) the denoised CCs, (bottom) the estimated VS (background noise-like)

As it is apparent from the above referenced examples, WT provides new opportunities in LS representation that allow construction of hybrid analysis tools. The latter stems from the beneficial advantages of WT and, by combining other efficient methods, introduces new approaches in LS analysis and appreciation. This becomes clearer in the succeeding section.

9.6 HOS and WT: Wavelet Higher-Order Spectrum (WHOS)

9.6.1 Rationale

As it was previously presented, wavelet analysis can be seen as a generalization of the Fourier analysis and, in many cases, permits a similar interpretation but amplifies it by adding time resolution—in a more fundamental way than is permitted by the short-time Fourier transform (STFT), since the latter does not remove the objection raised above against Fourier-type methods.

Signals containing coherent couplings have traditionally been analyzed by means of a normalized bispectrum, i.e., the bicoherence, as described in Sect. 9.4.2.1 (see (9.1)). The bicoherence, when defined properly, quantifies the fraction of power contained in the nonlinearity. However, when the available data have a nonstationary nature, traditional fast Fourier transform (FFT)-based methods may be inadequate due to the inability of the STFT to resolve short-lived transients properly [115, 135]. To circumvent such problem, the *wavelet bispectrum/bicoherence* was proposed [136–138], based on a combination of CWT with HOS.

For the analysis of nonstationary processes, the wavelet bispectrum has two main advantages compared to traditional FFT-based methods. First, since the CWT is a time-scale representation of a signal, thus, a time axis is introduced in a natural way. Second, wavelets have an inherent constant-Q filtering property and are consequently well suited for detection of transients.

The wavelet bicoherence technique detects QPC while reducing time averages to a minimum, thus permitting short-lived events, pulsed, and intermittency to be resolved [139]. Relatively short data sequences are sufficient to perform an analysis, in contrast to the Fourier bicoherence that needs long-time series to obtain both sufficient frequency resolution and statistics. Estimates of the noise contribution and error level of the wavelet bicoherence provide a criterion for the reliability of the results. A powerful noise reduction is an integral part of the standard technique: as noncoherent contributions are averaged out, weak coherent signals can be detected in very noisy data. Moreover, the wavelet bicoherence is more independent of the frame of reference and may be expected to be more useful in experiments where measurement in the local frame of reference is difficult [138].

9.6.2 Epitomized Definitions and Examples of WHOS-Based Analysis of LSs

By analogy to the definition of the bispectrum in Fourier terms (see (9.3)), the *wavelet bispectrum* (WBS) is defined as [139]

$$B_{\mathrm{w}}\left(a_1,a_2\right)=\int_T W_x^*\left(a,\tau\right)W_x\left(a_1,\tau\right)W_x\left(a_2,\tau\right)\mathrm{d}\tau, \tag{9.11}$$

where $W_x(a_i,\tau)$, $i = 1, 2$, denotes the CWT defined in (9.7) and the integration is performed over a finite time interval $T: \tau_0 \leq \tau \leq \tau_1$, and a, a_1, a_2 satisfy the following rule:

$$\frac{1}{a}=\frac{1}{a_1}+\frac{1}{a_2}. \tag{9.12}$$

The WBS expresses the amount of QPC in the interval T, which occurs between wavelet components of scale lengths a_1, a_2 and a of $x(t)$, such that the sum rule of (9.12) is satisfied. By interpreting the scales as inverse frequencies, i.e., $\omega=\frac{2\pi}{a}$, the WBS can be interpreted as the coupling between wavelets of frequencies that satisfy $\omega = \omega_1 + \omega_2$ within the given frequency resolution.

Similarly to the definition of bicoherence (see (9.1)), the *wavelet bicoherence* (WBC) can be defined as the normalized WBS, i.e.,

$$b_{\mathrm{w}}\left(a_1,a_2\right)=\frac{B_{\mathrm{w}}\left(a_1,a_2\right)}{\left\{\left[\int_T\left|W_x\left(a_1,\tau\right)W_x\left(a_2,\tau\right)\right|^2\mathrm{d}\tau\right]\left[\int_T\left|W_x\left(a,\tau\right)\right|^2\mathrm{d}\tau\right]\right\}^{1/2}},\qquad(9.13)$$

and its magnitude, i.e., $|b_{\mathrm{w}}(a_1,a_2)|$, namely, *wavelet bicoherence index*, can attain values between 0 and 1.

Since the WBC defined in (9.13) refers to a certain time interval T, its value is corresponded to the center of this interval, i.e., $t_0 = T/2$. Consequently, the evolutionary WBC (EWBC) can be defined as

$$\begin{aligned}&\mathbf{b}_{\mathrm{w}}\left(\omega_1,,\omega_2,,t\right)=\left\{b_{\mathrm{w}}\left(\omega_1,\omega_2\right)\Big|_{t=t_0+k\Delta T_1}\right\}\\&\Delta T_1\geq\frac{2\pi}{\omega_{\mathrm{s}}}\wedge k\Delta T_1\leq T_{\mathrm{total}}-2t_0,k=0,1,2,\ldots,\end{aligned}\qquad(9.14)$$

where T_{total} is the total time duration of the analyzed signal $x(t)$. When using EWBC, the evolution of the nonlinearities across time can be represented, within a time resolution controlled by the selection of the ΔT_1 value.

Due to the nature of wheezes, the notion of QPC detection examined in Sect. 9.4.2.1 is expanded by employing wavelet bispectrum and wavelet bicoherence as a means to track and quantify the evolution of the nonlinear characteristics of wheezes within the breathing cycle. To this end, the combination of wavelet transform with third-order statistics/spectra introduces the nonlinear analysis of wheezes in the time-bi-frequency domain. This was investigated in [78, 79], where breath sound signals from asthmatic patients were analyzed using CWT-HOS-based parameters.

The variation in the time-frequency characteristics of wheezes justifies the necessity of using wavelet-based higher-order statistics/spectra to reveal their nonlinearities. Figure 9.4 (top-a) depicts one breathing cycle of a breath sound signal along with the normalized airflow (superimposed with a dotted line) recorded from an asthmatic patient. The positive and negative airflow values indicate inspiratory and expiratory phases, respectively. As it can be seen from Fig. 9.4 (top-a), the expiratory phase is prolonged compared to the inspiratory one; this is due to the existence of asthma. Similarly, the breath sound signal exhibits a profound high-amplitude section (~1.2–2.8 s) corresponding to inspiratory wheeze, whereas an extended expiratory wheeze (~3.7–6.3 s) with decaying amplitude dominates the expiratory phase.

Figure 9.4 (top-b) shows the representation of the signal in the time-frequency domain via the CWT of the signal. From this figure, the harmonic character of wheezes (both inspiratory and expiratory) is apparent. Clearly, there are coexisting distinct spectral peaks within the area of 150–500 Hz that emerge during the appearance of wheezes, revealing their polyphonic character (like a chord). In addition, a frequency sweep from low to high frequencies and vice versa can be noticed, mainly at the beginning and the end of wheezes, due to the increase or decrease of the airflow signal, respectively. Moreover, the spectral peak within 200–400 Hz that sustains its high amplitude during the inspiratory wheeze is subsided in the expiratory one, where the spectral peak around 200 Hz seems to be the most evident one.

Figure 9.4 (bottom) illustrates a graphical representation of the ESWBC for whole breath sound signal shown in Fig. 9.4 (top-a). In this way, the evolution of the nonlinearities in breath sound signal that contains wheezes is demonstrated. From this figure, it is apparent that QPC occurs in both breathing phases only at the time instances where the wheezes exist. Moreover, the main frequency pair with QPC $[(f_1, f_2) \approx (200, 200)$ Hz] is sustained, both in inspiratory and expiratory wheezes; however, additional pairs at higher frequencies with QPC emerge during the expiratory wheeze. This relates to the pathology of asthma, as it affects the expiratory phase more than the inspiratory one of asthmatic patients [140].

The CWT-HOS-based analysis of wheezes presented here could be expanded to different types of wheezes, as a means to characterize them according to the nonlinear properties they exhibit as they evolve within the breathing cycle. This would shed light upon the differences between different categories of wheezes (e.g., monophonic vs. polyphonic) and different pathologies (e.g., COPD and

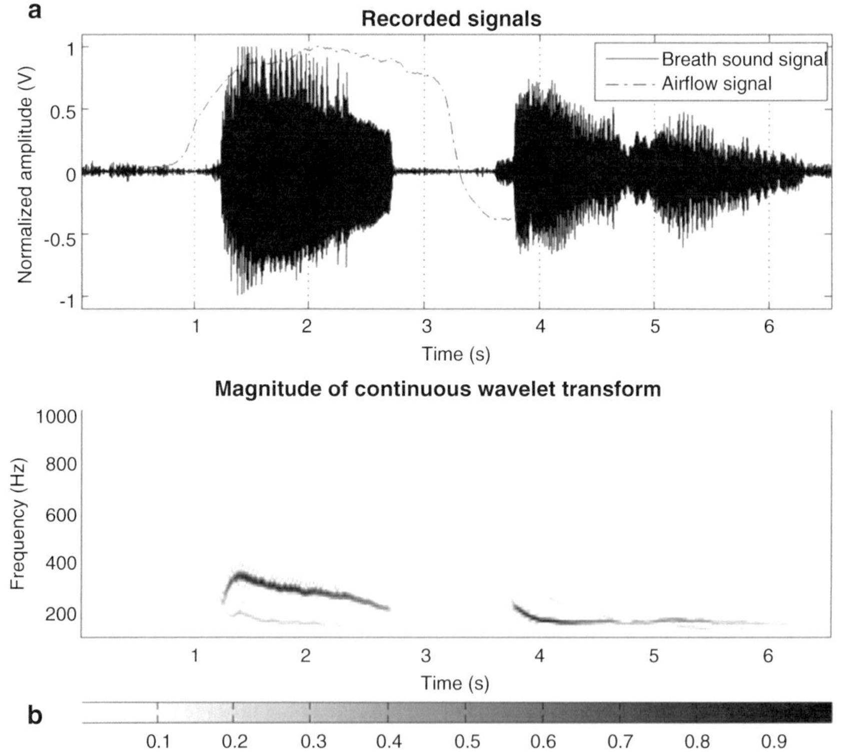

Fig. 9.4 Top-(**a**): One breathing cycle of a breath sound recording from an asthmatic patient with two dominant wheezes (one inspiratory and one expiratory). Top-(**b**): the CWT of the analyzed signal. Bottom: the corresponding ESWBC. The time axis includes one breathing cycle [79]

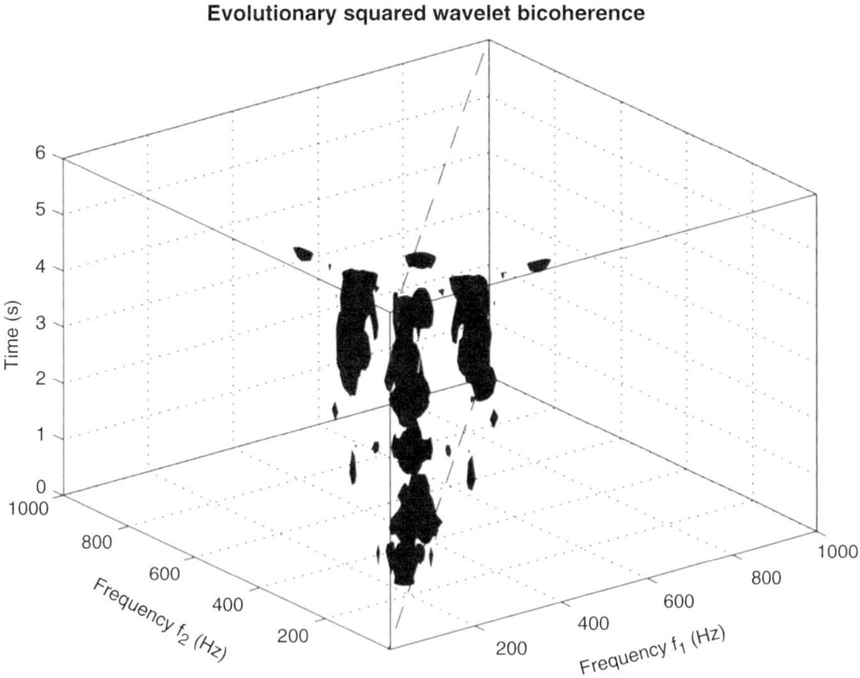

Fig. 9.4 (continued)

asthma). In either case, CWT-HOS provides an efficient hybrid analysis tool that allows enhancement of significant details in the LS interpretation, which could not be solely perceived by auscultation.

9.7 Empirical Mode Decomposition (EMD)

9.7.1 Rationale

To accommodate the nonstationarity of the LS signals, the corresponding analysis could be applied to either a moving data window or adaptively giving more weight to more current data as a means for summarizing a time dependent oscillation pattern. Nevertheless, a more efficient approach lies in the field of *empirical mode decomposition* (EMD), proposed by Huang et al. [141]. EMD decomposes the signal into components with well-defined instantaneous frequency. Each characteristic oscillatory mode extracted, namely, *intrinsic mode function* (IMF), is symmetric and has a unique local frequency, and different IMFs do not exhibit the same frequency at the same time [141].

The EMD method is necessary to deal with both nonstationary and nonlinear data, and, contrary to almost all the previous methods, EMD is intuitive; that is, the basis of the expansion is generated in a direct, a posteriori, and adaptive way, derived from the data [141]. The main idea behind EMD is that all data consist of different simple intrinsic modes of oscillations, represented by the IMFs. An IMF represents a simple oscillatory mode as a counterpart of the simple harmonic function, yet it allows amplitude and frequency modulation; thus, it is much more general. The EMD method considers the signals at their local oscillation scale, subtracts the faster oscillation, and iterates the residual. EMD can also be viewed as an expansion of the data in terms of the IMFs. Then, these IMFs, based on and derived from the data, can serve as the basis of that expansion which can be linear or nonlinear as dictated by the data, and it is complete and almost orthogonal. Most important of all, it is adaptive,and, therefore, highly efficient.

Representation of LS in the EMD domain reveals their intrinsic characteristics, as these are reflected in the IMFs, and provides a new analysis space where detailed exploitation of LS diagnostic information is feasible.

9.7.2 Epitomized Definitions and Examples of EMD-Based Analysis of LSs

EMD is formed through the estimation of the IMFs, which each one satisfies two conditions [141]: (1) in the whole dataset, the number of extrema and the number of zero-crossings must either equal or differ at most by one; and (2) at any point, the mean value of the envelope defined by the local maxima and the envelope defined by the local minima is zero. A sifting process adopted [141] results in a decomposition of the data into empirical modes and a residue which can be either a monotonic function or a single cycle, i.e.,

$$x(t) = \sum_{i=1}^{N} c_i(t) + r_N(t), \tag{9.15}$$

where $c_i(t)$ is the ith IMF and $r_N(t)$ the final residue.

It is noteworthy that, in order to apply the EMD method, there is no need for a mean or zero reference; EMD only needs the locations of the local extrema to generate the zero reference for each component (except for the residue) through the shifting process. Moreover, using the IMF components, a time-space filtering can be devised simply by selecting a specific range of them in the reconstruction procedure (e.g., in (9.15), for high-pass filtering, $i = 1 : k$, $k < N$ or for band-pass one, $i = b : k$, $1 < b, k < N$). This time-space filtering has the advantage that its results preserve the full nonlinearity and nonstationarity in the physical space [142].

The process of finding IMFs is indeed like sifting: to separate the finest local mode from the data first based only on the characteristic time scale. The sifting process, however, has two effects: (1) to eliminate riding waves and (2) to smooth uneven amplitudes. While the first condition is absolutely necessary for the instantaneous frequency to be meaningful, the second condition is also necessary in case the neighboring wave amplitudes have too large a disparity. Unfortunately, the second effect, when carried to the extreme, could obliterate the physically meaningful amplitude fluctuations. Therefore, the sifting process should be applied with care, for carrying the process to an extreme could make the resulting IMF a pure frequency-modulated signal of constant amplitude. One of the possible drawbacks of EMD is the occasional appearance of *mode mixing*, which is defined as a single IMF consisting of either signals of widely disparate scales or a signal of a similar scale residing in different IMF components. Mode mixing is a consequence of signal intermittency. Recently, a new sifting approach was proposed, namely, *Ensemble EMD* (EEMD) [143, 144], that successfully deals with the mode mixing problem. This new approach consists of sifting an ensemble of white noise-added signal and treats the mean as the final true result. Finite, not infinitesimal, amplitude white noise is necessary to force the ensemble to exhaust all possible solutions in the sifting process, thus making the different scale signals to collate in the proper IMFs dictated by the dyadic filter banks. An extension to the EEMD was proposed by Yeh et al. [145], with the purpose of removing the residue of added white noises. They modified the EEMD method by using the complementary sets of added white noises to remove residue of added white noises. This modified EEMD, namely, *complementary* EEMD (CEEMD), was also developed as a new technique to overcome intermittence [145], hence mode mixing. CEEMD extents the concept of EEMD method by generating two sets of averaged IMFs, i.e., averaged IMFs with positive and negative residues of added white noises.

An example of the application of the EMD and EEMD to recorded CC is illustrated in Fig. 9.5a, b, respectively. In particular, the recorded LS signal along with the first nine IMFs is depicted, showing the distribution of the vesicular sound and CC waveforms across the decomposition levels. When comparing the morphology of the IMFs between the two decompositions, some differences can be identified. In particular, IMF_1 clearly differs from the original signal in the case of EMD (Fig. 9.5a), whereas in the case of EEMD (Fig. 9.5b), it exhibits strong similarity with the original signal. CC are more isolated in the first four EMD-IMFs, whereas CC dominate in the third and fourth EEMD-IMFs. Clearly, EEMD-IMF_2 corresponds to the additive noise used in the EEMD realization. In general, EEMD-IMFs seem to better represent CC than the EMD-IMFs, despite the domination of noise in some IMFs, as EEMD reduces the mode-mixing effect (e.g., at IMF_3 and IMF_4 level).

A similar approach was attempted for discriminating between fine and coarse crackles in [146]. They reported that the EMD technique improved the visual identification of crackles embedded in respiratory sound. Although crackles and respiratory sound were mixed, their respective oscillations were able to be identified at different IMFs.

In their work, Lozano et al. [147] present a new classifier that automatically distinguishes normal sounds from CAS, based on the multi-scale analysis of instantaneous frequency (IF) and instantaneous envelope (IE) calculated after the use of EEMD. The classifier was based on the fact that the IF dispersion of respiratory signals markedly decreases when CAS appear in respiratory cycles. Therefore, CAS were detected by using a moving window to calculate the dispersion of IF sequences. The study dataset contained 1494 LS segments extracted from 870 inspiratory cycles recorded from 30 patients with asthma. All cycles and their LS segments were previously classified as containing normal sounds or CAS by a highly experienced physician to obtain a gold standard classification. A SVM classifier was trained and tested using an iterative procedure in which the dataset was randomly divided into training (65%) and testing (35%) sets inside a loop. The SVM classifier was also tested on 4592 simulated CAS cycles. High total accuracy was obtained with both recorded (94.6% ± 0.3%) and simulated (92.8% ± 3.6%) signals, showing that the proposed method sets an efficient approach in LS analysis and classification.

EMD analysis has also been used in a DAS denoising process, as thoroughly is described in [56].

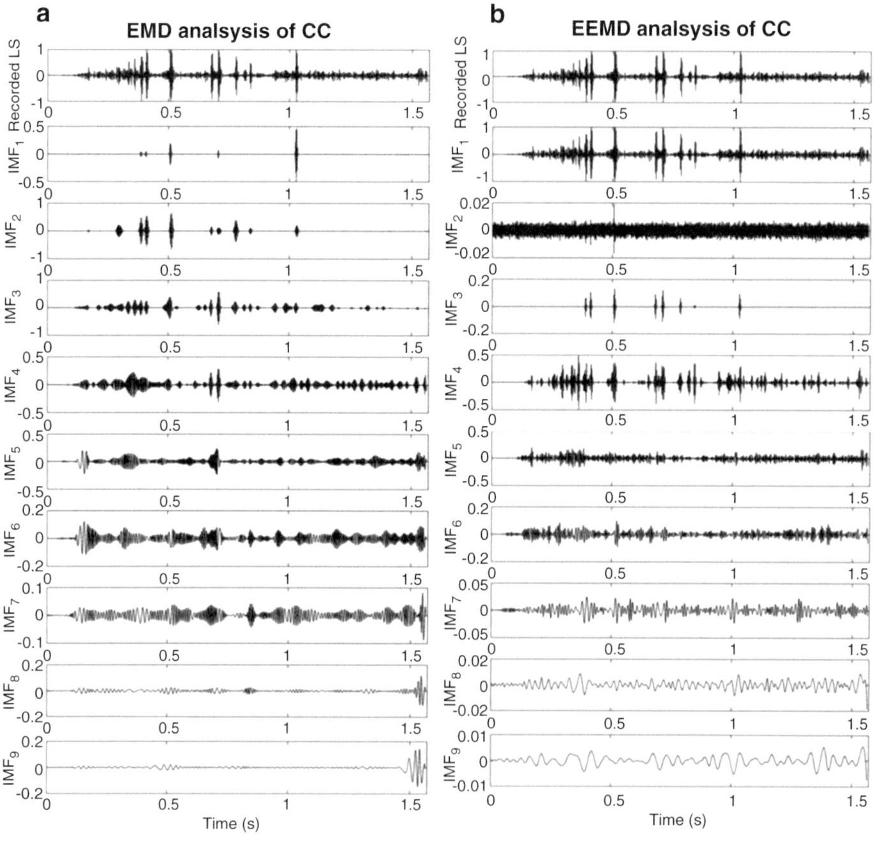

Fig. 9.5 Application of (**a**) EMD and (**b**) EEMD to LS containing CC superimposed on vesicular LS. In both cases, the recorded LS signal along with the first nine IMFs are depicted, respectively

9.8 Other Approaches

9.8.1 Back to Lower-Order Statistics (LOS)

A broad class of non-Gaussian phenomena encountered in practice can be characterized as impulsive. Signals and/or noise in this class tend to produce large-amplitude excursions from the average value more frequently than Gaussian signals. They are more likely to exhibit sharp spikes or occasional bursts of outlying observations than one would expect from normally distributed signals. As a result, their density function decays in the tails less rapidly than the Gaussian density function [148]. Among the different kinds of LS, there are some that seem to belong in the aforementioned class, occurring with a different degree of impulsiveness. Since modeling based on α-stable distribution related to lower-order statistics (LOS) is appropriate for enhanced description of impulsive processes (ibid), its use could provide a useful processing tool for analysis of impulsive LS.

Analysis of LS with explosive character, like crackles, by means of LOS-based modeling provides an innovating perception in the analysis of impulsive LS, suggesting a new field in their processing for diagnostic feature extraction. Following this approach, impulsive LS (i.e., DAS) with explosive character can be modeled by means of LOS [86]. From the estimated parameters of the symmetric α-stable ($S\alpha S$) distribution of the analyzed impulsive LS using the log $| S\alpha S|$ method [148], it is derived that the *covariation coefficient* calculated for the cases of the sound sources of squawks (SQ) and FC [86] shows an almost 50% correlation between the SQ and FC, confirming the accepted theory that SQ are produced by the explosive opening, due to a FC, and decaying fluttering of an unstable airway [18]. Moreover, by estimating the characteristic exponent α for each category (crackles, background noise, and artifacts), based again on the log $| S\alpha S|$ method (Nikias and Shao 1995), a classification criterion could be established, according to the estimated alpha values. This approach has been adopted in [149], from where it is deduced that FC follow approximately a Cauchy distribution (mean $\alpha = 0.92$, which is close to $\alpha = 1.0$ that holds in the case of the Cauchy distribution), while the CC deviate both from Cauchy and Gaussian distributions (mean $\alpha = 1.33$); the artifacts have high impulsiveness with values of $\alpha \ll 1.0$. The events that resemble the vesicular sound are seen as background noise and are modeled as Gaussian processes (values of $\alpha > 1.8$ or very close to 2.0, which hold in the case of the Gaussian distribution). Using this approach, disputed sounds that could not be classified by the doctor could be clearly classified.

9.8.2 Higher-Order Crossings (HOC)

Apart from the transform-based approach presented so far, time characteristics of LS could also be considered as a focus field. Taking into consideration that almost all observed time series are oscillatory, displaying local and global up and down movements as time progresses, proper time series analysis could "capture" these oscillatory patterns and use them as a new domain of representation. This is done here by the concept of higher-order crossings (HOC) [150]. HOC analysis of time series is a way to study oscillation of stochastic processes combinatorically by counting and provides an alternative to commonly used spectral methods.

Time ordering makes it possible to apply to a time-series linear filtering, one of the most indigenous elements of time series analysis. This filtering, in fact, changes the time-series oscillations, and this can be reflected in the change in the zero-crossing count effected by the filtering procedure. The application of a specific sequence of filters (or family of filters) to a time series forms the corresponding sequence (or family) of zero-crossing counts, namely, HOC, and, thus, provides a summary of the oscillation "history" observed in the time series and its filtered versions.

Following the properties of HOC estimated from different LS signals, new discrimination features could be established that provide successful differentiation among LS with similar acoustic behavior. In this vein, HOC have been used to perform a discrimination analysis of DAS, especially FC, CC, and SQ [87]. In fact, HOC assesses the changes in oscillatory pattern of DAS according to their type, by estimating the relevant HOC sequence. Based on the connection between filtering and zero-crossings, the proposed method constitutes a possible tool for DAS discrimination analysis, namely, HOC-DA, which is quite attractive due to its simplicity in the evaluation of the HOC sequence and its ability to provide simple discrimination criteria between the examined LS classes [87].

9.8.3 Fractality/Lacunarity (F/L)

The term "fractal dimension" (FD) can more generally refer to any of the dimensions commonly used for fractal characterization (e.g., capacity dimension, correlation dimension, information dimension, Lyapunov dimension, Minkowski–Bouligand dimension) [151]. In other words, FD is a measure of how "complicated" a self-similar figure is. To this end, the FD can be considered as a relative measure of the number of basic building blocks that form a pattern [152]. Consequently, the FD could reflect the signal complexity in the time domain. This complexity could vary with sudden occurrence of transient signals, such as explosive LS.

As Gnitecki and Moussavi [73] note, LS will possess valid FD values, based on their morphological properties. Most obviously, the signals do not self-cross. In physical systems, the property of self-similarity in pure fractal objects is not strict but is probabilistic, and there are minimum and maximum scaling limits [153]. In reality, an object occurring in nature, such as a physiological signal, that exactly duplicates itself over several scales does not exist. Thus, the fractality of LS is in the self-affine sense [73]. Furthermore, the LS exhibits clear quasi-periodicity because they emerge from natural biological processes, like breathing, which implies that they are not purely random [153]. Consequently, FD analysis could clearly shed light upon the understanding of LS from a functional point of view.

An analysis of LS with FD is presented in the work of Gnitecki and Moussavi [73], where they examined the fractality of LS from normal subjects reflected in the estimated values of FD. LS was sequestered corresponding to 85–100% of the maximum flow per inspiratory breath. Three sliding window sizes were used for each FD calculation across the signals, i.e., 50, 100, and 200 ms, respectively, shifted forward by 25 ms. In [73], apparent similarities, in terms of both morphology and overall variability, between three scalings of LS were found. Overall, FD showed an increase with airflow. From the characteristics of the FD analysis of the examined normal LS, a fractal character was identified; this finding, however, was not justified for the case of abnormal LS. FD was also used in the analysis of DAS for their detection and isolation from the vesicular sound combined with both WT [54, 55] and EMD [56] analyses.

Laennec in his attempt to develop a metalanguage of sound (as reported in his magnum opus Treatise [154]) defined a set of descriptions for the shape and texture of sounds that was independent of subjective experience (i.e., independently verifiable). By employing the texture of the LS in this codification, Laennec showed the importance of this sound property in the hydraulic hermeneutics of mediated auscultation. Following this pathway, LS texture could be approached through the concept of lacunarity. The latter was originally developed to describe a property of fractals [155–158] and to discriminate textures and natural surfaces that share the same FD. Gefen et al. [156] define lacunarity as the deviation of a fractal from translational invariance. Translational invariance can also be a property of non-fractal sets [155], and it is highly scale dependent; sets which are heterogeneous at small scales can be quite homogeneous when examined at larger scales or vice versa [159]. From this perspective, lacunarity can be considered a scale-dependent measure of heterogeneity or texture of an object, whether or not it is fractal [155]. Lacunarity features can be used to assess the largeness of gaps or holes of one- (signals) or two-dimensional sets (images). A set with low lacunarity is homogeneous and transitional invariant, whereas one with high lacunarity has gaps distributed across a broad range of sizes [160].

In the work of Hadjileontiadis [6, 88], lacunarity analysis was applied to two datasets of DAS exhibiting high-classification performance, resulting in a combined mean classification accuracy greater than 99.6% for all comparison groups (FC-CC; FC-SQ; CC-SQ; FC-CC-SQ) [88]. The randomized training and testing sections used in the evaluation of the lacunarity analysis augurs a promising performance of the LAC analysis under different case scenarios. The simplicity of the LAC analysis facilitates the customization of its computational environment under a real-time context, resulting in an easily implemented and user-friendly processing tool of DAS.

9.9 Emerging Approaches

9.9.1 Swarm Decomposition (SwD)–Swarm Transform (SwT)

In Sects. 9.5 and 9.7, the MRD–MRR and the EMD/EEMD multiresolution analysis schemes were referenced, respectively, as bases to build upon the analysis of LSs and derive new diagnostic features. The issue behind the use of MRD–MRR is the demand for an a priori selection of the analysis basis (wavelet) from a given library (e.g., Daubechies, Morlet), whereas in the EMD/EEMD case, this requirement is waived, as the analysis basis is produced from the signal itself, via the sifting process. Nevertheless, as the name of EMD/EEMD denotes, it is an empirical approach.

In the light of the aforementioned, a new multiresolution analysis scheme has been recently proposed [161], based on the swarm perception, namely, the *swarm decomposition* (SwD). The latter circumvents the empirical character of EMD by proposing a more deterministic approach to achieve effective multiresolution decomposition.

In the SwD, a swarming model is used as the analysis basis, where the processing is intuitively considered as a *virtual swarm–prey hunting*, where the prey is the signal itself. According to the state of the swarm, i.e., relations of its members, different oscillatory characteristics of the signal are revealed (e.g., its low/high frequencies when the swarm has low/high coherence between its members). To systematically use this type of filtering, the relations between the swarm parameters and particular responses are needed; these are derived using a genetic algorithm [161]. Eventually, the SwD is realized by iteratively applying the swarm filtering, where, at each iteration, it is properly parametrized, so as to result in an *oscillatory mode* (OM) sequence (roughly corresponding to the IMFs of the EMD/EEMD). The main advantage of the proposed swarm-based perspective is that SwD allows for the efficient decomposition of a signal into components that preserve physical meaning, likewise EMD/EEMD, being yet based on a rigid mathematical model [161]. By applying Hilbert transform to the resulted OM components, a time-frequency representation is formed, namely, *swarm transform* (SwT), which allows for better discrimination of the localization in time and frequency of the inherent oscillations of the input signal (e.g., pitched LSs, such as wheezes).

Figure 9.6a displays the OMs derived from the analysis of an asthmatic wheeze (first panel of Fig. 9.6a) using the SwD, whereas Fig. 9.6b displays the corresponding output of the EEMD analysis (first seven IMFs) of the same input LS signal (first panel of Fig. 9.6b). In addition, Fig. 9.7a displays the estimated SwT corresponding to the OMs from the SwD of Fig. 9.6a, whereas Fig. 9.7b shows the Hilbert–Huang spectrum, as the Hilbert transform of all derived IMFs via the EEMD displayed (in part) in Fig. 9.6b.

As it can be seen from the comparison of Fig. 9.6a, b, there is a more focused approach in the oscillatory characteristics of the wheeze components in the output of the SwD, compared to the one of the EEMD. In fact, in the SwD output (Fig. 9.6a), the wheezing parts (roughly identified within the time sections of [0–0.5 s], [0.5–1.8 s], and [1.8–3.16 s]) are clearly isolated across the identified OMs, whereas in the EEMD output (Fig. 9.6b), more general transitions from high- (IMF1) to low- (IMF7) frequency components are corresponded.

This is directly reflected in the corresponding SwT and Hilbert–Huang spectrum of Fig. 9.7a, b, respectively, as the multiphonic character of the recorded wheeze along with the frequency sweeping episodes (mostly at [1.8–3.16 s]) is clearly represented in the SwT (Fig. 9.7a) with parallel and sweeping ridges, whereas is in the Hilbert–Huang spectrum (Fig. 9.7b), more dispersed spectral information is

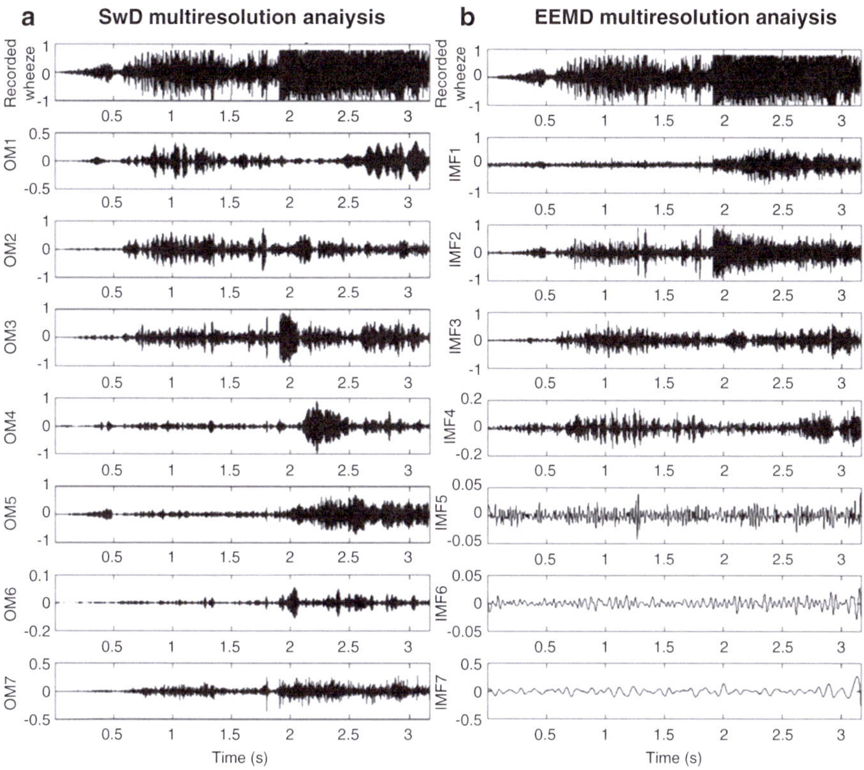

Fig. 9.6 Application of (**a**) SwD and (**b**) EEMD to an asthmatic wheeze recording. In both cases, the recorded LS signal along with the seven OMs and IMFs are depicted, respectively

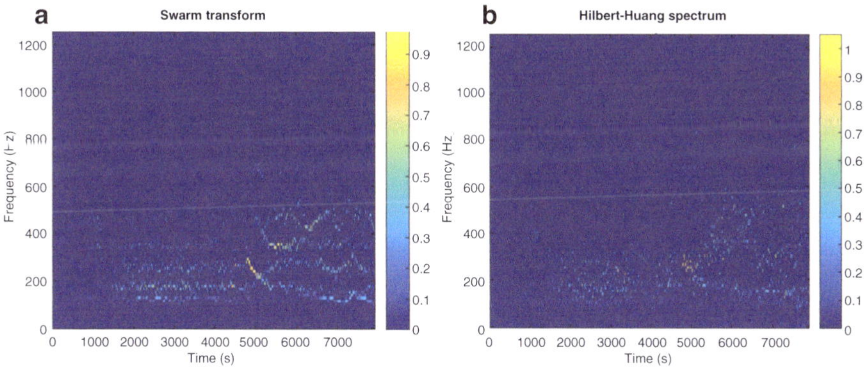

Fig. 9.7 The derived (**a**) SwT and (**b**) Hilbert–Huang spectrum, corresponding to the OMs and IMFs illustrated in Figs. 9.6a, b, respectively

displayed. The latter results in less distinct representation of the time-frequency characteristics of the wheeze, leaving unclear the interconnection of its harmonic content and the transition to different frequency bands across time, depending on the changes of the breathing airflow.

9.9.2 Deep Learning (DL)

In the analysis of LSs, the main pathway adopted for decades is the construction of a pattern-recognition or machine-learning system, based on the predesign of feature extractors that transform the raw data (LS recordings) into a suitable internal representation or feature vector, from which the learning subsystem, often a classifier, could detect or classify patterns in the input. Nevertheless, in a different course, *representation learning* (RL) could be adopted. In fact, RL is a set of methods that allows a machine to be fed with raw data and to automatically discover the representations needed for detection or classification. In the case of probabilistic models, a good representation is often one that captures the posterior distribution of the underlying explanatory factors for the observed input. A good representation is also one that is useful as input to a supervised predictor [162].

Deep learning (DL) methods are RL methods with multiple levels of representation, obtained by composing simple, but nonlinear, modules. Each of these models transforms the representation at one level (starting with the raw input) into a representation at a higher, slightly more abstract level [163]. By composing enough of such transformations, very complex functions can be learned, and the classification tasks are further enhanced, as higher layers of representation amplify aspects of the input that are important for discrimination and suppress irrelevant variations. The key aspect behind the DL is that these layers of features are not designed by human engineers, but they are learned from data using a general-purpose learning procedure [164].

Convolutional neural networks (CNNs), originated in the work of LeCun et al. [165], are often used in DL. CNNs use a special architecture which is particularly well adapted to classify images, as they try to take advantage of the spatial structure. CNNs use three basic ideas, i.e., *local receptive fields*, *shared weights*, and *pooling*. In a fully connected ANN, the inputs are considered in a vertical line of neurons. In a CNN, these inputs are organized as square of neurons connected to a layer of hidden neurons. This connection, however, is realized in small, localized regions of the input square, i.e., the *local receptive field*, for the hidden neuron. For each local receptive field, there is a different hidden neuron in the first hidden layer, and each connection learns a weight, and the hidden neuron learns an overall bias, as well, by learning to analyze its particular local receptive field. The map from the input layer to the hidden layer is referenced as a *feature map*, and the weights defining the feature map are the *shared weights*, whereas the bias defining the feature map in this way is the *shared bias*. The shared weights and bias are often said to define a *kernel* or *filter*. A big advantage of sharing weights and biases is that it greatly reduces the number of parameters involved in a convolutional network. A complete convolutional layer

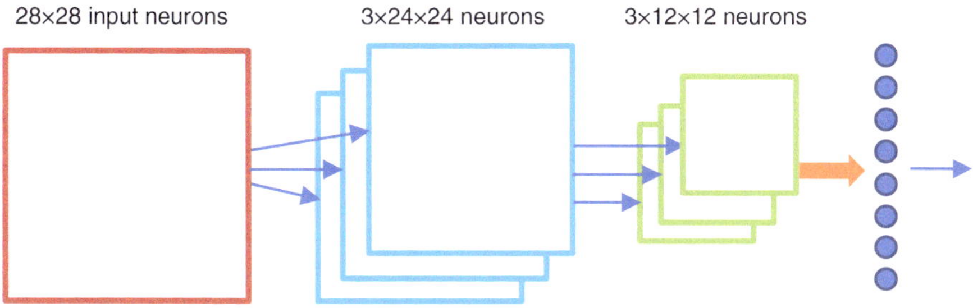

Fig. 9.8 An example of a CNN structure with 28 × 28 input neurons, 5 × 5 local receptive field and three feature maps, a max-pooling layer, applied to 2 × 2 region across each of the three feature maps, resulting in a layer of 3 × 12 × 12 hidden feature neurons that feed the fully connected layer (thick arrow) at the end of the CNN structure layer, which provides the final output from the eight possible classes

consists of several different feature maps. CNNs also contain *pooling layers*, which are usually used immediately after the convolutional layers to simplify the information in their output. A pooling layer takes each activation of the hidden neuron's output from the convolutional layer and prepares a condensed feature map. One common procedure for pooling is known as *max pooling*, where a pooling unit simply outputs the maximum activation in the small square (e.g., 2 × 2) input region. The process of max pooling is separately applied to each feature map. The intuition is that once a feature has been found, its exact location is not as important as its rough location relative to other features. In this way, there are many fewer pooled features, and the number of parameters needed in later layers is reduced. The final layer of connections in the CNN network is a *fully connected layer*, where *every* neuron from the max-pooled layer is connected to every one of the final output neurons.

An example of a CNN structure is shown in Fig. 9.8. This CNN consists of 28 × 28 input neurons, followed by a convolutional layer using a 5 × 5 local receptive field and three feature maps, resulting in a layer of 3 × 24 × 24 hidden feature neurons, followed by a max-pooling layer, applied to 2 × 2 regions, across each of the three feature maps, resulting in a layer of 3 × 12 × 12 hidden feature neurons that connect to the fully connected layer that provides the final output (eight possible classes).

The newly introduced concept of DL and CNNs reveals an emerging field for the analysis of LSs. An effort toward such direction has been proposed in the work of Chamberlain et al. [81], where they used a semi-supervised DL algorithm to automatically classify LS from 284 patients. The two classes considered were wheezes and crackles, and 11,627 sound files recorded from 11 different auscultation locations on these 284 patients with pulmonary disease were analyzed. Eight hundred and ninety of these sound files were labeled to evaluate the DL model. Each recorded sound file was converted to a spectrogram using the STFT, and the resulted STFT image was fed to the DL model. The latter was used as an *autoencoder* algorithm, which discovers the underlying structure of a dataset and maps it to a lower-dimensional representation. More specifically, they used the DL structure to create a *denoising autoencoder*, which uses randomly corrupted input data to find a lower-dimensional representation. Input data are corrupted and passed to the denoising autoencoder, which then seeks to recreate the original uncorrupted data. This random corruption helps to remove the effects of random noise from the dataset and forces the algorithm to learn better features. By using layers of denoising autoencoders, robust high-level features can be learned from a dataset. The validation results, when using a subset of ten features from the DL process to train two SVMs (one to identify wheezes and one to identify crackles), have shown ROC curves with AUCs of 0.86 for wheezes and 0.74 for crackles. Although these results do not exhibit extreme high-classification performance, they demonstrate how semi-supervised DL can be used with larger data sets without requiring extensive labeling of data (less than 5%).

Another more recent approach in the same vein has been proposed in [166, 167]. In their work the authors proposed the use of the CWT to represent the respiratory cycles as time-scale diagrams (scalograms) that depict the presence or not of wheezes and/or crackles. Subsequently, a CNN is structured for image recognition, which, after training, is capable to distinguish the scalograms from different classes. The initial CNN consists of 32×32 input neurons, a 5×5 local receptive field, and 2×2 max pooling. This structure is repeated two more times, with the second one having 64×64 input neurons, followed with a flattened layer that leads to a 64 fully connected layer. Validation results from the analysis of 2364 breathing cycles, which with a noise-driven data augmentation process resulted in 21,000 breathing cycles, have shown an 84% and 87% accuracy for the cases of crackles and wheezes, respectively. The use of the CWT-based scalograms, instead of the STFT-based images used in Chamberlain et al. [81], to feed the CNN, was motived by the fact that scalograms, unlike the STFT, could better represent the nonstationarities in the acquired LS signals, as STFT has an inherent resolution trade-off; hence, scalograms as input to the CNN more accurately represent the nature of the LSs, facilitating efficient CNN feature encoding.

Clearly, increase in the size of LS databases toward the big data concept would further enhance the efficiency of DL techniques.

9.10 Concluding Remarks and Future Trends

In this chapter, a variety of approaches in the area of LSs analysis have been presented. Despite their differences, all these approaches share a common aim: *to enhance the underlying diagnostic value of breath sounds*. The simplicity of the auscultation makes it appealing; the subjectivity in its interpretation and its noise susceptibility, though, make it challenging for the processing approaches. Apparently, the evolution of available processing capabilities is related to a series of parallel developments, such as technology growth, introduction of new theories, better understanding of the mechanisms of biological functionality, and gradual integration of the biomedical engineering research findings in clinical practice. In fact, clinical validation, real-time implementation, generalization, noise robustness, and appropriate training are some of the key issues that need to be considered for a realistic scenario of intelligent auscultation systems. Although the signal processing methods described in this book do not account for all these issues, they create a strong basis for more pragmatic exploitation of breath sounds and contribute toward the enhancement of their diagnostic value.

The emerging techniques of SwD and DL, briefly presented here, demonstrate the potentiality of how biologically inspired techniques could be used for explaining more complex structures that better reveal the connection of the pathology with the acquired signals. For instance, a combination of SwD with DL could be attempted, as the derived OMs could facilitate the transition from the raw data space to the image space with an enhanced representation of the characteristics of the signal's inherent oscillations. A first effort toward this direction with very promising results has already been attempted for the case of EEG raw data [168].

Moreover, a combination of CNNs with recurrent neural networks (RNNs) that use reinforcement learning could further enhance learning and decision-making. This is due to the nature of RNNs, in which connections between units form a directed cycle and allow them to exhibit dynamic temporal behavior and use their internal memory to process arbitrary sequences of inputs [169]. Furthermore, DL, and in a more general perspective RL, could be combined with complex reasoning, in which rule-based manipulation of symbolic expressions could be replaced by operations on large vectors [170].

From the flipped side of the coin, regulatory agencies, such as the Food and Drug Administration, as well as industry and clinicians, would be able to compare new algorithms of LSs analysis to existing ones, revealing incremental improvements and validating the performance claims. Their acceptable accuracy in clinical practice would reduce variability inherent in unassisted auscultation, contributing to avoiding unnecessary and costly referrals and diagnostic testing. This is supported by Reid Thompson's [171] view, who coins:

> Using technology, we are now poised to improve auscultation skills, set standards for proficiency and develop automated pathologic (heart) sound detection algorithms to assist the busy clinician or the underserved area without access to trained healthcare workers or advanced technology. The future of auscultation, like its past, is starting to sound glorious (p. 46).

Overall, the ample space for new discoveries and optimization is the driving force that keeps bioacoustic research alive. The latter could also be extended to a more immersive perception, in which visual and auditory information of the human body status are merged in a unified medium that fosters experiential perception of the diagnostic information. The latest advances in the *augmented* (e.g., Microsoft HoloLens) and *virtual reality* (e.g., Oculus) provide the technological means for realization of such ideas in practice, as exemplified in Fig. 9.9.

Last but not least, we should bear in mind that all breath sound analysis techniques require physicians' support and collaboration; only joint efforts could really catalyze and guarantee the success of such endeavors, truly adding to the global health.

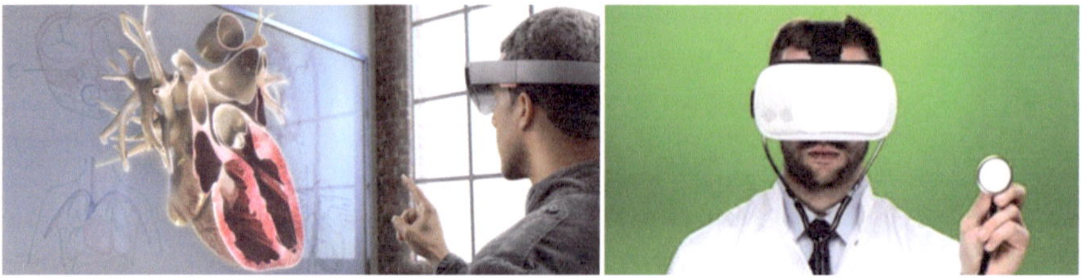

Fig. 9.9 The concept of immersive environment (HoloLens (left) (https://diendanthucteaoweb.files.wordpress.com/2016/06/medical.png?w=990) and Oculus (right) (https://www.videoblocks.com/video/doctor-wearing-virtual-reality-glasses-conducts-research-stethoscope-r8ney-xxxi-w8y136n/)) combined with the process of more experiential clinical examination

References

1. McKusick VS (1958) Cardiovascular sound in health and disease. Williams & Wilkins, Baltimore, MD
2. Rapoport J (1986) Laennec and the discovery of auscultation. Israel J Med 22:597–601
3. Foucault M (1973) The birth of the clinic: an archaeology of medical perception (A. M. Sheridan Smith, Trans.). Pantheon Books, New York, NY
4. Sterne J (2001) Mediate auscultation, the stethoscope, and the 'autopsy of the living': medicine's acoustic culture. J Med Humanities 22(2):115–136
5. Davis AB (1981) Medicine and its technology: an introduction to the history of medical instrumentation. Greenwood Press, Westport, CT, pp 88–89
6. Hadjileontiadis LJ (2009a) Lung sounds: an advanced signal processing perspective (Volume 9 of Synthesis lectures on biomedical engineering). Williston, VT: Morgan & Claypool Publishers
7. Crary J (1990) Techniques of the observer: on vision and modernity in the nineteenth century. MIT Press, Cambridge, MA, pp 89–90
8. Kraman SS (1985) Vesicular (normal) lung sounds: how are they made, where do they come from and what do they mean? Semin Respir Med 6:183–191
9. Thacker RE, Kraman SS (1982) The prevalence of auscultatory crackles in subjects without lung disease. Chest 81(6):672–674
10. Workum P, Holford SK, Delbono EA, Murphy RLH (1982) The prevalence and character of crackles (rales) in young women without significant lung disease. Am Rev Respir Dis 126(5):921–923
11. Robertson AJ (1957) Rales, rhonchi, and Laennec. Lancet 1:417–423
12. Bohadana A, Izbicki G, Kraman SS (2014) Fundamentals of lung auscultation. N Engl J Med 370(8):744–751
13. Cugell DW (1987) Lung sound nomenclature. Am Rev Respir Dis 136:1016
14. Kraman SS (1983) Lung sounds: an introduction to the interpretation of auscultatory findings (workbook). American College of Chest Physicians, Northbrook, IL
15. Murphy RLH (1985) Discontinuous adventitious lung sounds. Semin Respir Med 6:210–219
16. Sovijarvi ARA, Dalmasso F, Vanderschoot J, Malmberg LP, Righini G, Stoneman SAT (2000) Definition of terms for applications of respiratory sounds. Eur Respir Rev 10:597–610
17. Earis JE, Marsh K, Rearson MG, Ogilvie CM (1982) The inspiratory squawk in extrinsic allergic alveolitis and other pulmonary fibroses. Thorax 37(12):923–936
18. Gavriely N, Cugell DW (1995) Breath sounds methodology. CRC Press, Boca Raton, FL, p 2
19. Gavriely N, Palti Y, Alroy G (1981) Spectral characteristics of normal breath sounds. J Appl Physiol 50:307–314

20. Katila T, Piirila P, Kallio K, Paajanen E, Rosqvist T, Sovijarvi ARA (1991) Original waveform of lung sound crackles: a case study of the effect of high-pass filtration. J Appl Physiol 71(6):2173–2177
21. Murphy RLH, Holford SK, Knowler WC (1978) Visual lung-sound characterization by time-expanded wave-form analysis. N Engl J Med 296:968–971
22. Holmes MS, Seheult JN, Geraghty C, D'Arcy S, O'Brien U, O'Connell GC et al (2013) A method of estimating inspiratory flow rate and volume from an inhaler using acoustic measurements. Physiol Meas 34(8):903–914
23. Huq S, Moussavi Z (2012) Acoustic breath-phase detection using tracheal breath sounds. Med Biol Eng Comput 50(3):297–308
24. Moussavi Z, Leopando MT, Pasterkamp H, Rempel G (2000) Computerized acoustical respiratory phase detection without airflow measurement. Med Biol Eng Comput 38(2):198–203
25. Nam Y, Reyes BA, Chon KH (2016) Estimation of respiratory rates using the built-in microphone of a smartphone or headset. IEEE J Biomed Health Informatics 20(6):1493–1501
26. Palaniappan R, Sundaraj K, Sundaraj S (2017) Adaptive neuro-fuzzy inference system for breath phase detection and breath cycle segmentation. Comput Methods Prog Biomed 145:67–72
27. Yadollahi A, Moussavi Z (2006) A robust method for estimating respiratory flow using tracheal sound entropy. IEEE Trans Biomed Eng 53(4):662–668
28. Yadollahi A, Moussavi ZM (2007) Acoustical respiratory flow. IEEE Eng Med Biol Mag 26(1):56–61
29. Yadollahi A, Montazeri A, Azarbarzin A, Moussavi Z (2013) Respiratory flow–sound relationship during both wakefulness and sleep and its variation in relation to sleep apnea. Ann Biomed Eng 41(3):537–546
30. Ahlstrom C, Liljefeldt O, Hult P, Ask P (2005) Heart sound cancellation from lung sound recordings using recurrence time statistics and nonlinear prediction. IEEE Signal Process Lett 12(12):812–815
31. Falk TH, Chan WY (2008) Modulation filtering for heart and lung sound separation from breath sound recordings. In: 30th Annual international conference of the IEEE engineering in medicine and biology society, EMBS 2008, pp 1859–1862
32. Floras D, Moussavi Z, Thomas G (2007) Heart sound cancellation based on multiscale product and linear prediction. IEEE Trans Biomed Eng 54(2):234–243
33. Ghaderi F, Mohseni HR, Sanei S (2011) Localizing heart sounds in respiratory signals using singular spectrum analysis. IEEE Trans Biomed Eng 58(12):3360–3367
34. Gnitecki J, Hossain I, Moussavi Z, Pasterkamp H (2005a) Qualitative and quantitative evaluation of heart sound reduction from lung sound recordings. IEEE Trans Biomed Eng 52(10):1788–1792
35. Hadjileontiadis LJ, Panas SM (1997c) Adaptive reduction of heart sounds from lung sounds using fourth-order statistics. IEEE Trans Biomed Eng 44(7):642–648
36. Hadjileontiadis LJ, Panas SM (1998a) A wavelet-based reduction of heart sound noise from lung sounds. Int J Med Inform 52:183–190
37. Hossain I, Moussavi Z (2003) An overview of heart-noise reduction of lung sound using wavelet transform based filter. In: Proc. 25th IEEE Eng. Med. Biol. Soc. (EMBS), pp 458–461
38. Iyer VK, Ramamoorthy PA, Fan H, Ploysongsang Y (1986) Reduction of heart sounds from lung sounds by adaptive filtering. IEEE Trans Biomed Eng 33(12):1141–1148
39. Li T, Tang H, Qiu T, Park Y (2013) Heart sound cancellation from lung sound record using cyclostationarity. Med Eng Phys 35(12):1831–1836
40. Mondal A, Banerjee P, Somkuwar A (2017) Enhancement of lung sounds based on empirical mode decomposition and Fourier transform algorithm. Comput Methods Prog Biomed 139:119–136
41. Nersisson R, Noel MM (2017) Heart sound and lung sound separation algorithms: a review. J Med Eng Technol 41(1):13–21

42. Pourazad MT, Moussavi Z, Thomas G (2006) Heart sound cancellation from lung sound recording using time-frequency filtering. J Med Biol Eng 44(3):216–225
43. Sathesh K, Muniraj NJR (2014) Real time heart and lung sound separation using adaptive line enhancer with NLMS. J Theor Appl Inf Technol 65(2):559–564
44. Tsalaile T, Naqvi SM, Nazarpour K, Sanei S, Chambers JA (2008) Blind source extraction of heart sound signals from lung sound recordings exploiting periodicity of the heart sound. In: IEEE international conference on acoustics, speech and signal processing, ICASSP, pp 461–464
45. Zivanovic M, González-Izal M (2013) Quasi-periodic modeling for heart sound localization and suppression in lung sounds. Biomed Signal Process Control 8(6):586–595
46. Emmanouilidou D, McCollum ED, Park DE, Elhilali M (2017) Computerized lung sound screening for pediatric auscultation in noisy field environments. IEEE Trans Biomed Eng. https://doi.org/10.1109/TBME.2017.2717280
47. Grønnesby M, Solis JCA, Holsbø E, Melbye H, Bongo LA (2017) Machine learning based crackle detection in lung sounds. arXiv preprint arXiv:1706.00005
48. Hadjileontiadis LJ, Panas SM (1996) Nonlinear separation of crackles and squawks from vesicular sounds using third-order statistics. In: Proc. IEEE 18th EMBS Conf. (EMBS), vol 5, pp 2217–2219
49. Hadjileontiadis LJ, Panas SM (1997d) Separation of discontinuous adventitious sounds from vesicular sounds using a wavelet-based filter. IEEE Trans Biomed Eng 44(12):1269–1281
50. Hadjileontiadis LJ, Patakas DA, Margaris NJ, Panas SM (1998) Separation of crackles and squawks from vesicular sounds using a wavelet-based filtering technique. COMPEL 17(5/6):649–657
51. Hadjileontiadis LJ, Panas SM (1998c) Enhanced separation of crackles and squawks from vesicular sounds using nonlinear filtering with third-order statistics. J Tennessee Acad Sci 73(1–2):47–52
52. Hadjileontiadis LJ, Tolias YA, Panas SM (2002) Intelligent system modeling of bioacoustic signals using advanced signal processing techniques. In: Leondes CT (ed) Intelligent systems: technology and applications, vol 3. CRC Press, Boca Raton, FL, pp 103–156
53. Hadjileontiadis LJ, Rekanos IT (2003) Detection of explosive lung and bowel sounds by means of fractal dimension. IEEE Signal Process Lett 10(10):311–314
54. Hadjileontiadis LJ (2005a) Wavelet-based enhancement of lung and bowel sounds using fractal dimension thresholding-Part I: Methodology. IEEE Trans Biomed Eng 52(6):1143–1148
55. Hadjileontiadis LJ (2005b) Wavelet-based enhancement of lung and bowel sounds using fractal dimension thresholding—Part II: Application results. IEEE Trans Biomed Eng 52(6):1050–1064
56. Hadjileontiadis LJ (2007) Empirical mode decomposition and fractal dimension filter: a novel technique for denoising explosive lung sounds. IEEE Eng Med Biol Mag 26(1):30–39
57. Jin F, Krishnan S, Sattar F (2011) Adventitious sounds identification and extraction using temporal–spectral dominance-based features. IEEE Trans Biomed Eng 58(11):3078–3087
58. Li Z, Wu X (2013) Pulmonary crackle detection based on fractional Hilbert Transform. In: World Congress on medical physics and biomedical engineering, May 26–31, 2012, Beijing, China, pp 578–580
59. Lu X, Bahoura M (2008) An integrated automated system for crackles extraction and classification. Biomed Signal Process Control 3(3):244–254
60. Maruf SO, Azhar MU, Khawaja SG, Akram MU (2015) Crackle separation and classification from normal Respiratory sounds using Gaussian Mixture Model. In: IEEE 10th international conference on industrial and information systems (ICIIS), pp 267–271
61. Mastorocostas PM, Tolias YA, Theocharis JB, Hadjileontiadis LJ, Panas SM (1997) An orthogonal least squares-based fuzzy filter for real time analysis of lung sounds. IEEE Trans Biomed Eng 47(9):1165–1176
62. Ono M, Arakawa K, Mori M, Sugimoto T, Harashima H (1989) Separation of fine crackles from vesicular sounds by a nonlinear digital filter. IEEE Trans Biomed Eng 36(2):286–291

63. Pinho C, Oliveira A, Jácome C, Rodrigues JM, Marques A (2016) Integrated approach for automatic crackle detection based on fractal dimension and box filtering. Int J Reliable Qual E-Healthcare 5(4):34–50
64. Rekanos IT, Hadjileontiadis LJ (2006) An iterative kurtosis-based technique for the detection of nonstationary bioacoustic signals. Signal Process 86:3787–3795
65. Serbes G, Sakar CO, Kahya YP, Aydin N (2013) Pulmonary crackle detection using time–frequency and time–scale analysis. Digital Signal Process 23(3):1012–1021
66. Tolias YA, Hadjileontiadis LJ, Panas SM (1997) A fuzzy rule-based system for real-time separation of crackles from vesicular sounds. In: Proc. 19th IEEE Eng. Med. Biol. Soc. (EMBS), pp 1115–1118
67. Tolias YA, Hadjileontiadis LJ, Panas SM (1998) Real-time separation of discontinuous adventitious sounds from vesicular sounds using a fuzzy rule-based filter. IEEE Trans Inf Technol Biomed 2(3):204–215
68. Zhang K, Wang X, Han F, Zhao H (2015) The detection of crackles based on mathematical morphology in spectrogram analysis. Technol Health Care 23(s2):S489–S494
69. Ahlstrom C, Johansson A, Hult P, Ask P (2006) Chaotic dynamics of respiratory sounds. J Chaos Soliton Fractals 29:1054–1069
70. Charleston-Villalobos S, Albuerne-Sanchez L, Gonzalez-Camarena R, Mejia-Avila M, Carrillo-Rodriguez G, Aljama-Corrales T (2013) Linear and nonlinear analysis of base lung sound in extrinsic allergic alveolitis patients in comparison to healthy subjects. Methods Inf Med 52(3):266–276
71. Conte E, Vena A, Federici A, Giuliani R, Zbilut JP (2004) A brief note on possible detection of physiological singularities in respiratory dynamics by recurrence quantification analysis of lung sounds. J Chaos Soliton Fractals 21:869–877
72. Gnitecki J, Moussavi Z, Pasterkamp H (2004) Classification of lung sounds during bronchial provocation using waveform fractal dimensions. In: Proc. 26th IEEE Eng. Med. Biol. Soc. (EMBS), pp 3844–3847
73. Gnitecki J, Moussavi Z (2005) The fractality of lung sounds: a comparison of three waveform fractal dimension algorithms. J. Chaos Soliton Fractals 26(4):1065–1072
74. Gnitecki J, Moussavi Z, Pasterkamp H (2005b) Geometrical and dynamical state space parameters of lung sounds. In 5th international workshop on biosignal interpretation (BSI), pp 113–116
75. Hadjileontiadis LJ, Panas SM (1997a) Autoregressive modeling of lung sounds using higher-order statistics: estimation of source and transmission. In: Proc. IEEE signal processing workshop on higher-order statistics (SPW-HOS), pp 4–8
76. Hadjileontiadis LJ, Panas SM (1997b) Nonlinear analysis of musical lung sounds using the bicoherence index. In: Proc. 19th IEEE Eng. Med. Biol. Soc. (EMBS), pp 1126–1129
77. Reyes BA, Charleston-Villalobos S, Gonzalez-Camarena R, Aljama-Corrales T (2008) Analysis of discontinuous adventitious lung sounds by Hilbert-Huang spectrum. In 30th Annual international conference of the IEEE, Engineering in Medicine and Biology Society, 2008, EMBS 2008, pp 3620–3623
78. Taplidou SA, Hadjileontiadis LJ (2007) Nonlinear analysis of wheezes using wavelet bicoherence. Comput Biol Med 37(4):563–570
79. Taplidou SA, Hadjileontiadis LJ (2010) Analysis of wheezes using wavelet higher order spectral features. IEEE Trans Biomed Eng 57(7):1596–1610
80. Bahoura M (2009) Pattern recognition methods applied to respiratory sounds classification into normal and wheeze classes. Comput Biol Med 39(9):824–843
81. Chamberlain D, Kodgule R, Ganelin D, Miglani V, Fletcher RR (2016) Application of semi-supervised deep learning to lung sound analysis. In: IEEE 38th annual international conference of the engineering in medicine and biology society (EMBC), pp 804–807)
82. Charleston-Villalobos S, Martinez-Hernandez G, Gonzalez-Camarena R, Chi-Lem G, Carrillo JG, Aljama-Corrales T (2011) Assessment of multichannel lung sounds parameterization for two-class classification in interstitial lung disease patients. Comput Biol Med 41(7):473–482

83. Cohen A (1990) Signal processing methods for upper airway and pulmonary dysfunction diagnosis. IEEE Eng Med Biol Mag 9(1):72–75
84. Dokur Z (2009) Respiratory sound classification by using an incremental supervised neural network. Pattern Anal Applic 12(4):309–319
85. Göğüş FZ, Karlik B, Harman G (2015) Classification of asthmatic breath sounds by using wavelet transforms and neural networks. Int J Signal Process Syst 3:106–111
86. Hadjileontiadis LJ, Panas SM (1998b) On modeling impulsive bioacoustic signals with symmetric alpha-stable distributions: application in discontinuous adventitious lung sounds and explosive bowel sounds. In: Proc. 20th IEEE Eng. Med. Biol. Soc. (EMBS), vol 1, pp 13–16
87. Hadjileontiadis LJ (2003) Discrimination analysis of discontinuous breath sounds using higher-order crossings. Med Biol Eng Comput 41(4):445–455
88. Hadjileontiadis LJ (2009b) A texture-based classification of crackles and squawks using lacunarity. IEEE Trans Biomed Eng 56(3):718–732
89. Hoevers J, Loudon RG (1990) Measuring crackles. Chest 98(5):1240–1243
90. İçer S, Gengeç Ş (2014) Classification and analysis of non-stationary characteristics of crackle and rhonchus lung adventitious sounds. Digital Signal Process 28:18–27
91. Jin F, Sattar F, Goh DY (2014) New approaches for spectro-temporal feature extraction with applications to respiratory sound classification. Neurocomputing 123:362–371
92. Kahya YP, Yilmaz CA (2000) Modeling of respiratory crackles. In: Proc. 22nd IEEE Eng. Med. Biol. Soc. (EMBS), vol 1, pp 632–634
93. Kahya YP, Yeginer M, Bilgic B (2006) Classifying respiratory sounds with different feature sets. In: EMBS'06. 28th Annual international conference of the IEEE, Engineering in Medicine and Biology Society, 2006, pp 2856–2859
94. Kandaswamy A, Kumarb CS, Ramanathan RP, Jayaraman S, Malmurugan N (2004) Neural classification of lung sounds using wavelet coefficients. Comp Biol Med 34:523–537
95. Matsunaga S, Yamauchi K, Yamashita M, Miyahara S (2009). Classification between normal and abnormal respiratory sounds based on maximum likelihood approach. In: IEEE international conference on acoustics, speech and signal processing (ICASSP 2009), pp 517–520
96. Munakata M, Ukita H, Doi I, Ohtsuka Y, Masaki Y, Homma Y, Kawakami Y (1991) Spectral and waveform characteristics of fine and coarse crackles. Thorax 46(9):651–657
97. Naves R, Barbosa BH, Ferreira DD (2016) Classification of lung sounds using higher-order statistics: a divide-and-conquer approach. Comput Methods Prog Biomed 129:12–20
98. Oweis RJ, Abdulhay EW, Khayal A, Awad A (2015) An alternative respiratory sounds classification system utilizing artificial neural networks. Biomed J 38:153–161
99. Palaniappan R, Sundaraj K, Sundaraj S, Huliraj N, Revadi SS, Archana B (2014) Pulmonary acoustic signal classification using autoregressive coefficients and k-nearest neighbor. Appl Mech Mater 591:211–214
100. Pesu L, Helistö P, Ademovic E, Pesquet JC, Saarinen A, Sovijarvi AR (1998) Classification of respiratory sounds based on wavelet packet decomposition and learning vector quantization. Technol Health Care 6(1):65–74
101. Sankur B, Kahya YR, Güler EC, Engin TS (1994) Comparison of AR-based algorithms for respiratory sounds classification respiratory disease diagnosis using lung sounds. Comput Biol Med 24(1):67–76
102. Sosa GD, Cruz-Roa A, González FA (2015) Automatic detection of wheezes by evaluation of multiple acoustic feature extraction methods and C-weighted SVM. In: 10th International symposium on medical information processing and analysis, International Society for Optics and Photonics, pp 928709–928709
103. Taketoshi O, Hayaru S, Shoji K (2006) Discrimination of lung sounds using a statistics of waveform intervals. IPSJ SIG Technical Reports, 2006(68(MPS-60)), pp 1–4
104. Ulukaya S, Serbes G, Sen I, Kahya YP (2016) A lung sound classification system based on the rational dilation wavelet transform. In: IEEE 38th annual international conference of the engineering in medicine and biology society (EMBC), pp 3745–3748

105. Xie S, Jin F, Krishnan S, Sattar F (2012) Signal feature extraction by multi-scale PCA and its application to respiratory sound classification. Med Biol Eng Comput 50(7):759–768
106. Yilmaz CA, Kahya YP (2005) Modeling of pulmonary crackles using wavelet networks. In: Proc. 27th IEEE Eng. Med. Biol. Soc. (EMBS), pp 7560–7563
107. Yilmaz CA, Kahya YP (2006) Multi-channel classification of respiratory sounds. In: Proc. 28th IEEE Eng. Med. Biol. Soc. (EMBS), vol 1, pp 2864–2867
108. Murphy RLH, Holford SK, Knowler WC (1977) Visual lung sound characterization by time-expanded waveform analysis. New Eng J Med 296:968–971
109. Palaniappan R, Sundaraj K, Ahamed NU (2013) Machine learning in lung sound analysis: a systematic review. Biocybernetics Biomed Eng 33(3):129–135
110. Mendel JM (1991) Tutorial on higher-order statistics (spectra) in signal processing and system theory: theoretical results and some applications. Proc IEEE 79(3):278–305
111. Nikias CL, Petropulu AP (1993) Higher-order spectra analysis: a nonlinear signal processing framework. Prentice-Hall, Englewood Cliffs, NJ
112. Huber PJ, Kleiner B, Gasser T, Dumermuth G (1971) Statistical methods for investigating phase relations in stationary stochastic processes. IEEE Trans Audio Electracoust 19:78–86
113. Iyer VK, Ramamoorthy PA, Ploysongsang Y (1989) Autoregressive modeling of lung sounds: characterization of source and transmission. IEEE Trans Biomed Eng 36(11):1133–1137
114. Raghuveer MR, Nikias CL (1985) Bispectrum estimation: a parametric approach. IEEE Trans Acoustics Speech Signal Process 33(4):1213–1230
115. Nikias CL, Raghuveer MR (1987) Bispectrum estimation: a digital signal processing framework. Proc IEEE 75(7):869–891
116. Gavriely N, Palti Y, and Alroy, G "Spectral characteristics of normal breath sounds," J. Appl. Physiol., Vol.50, pp. 307–314, 1981
117. Hadjileontiadis LJ (1997) Analysis and processing of lung sounds using higher-order statistics-spectra and wavelet transform. PhD dissertation, Aristotle University of Thessaloniki, Thessaloniki, Greece, pp 139–175
118. Li S, Liu Y (2010) Feature extraction of lung sounds based on bispectrum analysis. In: Third international symposium on information processing (ISIP), pp 393–397
119. Grossmann A, Morlet J (1984) Decomposition of Hardy functions into square integrable wavelets of constant shape. SIAM J Math Anal 15:723–736
120. Addison PS (2017) The illustrated wavelet transform handbook: introductory theory and applications in science, engineering, medicine and finance. CRC press, Cleveland, OH
121. Astafieva NM (1996) Wavelet analysis: basic theory and some applications. Physics-Uspekhi 39(11):1085–1108
122. Mallat SG (1989) A theory for multiresolution signal decomposition: the wavelet representation. IEEE Trans Pattern Anal Machine Intell 11(7):674–693
123. Daubechies I (1988) Orthonormal bases of compactly supported wavelets. Commun Pure Appl Math 41:909–996
124. Daubechies I (1991) Ten lectures on wavelets, CBMS lecture notes series. SIAM, Philadelphia, PA
125. Mallat SG (1996) Special issue on wavelets. Proc IEEE 84(4):507–686
126. Mallat SG (1998) A wavelet tour of signal processing. Academic, San Diego
127. Vetterli M, Kovačević J (1995) Wavelets and subband coding, ch. 4. Prentice-Hall, Englewood Cliffs, NJ, pp 201–298
128. Gross V, Penzel T, Hadjileontiadis LJ, Koehler U, Vogelmeier C (2002) Electronic auscultation based on wavelet transformation in clinical use. In: Proc. 24th IEEE Eng. Med. Biol. Soc. (EMBS), pp 1531–1532)
129. Gross V, Penzel T, Fachinger P, Fröhlich M, Sulzer J, von Wichert P (1999) A simple method for detecting pneumonia with using wavelet-transformation. In: Proc. Med. and Biol. Eng. and Comp. (EMBEC), vol 37, Suppl 2, pp 536–537
130. Ayari F, Alouani AT, Ksouri M (2008) Wavelets: an efficient tool for lung sounds analysis. Proc. IEEE computer systems and applications (AICCSA):875–878

131. Ke L, Houjun W (2007) A novel wavelet transform modulus maxima based method of measuring Lipschitz exponent. In: Proc. International conference communications, circuits and systems (ICCCAS), pp 628–632
132. Mallat SG, Hwang WL (1992) Singularity detection and processing with wavelets. IEEE Trans Inf Theory 38(2):617–643
133. Riedmiller M, Braun H (1993) A direct adaptive method for faster backpropagation learning: the RPROP algorithm. In: Ruspini H (ed) Proc. IEEE international conference on neural networks (ICNN), pp 586–591
134. Bayram I, Selesnick IW (2009) Frequency-domain design of overcomplete rational-dilation wavelet transforms. IEEE Trans Signal Process 57(8):2957–2972
135. Birkelund Y, Hanssen A (1999) Multitaper estimators for bispectra. In: Proc. IEEE SP workshop on higher-order (SPW-HOS), pp 207–213
136. Dudok de Wit T, Krasnosel'Skikh VV (1995) Wavelet bicoherence analysis of strong plasma turbulence at the earth's quasiparallel bow shock. Phys Plasmas 2(11):4307–4311
137. Larsen Y, Hanssen A (2000) Wavelet-polyspectra: analysis of non-stationary and non-Gaussian/non-linear signals. In: Proc. IEEE workshop on statistical signal and array processing (WSSAP), pp 539–543
138. van Milligen BP, Sánchez E, Estrada T, Hidalgo C, Brañas B, Carreras B, Garcia L (1995a) Wavelet bicoherence: a new turbulence analysis tool. Phys Plasmas 2(8):3017–3032
139. van Milligen BP, Hidalgo C, Sánchez E (1995b) Nonlinear phenomena and intermittency in plasma turbulence. Phys Rev Lett 74(3):395–398
140. Duke JR Jr, Good JT Jr, Hudson LD, Hyers TM, Iseman MD, Mergenthaler DD, Murray JF, Petty TL, Rollins DR (2000) Frontline assessment of common pulmonary presentations. In: Murray JF, Hudson LD, Petty TL (eds) A monograph for primary care physicians. Snowdrift Pulmonary Conference, Inc, Denver, CO. http://www.lungcancerfrontiers.org/pdf-books/asmnt_cmn_pulmryPrsntn.pdf
141. Huang NE, Shen Z, Long SR, Wu ML, Shih HH, Zheng Q, Yen NC, Tung CC, Liu HH (1998) The empirical mode decomposition and Hilbert spectrum for nonlinear and nonstationary time series analysis. Proc R Soc Lond A 454(1971):903–995
142. Gloersen P, Huang NE (2003) Comparison of interannual intrinsic modes in hemispheric sea ice covers and other geophysical parameters. IEEE Trans GeosciRemote Sens 41(5):1062–1074
143. Wu Z, Huang NE (2004) A study of the characteristics of white noise using the empirical mode decomposition method. Proc Roy Soc London 460A:1597–1611
144. Wu Z, Huang NE (2009) Ensemble empirical mode decomposition: a noise-assisted data analysis method. Adv Adapt Data Anal 1(01):1–41
145. Yeh JR, Lin TY, Shieh JS, Chen Y, Huang NE, Wu Z, Peng CK (2008) Investigating complex patterns of blocked intestinal artery blood pressure signals by empirical mode decomposition and linguistic analysis. J Phys Conf Ser 96:1–7. https://doi.org/10.1088/1742-6596/96/1/012153
146. Villalobos SC, Camarena RG, Lem GC, Corrales TA (2007) Crackle sounds analysis by empirical mode decomposition: nonlinear and nonstationary signal analysis for distinction of crackles in lung sounds. IEEE Eng Med Biol Mag 26(15):40–47
147. Lozano M, Fiz JA, Jané R (2016) Automatic differentiation of normal and continuous adventitious respiratory sounds using ensemble empirical mode decomposition and instantaneous frequency. IEEE J Biomed Health Informatics 20(2):486–497
148. Nikias CL, Shao M (1995) Signal Processing with Alpha-Stable Distributions and Applications. Wiley & Sons, Inc., USA, New York
149. Hadjileontiadis LJ, Giannakidis AJ, Panas SM (2000) a-Stable modeling: a novel tool for classifying crackles and artifacts. In: Pasterkamp H (ed) Proc. 25th international lung sounds association conference (ILSA), Chicago, IL
150. Kedem B (1994) Time series analysis by higher-order crossings. IEEE Press, Piscataway, NJ
151. Rasband SN (1997) Fractal dimension, Ch. 4. In: Chaotic dynamics of nonlinear systems. Wiley-Interscience, New York, pp 71–83

152. Esteller R, Vachtsevanos G, Echauz J, Henry T, Pennell P, Epstein C, Bakay R, Bowen C, Litt B (1999). Fractal dimension characterizes seizure onset in epileptic patients. In: Proc. IEEE international conference on acoustics, speech & signal processing (ICASPP), 1999, vol 4, Phoenix, AZ, pp 2343–2346
153. Kinsner W (1994) Batch and real-time computation of a fractal dimension based on variance of a time series. Technical Report, DEL94-6, Dept. of Electrical & Computer Eng., University of Manitoba
154. Laennec RTH (1830) A treatise on the diseases of the chest and on mediate auscultation (J. Forbes, Trans.), 3rd edn. Samuel Wood and Sons, and Collins and Hannay, New York
155. Allain C, Cloitre M (1991) Characterizing the lacunarity of random and deterministic fractal sets. Phys Rev A 44(6):3552–3558
156. Gefen Y, Meir Y, Mandelbrot BB, Aharony A (1983) Geometric implementation of Hypercubic lattices with non-integer dimensionality by use of low lacunarity fractal lattices. Phys Rev Lett 50(3):145–148
157. Lin B, Yang ZR (1986) A suggested lacunarity expression for Sierpinski carpets. J Phys A 19(2):L49–L52
158. Mandelbrot BB (1983) The fractal geometry of nature. Freeman, New York
159. Plotnick RE, Gardner RH, Hargrove WW, Prestegaard K, Perlmutter M (1996) Lacunarity analysis: a general technique for the analysis of spatial patterns. Phys Rev E 53(5):5461–5468
160. Du G, Yeo TS (2002) A novel lacunarity estimation method applied to SAR image segmentation. IEEE Trans Geosci Remote Sens 40(12):2687–2691
161. Apostolidis GK, Hadjileontiadis LJ (2017) Swarm decomposition: a novel signal analysis using swarm intelligence. Signal Process 132:40–50
162. Bengio Y, Courville A, Vincent P (2013) Representation learning: a review and new perspectives. IEEE Trans Pattern Anal Mach Intell 35(8):1798–1828
163. Hinton GE, Osindero S, Teh YW (2006) A fast learning algorithm for deep belief nets. Neural Comput 18(7):1527–1554
164. LeCun Y, Bengio Y, Hinton G (2015) Deep learning. Nature 521(7553):436–444
165. LeCun Y, Bottou L, Bengio Y, Haffner P (1998) Gradient-based learning applied to document recognition. Proc IEEE 86(11):2278–2324
166. Mavrodis K (2017) Identification of crackles and wheezes in recordings of respiratory cycles, utilizing advanced signal processing techniques, machine learning and convolutional neural networks. Diploma Thesis, Dept. of Electrical & Computer Engineering, Aristotle University of Thessaloniki, July 2017, Thessaloniki, Greece
167. Mavrodis K, Hadjileontiadis LJ (2017) Detection of wheezes and crackles using deep learning. IEEE Trans Biomed Eng [in process]
168. Baltatzis V, Bintsi K-M, Apostolidis GK, Hadjileontiadis LJ (2017) Bullying incidences identification within an immersive environment using HD EEG-based analysis: a swarm decomposition and deep learning approach. Nature Sci Rep. https://doi.org/10.1038/s41598-017-17562-0
169. Schmidhuber J (2015) Deep learning in neural networks: an overview. Neural Netw 61:85–117
170. Bottou L (2014) From machine learning to machine reasoning. Mach Learn 94:133–149
171. Thompson WR (2017) In defence of auscultation: a glorious future? Heart Asia 9:44–47

Part III

Respiratory Sounds

10 Normal Versus Adventitious Respiratory Sounds

Alda Marques and Ana Oliveira

10.1 Normal Respiratory Sounds

Normal respiratory sounds are nonmusical sounds produced from breathing and heard over the trachea (i.e., normal tracheal sounds) and chest wall (i.e., normal lung sounds) [1].

Normal tracheal sounds can be heard at the suprasternal notch and are generated by turbulent airflow in upper airways, including pharynx, glottis, and subglottic regions [2]. These sounds are strong, easy to hear, and with distinguish respiratory phases, as the distance from the sound source to the sensor is short and there is no lung filter [2]. Acoustically, normal tracheal sounds cover a wide range of frequencies, from less than 100 Hz to 5000 Hz with a sharp drop in power at frequencies above 800 Hz and little energy beyond 1500 Hz [3]. Expiratory tracheal spectra has higher mean frequencies than the inspiratory spectra, and increases in tracheal sound mean frequencies are closely related to increases in airflow until flows of 0.75 L/s [4]. Measurements of tracheal sounds are not frequently performed but may provide valuable clinical respiratory information in particular cases, such as in upper airway flow obstruction (e.g., to monitor apnea in adults [5–8] and children [9, 10]), or in the presence of lung consolidation, as tracheal sounds are similar to the abnormal bronchial breathing in these patients.

The sounds heard over the chest wall, normal lung sounds, are generally only heard during inspiration and early part of expiration [11]. It is believed that normal lung sounds at frequencies above 300 Hz are generated by turbulent airflow

A. Marques (✉) · A. Oliveira
Lab 3R—Respiratory Research and Rehabilitation Laboratory, School of Health Sciences, University of Aveiro (ESSUA), Aveiro, Portugal

Institute for Research in Biomedicine (iBiMED), University of Aveiro, Aveiro, Portugal
e-mail: amarques@ua.pt; alao@ua.pt

K. N. Priftis et al. (eds.), *Breath Sounds*, https://doi.org/10.1007/978-3-319-71824-8_10

vortices; however the generation of sounds heard below 300 Hz is not clear [12]. It seems well established that the sound heard during inspiration is produced primarily within the lobar and segmental airways, whereas the sound produced during expiration seems to be originated in more proximal airways [13–15]. Normal lung sounds have a median frequency (F50) around 500 Hz (131–552.5 Hz), their intensity peaks at about 100—200 Hz [11, 16] and there is an energy drop above 300 Hz [12]. Therefore, normal lung sounds may be difficult to hear, as their sound frequencies are mixed with muscle and cardiovascular sounds [2]. Nevertheless, much higher respiratory sound frequencies, above 1 kHz [17], can be heard if an adequate microphone is used.

Characteristics of normal respiratory sounds change from individual to individual because airway dimensions are a function of body height [18]. But there are other factors, such as gender, chest location where it is heard, body position, and airflow, that affect normal respiratory sounds [11], being particularly different between children and adults [17] and in the presence of a respiratory condition. Normal lung sounds heard over the chest wall of a newborn, infant, or children present louder inspiratory and expiratory sound and higher median frequencies than those found in adults [17]. This sound pattern corresponds to normal bronchial breathing and is generally attributed to acoustic transmission through smaller lungs, thinner chest walls, and less contribution of low-frequency muscle noise [2].

In the presence of a respiratory condition, normal lung sounds may be classified as "abnormal" if heard at inappropriate locations. Bronchial breathing involves a prolonged and loud expiratory phase with frequency components up to 600–1000 Hz [19], and it is abnormal if heard at the lung periphery of an adult. This would be typically heard in the presence of lung consolidation, as there is an increase in the transmission of higher frequencies from central airway to the chest wall and absorption of low frequencies due to the reduction of filtering effect.

We will now describe in detail normal tracheal and lung sounds in healthy people and in people with a respiratory condition. A summary of normal respiratory sounds, from their mechanisms to clinical interpretation, is presented in Table 10.4.

10.1.1 Normal Tracheal Sound

Normal tracheal sound has been reported as having higher frequency and intensity than normal lung sounds.

10.1.1.1 Frequency

In Healthy People

The highest normal respiratory sound frequencies have been reported at the trachea, where inspiratory values of 447 to 766 Hz at F50 [20, 21] and of 1323 ± 192 Hz at 75% of the total spectral power (F75) have been described [20]. Expiratory sounds have been found to be slightly lower, i.e., 540 ± 174 Hz at F50 [21]. Values of frequency at maximum power (Fmax) at the trachea between 93 and 154 Hz during inspiration and 99 ± 8 Hz during expiration have been found [20, 21]. A synthesis of normal respiratory sound features in healthy people can be found in Table 10.1.

In the Presence of a Respiratory Condition

Slightly higher frequency values of normal tracheal sound have been found when a respiratory condition is present compared to people without respiratory conditions. For F50, inspiratory frequencies of 753 ± 177 Hz in chronic obstructive pulmonary disease (COPD) [20] and 507 ± 153 Hz in asthma [21] and expiratory frequencies of 546 ± 117 Hz in asthma [21] have been reported. For F75, inspiratory frequencies of 1239 ± 186 Hz in patients with COPD [20] have also been reported. In COPD, inspiratory sound power tends to peak at 228 ± 340 Hz [20] and at 106 ± 47 Hz in asthma [21], while expiratory sound peaks at about 92 ± 7 Hz in asthma.

A decrease in the centroid frequency (defined as frequency that includes half of the total power of the spectrum) of the tracheal sound, from 273 to 552 Hz, has been observed in patients with asthma [34] after a bronchodilator administration. A synthesis of normal respiratory sound features in people with respiratory conditions can be found in Table 10.1.

10.1.1.2 Intensity

In Healthy People

Studies on intensity of normal tracheal sounds have focused on healthy people. Intensity values between 34.6 and 83.1 dB during inspiration [12, 20, 22] and between 45.4 and 85.1 dB during expiration [12, 22] have been found. Some studies have also measured respiratory sound intensity in amplitude, and values of 67 ± 24 mV have been reported for people without respiratory conditions [21]. A synthesis of normal respiratory sound features in healthy people can be found in Table 10.1.

In the Presence of a Respiratory Condition

Tracheal sound intensity has not been commonly used as an indicator of pathology in respiratory conditions. No differences in inspiratory tracheal sound intensity/amplitude have been reported among patients with stable asthma (84.7 ± 3.7 dB; 56 ± 44 mV), stable COPD (82.6 ± 3.1 dB), and people without respiratory conditions (83.1 ± 3.7 dB; 67 ± 24 mV) [20, 21]. Similarly, no significant differences in expiratory tracheal sound amplitude have been found between patients with stable asthma (64 ± 42 mV) and people without respiratory conditions (117 ± 103 mV) [21].

During histamine challenges, higher inspiratory and lower expiratory sound amplitude has been reported in patients with asthma (inspiration, 97 ± 31 mV;

expiration, 94 ± 26 mV) compared to people without respiratory conditions (inspiration, 68 ± 34 mV; expiration, 124 ± 113 mV) [21]. However, after the administration of bronchodilators in both groups, sound amplitude is significantly lower in both respiratory phases in patients with asthma (inspiration, 58 ± 36 mV; expiration, 61 ± 17 mV) than in people without respiratory conditions (inspiration, 77 ± 23 mV; expiration, 118 ± 95 mV) [21]. Changes in the asthmatic tracheal sound group may be due to changes in airway diameter caused by bronchoconstriction after histamine and bronchodilator administration. A synthesis of normal respiratory sound features in people with respiratory conditions can be found in Table 10.1.

10.1.2 Normal Lung Sounds

Normal lung sounds present higher inspiratory frequency and intensity values than expiratory sounds. Most studies have been focusing on analyzing lung sound frequencies in healthy people and in people with respiratory conditions.

10.1.2.1 Frequency

In Healthy People

Frequency of normal respiratory sounds in healthy people has been revised as shown in Oliveira and Marques [11]. It has been reported that lung sound frequencies are higher in women than in men at Fmax (444–999 Hz vs. 426 to 826 Hz; $p < 0.01$) [17] and in children than in adults at 25% of the total spectral power (F25, 125 ± 6 Hz; 139 ± 15 Hz, $p = 0.02$), F50 (169 ± 14 Hz; 194 ± 26 Hz, $p = 0.03$), 95% of the total spectral power (F95: 527 ± 52 Hz; 467 ± 45 Hz, $p = 0.02$), and Fmax (1040–1595 Hz vs. 104–1735 Hz; $p < 0.01$). Also, decreases in frequency quartiles have been reported to be dependent not only on people's age but also on their height ($p < 0.001$) [23].

During inspiration, values of Fmax of 822–999 Hz at right upper anterior chest [3], of 106–843 Hz at right lower posterior chest [3, 17, 20, 21, 23, 24], and of 236.6–885 Hz at left lower posterior chest have been reported [3, 24]. Lower Fmax values have been reported for the same locations during expiration, i.e., Fmax of 604–794 Hz at right upper anterior chest [3], 104–420 Hz at right lower posterior chest [3, 17, 21, 24], and 172.6–480.1 Hz at left lower posterior chest [3, 24].

Frequency at maximum power has also been found to change with the body position. The highest values of Fmax have been reported during inspiration at the right lung when it is in the dependent side-lying position (278.4 ± 42.3 Hz). Inspiratory Fmax then decreases in the sitting position (244.5 ± 51.9 Hz), and the lowest values have been found when the right lung is in the nondependent side-lying position (201.6 ± 57.6 Hz) ($p < 0.001$) [24]. No significant differences have been found for the left lung.

Therefore, it seems established that normal lung sound frequencies are higher in children than in adults, in women than in men, and in inspiration than in expiration and change with body position, being progressively lower from dependent side-lying, sitting, and nondependent side-lying positions. A synthesis of normal respiratory sound features in healthy people can be found in Table 10.1.

In the Presence of a Respiratory Condition

A similar lung sound pattern to the one described for healthy people has been observed in patients with respiratory conditions. Values of F25 of 153.8 ± 42.8 Hz in interstitial pneumonia [32] and of 131.9 ± 16.3 Hz in asbestos [33] during inspiration and of 111.2 ± 10.6 Hz in asbestos [33] during expiration have been reported. For F50, values of 165 ± 18 Hz in asthma [21], 190.3 ± 26.6 Hz in asbestos [33], and 231.9 ± 104.7 Hz in interstitial pneumonia [32] during inspiration and of 143 ± 20 Hz in asthma [21] and 158.4 ± 22.4 in asbestos [33] during expiration have been found. For F75, values of 335.2 ± 142.7 Hz in interstitial pneumonia [32] and of 278.0 ± 53.5 Hz in asbestos [33] during inspiration and of 235.6 ± 34.8 Hz in asbestos [33] during expiration have been reported. Values of Fmax of 113 ± 30 Hz [20] and 130 ± 17 Hz [30] in COPD, 101 ± 17 Hz in asthma [21], 141.0 ± 29.8 Hz in asbestos [33], and 168.1 ± 99.8 Hz in interstitial pneumonia [32] during inspiration and of 100 ± 20 Hz in COPD [30], 95 ± 8 Hz in asthma [21], and 116.9 ± 32.2 Hz in asbestos [33] during expiration have been reported. Nevertheless, Fmax seems to be increased during histamine challenges in patients with asthma and COPD [33] compared with people without respiratory conditions, due to airway narrowing. Increased values of inspiratory Fmax have also been found in smokers compared to nonsmokers (117 ± 16.2 Hz vs. 106.4 ± 21.6 Hz; $p = 0.0081$) and may be an early sign of airway obstruction. A synthesis of normal respiratory sound features in people with respiratory conditions can be found in Table 10.1.

10.1.2.2 Intensity

Sound intensity varies considerably over the chest [35, 36] as they are regional- and volume-dependent. In frequencies below 300 Hz (main frequencies of normal lung sounds), the sounds are loudest over the best ventilated airways [37].

In Healthy People

Intensity of normal lung sounds in healthy people has also been revised as discussed in Oliveira and Marques [11]. Overall intensity (measure in amplitude values) between 1.2 and 1.7 V has been reported, being higher at left upper anterior chest and lower at right lower posterior chest [38].

Values for inspiratory sound intensity between 4.7 and 68.6 dB at right upper anterior chest [3, 22, 25], 79.1 ± 4.3 dB at left upper anterior chest [25], 4.3–72.8 dB at right lower posterior chest [3, 17, 22, 24, 25], and 5.7–76.6 dB at left lower posterior chest [3, 22, 24–27] have been found in the literature. Lower intensity values for expiratory sounds have been reported, i.e., 2.3 ± 1.3 dB at right upper anterior chest [3, 22], 1.9–11.2 dB at right lower posterior chest [3, 17, 22, 24], and 2.5–10.2 dB at left lower posterior chest [3, 22, 24].

Two studies have compared the intensity of lung sounds at different frequencies (150–300 and 300–600 Hz) between inspiration and expiration [26, 27] and found that inspiratory sounds were always louder than expiratory sounds. Also, the difference between the two respiratory phases was high in the frequency band of 300 to 600 Hz in both studies [26, 27]. The intensity of inspiratory sounds recorded over the posterior left chest was found to be higher than at the posterior right chest (left 25.6 dB vs. right 20.7 dB) [24, 26].

When comparing different chest locations, the sound intensity of both lungs has been reported as being significantly higher in sitting than in nondependent side-lying positions (inspiration, 20.7–25.6 dB vs. 15.7–19.7 dB; expiration 8.8–10.2 dB vs. 6.8–8.7 dB). Moreover, intensities have been found to be slightly lower (not statistically significant) in sitting than in the dependent side-lying positions (inspiration, 20.7–25.6 dB vs. 22.7–23.5 dB; expiration 8.8–10.2 dB vs. 9.3–11.2 dB). In side-lying, higher intensities of the dependent side vs. nondependent side have been reported (inspiration, 22.7–23.5 dB vs. 15.7–19.7 dB; expiration 9.3–11.2 dB vs. 6.8–8.7 dB) [24]. A synthesis of normal respiratory sound features in healthy people can be found in Table 10.1.

Thus, it seems established that intensity of normal lung sound is higher in upper regions of the chest than in lower regions, in the left than in the right lung, and in inspiration than in expiration. Also changes in body position cause sound intensity to be progressively lower from dependent side-lying to sitting to nondependent side-lying. Finally, lung sound intensity has been found to increase with higher frequency band and flows and to differ significantly among infants, children, and adults [17], i.e., higher flows imply lower sound intensity in infants and children (i.e., normal bronchial breathing) than in adults and vice versa [17]. A synthesis of normal respiratory sound features in healthy people can be found in Table 10.1.

In the Presence of a Respiratory Condition

Lung sound intensity has been studied in patients with asthma [20, 21, 31, 39, 40] and COPD [20, 28, 41, 42] in stable states and after allergen inhalation (i.e., *Dermatophagoides pteronyssinus* SQ502, methacholine, and histamine).

No differences have been found in the intensity of inspiratory sounds recorded at the right chest of patients with stable asthma (67.1 ± 4.5 dB; 129 ± 55 mV), stable COPD (63.5 ± 4.4 dB), and people without respiratory conditions (64.4 ± 4.4 dB; 84 ± 38 mV) [20, 21, 40]. Conflicting results have been reported for expiratory lung sound intensity in patients with asthma. Significant lower expiratory sound intensity at the right chest (upper, mid, and lower lobes) of patients with asthma than in healthy controls has been reported, being most evident at relatively low airflow values ($p < 0.005$) [40]. However, no significant differences have also been reported (asthmatic patients, 62 ± 27 mV vs. people without respiratory conditions, 104 ± 40 mV) [21].

During histamine challenges, no differences in lung sound amplitude have been reported between patients with asthma (inspiration, 86 ± 52 mV; expiration, 63 ± 33 mV) and people without respiratory conditions (inspiration, 136 ± 48 mV; expiration, 111 ± 36 mV) [21]. Different responses have however been observed during the course of responses to *Dermatophagoides pteronyssinus* SQ502 and methacholine challenges. After inhalation of *Dermatophagoides pteronyssinus* SQ502, expiratory lung sound intensity recorded over the right chest (upper, mid, and lower lobes) of patients with asthma showed a significant increase from the baseline (24.4 ± 3.1 dB) compared with the phases of airway obstruction (early asthmatic response, 30.7 ± 7.1 dB; late asthmatic response, 29.3 ± 7.1 dB, $p < 0.05$; and post-bronchodilator response, 26.6 ± 3.2 dB; $p < 0.05$) [31]. Similar results were observed in people without respiratory conditions and patients with asthma after inhalation of methacholine. During quiet inspiration and expiration, lung sounds were louder than at baseline in both subject groups ($p = 0.013$); however, the increase in intensity with airflow was greater in patients with asthma than in normal subjects during forced expiration ($p \leq 0.001$). In patients with asthma, during both quiet breathing ($p = 0.029$) and forced expiration ($p = 0.002$), expiratory sounds progressively increased with the decrease of FEV_1 (i.e., increase airway narrowing) [39]. These changes may suggest that the generation and/or transmission of lung sounds during asthmatic acute airway narrowing are modified by morphological abnormalities of the airway wall.

In patients with COPD, studies have found high lung sound intensities in tidal breathing, especially at the upper chest [41] and at higher frequency bands (>400 Hz) [28], than in people without respiratory conditions. Mean inspiratory lung sound intensities of 42.9 ± 4.9 dB in people with COPD and of 34.6 ± 2.4 dB in people without respiratory conditions have been reported independently of the respiratory phase and anatomical site of recording [28]. Nevertheless, at higher flow rates (1 to 2 L/s), no significant differences between patients with COPD and people without respiratory conditions have been found [20, 42]. At higher respiratory volumes, lower sound intensity, especially at lung bases, has been reported [41]. This diverse lung sound distribution in patients with COPD may be explained by several reasons, such as the altered ribcage and diaphragm configurations and movement due to hyperinflation and to the location and extent of emphysema areas [41]. Nevertheless, more studies with standardized airflows and volumes are needed to establish firm conclusions about the clinical utility of lung sound intensity in patients with COPD.

At high flow rates (i.e., 1.0–1.5 L/s), lower expiratory sound intensity has also been reported in smokers compared with nonsmokers without respiratory conditions both for maximum intensity (48.2 ± 3.8 dB vs. 50.9 ± 3.2 dB; $p = 0.001$) and mean intensity (31.2 ± 3.6 dB vs. 33.7 ± 3 dB $p = 0.001$, dz. = 0.75) [29]. These results may be an early sign of poorer pulmonary ventilation in smokers and should be further investigated. A synthesis of normal respiratory sound features in people with respiratory conditions can be found in Table 10.1.

Table 10.1 Synthesis of normal respiratory sound features in healthy people and in people with respiratory conditions

	Location	F50 (Hz)	Fmax (Hz)	Imean (dB)	Imax (dB)
Healthy [3, 12, 17, 20–29]	Trachea	Inspiration 447–766 Expiration 540 ± 174	Inspiration 93 and 154 Expiration 99 ± 8	Inspiration 34.6–83.1 Expiration 45.4–85.1	
	Chest	Inspiration 119.3–128.3 Expiration 91.3–104.5	Inspiration 90.4–885 Expiration 78.9–794	Inspiration 4.7–79.1 Expiration 1.9–37.7	Inspiration 52–58.8 Expiration 49.3–54.5
COPD [20, 21, 28, 30]	Trachea	Inspiration 753 ± 177	Inspiration 228 ± 340 Hz	Inspiration 82.6 ± 3.1	
	Chest		Inspiration 113–130 Expiration 100 ± 20	Inspiration 42.9–63.5	
Asthma [21, 31]	Trachea	Inspiration 507 ± 153 Expiration 546 ± 117	Inspiration 106 ± 47 Expiration 92 ± 7	Inspiration 84.7 ± 3.7	
	Chest	Inspiration 165 ± 18 Expiration 143 ± 20	Inspiration 101 ± 17 Hz Expiration 95 ± 8	Inspiration 67.1 ± 4.5 dB Expiration 24.4 ± 3.1	
Interstitial pneumonia [32]	Trachea				
	Chest	Inspiration 231.9 ± 104.7	Inspiration 168.1 ± 99.8		
Asbestos [33]	Trachea				
	Chest	Inspiration 190.3 ± 26.6 Expiration 158.4 ± 22.4	Inspiration 141.0 ± 29.8 Expiration 116.9 ± 32.2		

Values are presented as mean or as mean ± standard deviation per respiratory phase (inspiration or expiration)

F50, median frequency; Fmax, frequency at maximum power; Imean, mean intensity; Imax, maximum intensity

10.2 Adventitious Respiratory Sounds

Adventitious respiratory sounds are additional respiratory sounds superimposed to normal respiratory sounds. They are mainly composed by discontinuous (e.g., crackles) and continuous (e.g., wheezes) sounds. A summary of adventitious respiratory sounds, from their mechanisms to clinical interpretation, is presented in Table 10.4

10.2.1 Crackles

Crackles are discontinuous adventitious respiratory sounds. They are intermittent, nonmusical, brief, and explosive sounds thought to be caused by the sudden opening and closing of abnormally closed airways [43–45]. Paul Forgacs was the first to theorize that crackles were generated during inspiration as a result of sudden opening of the airways [45]. Despite almost four decades of subsequent research, this theory has never been refuted. A few years later, it was explained that these events could be modeled quantitatively on the basis of a stress-relaxation quadrupole [46]. In simple terms, it was found that the sudden airway opening and sudden airway closing originated stressed waves which were then propagated in the lung parenchyma, originating crackles. Currently, a crackle sound is believed to be originated from multiple events, such as the acoustic energy generated by pressure equalization, changes in elastic stress after a sudden opening or closing of airways [19, 47], when there is inflammation/edema in the lungs [48], or produced by boluses of gas passing through airways as they open and close intermittently [45] or, less frequently, by abundant secretions [16]. Recently, it has also been found that the events responsible for crackle generation must be as fast in expiration, due to sudden airway closing, as they are in inspiration, due to sudden airway reopening, even if the former is less energetic than the latter [49].

Frequency of crackles ranges from 100 to 2000 Hz [19] depending on the diameter of the airways (i.e., low diameter airways produce high-frequency crackles and vice versa), which are usually affected by the pathophysiology of the surrounding tissue. The short duration of crackles (<20 ms) and their often low intensity make its discrimination and characterization by conventional auscultation difficult [47]. The difficulty to detect crackles is aggravated when other respiratory sounds of greater intensity are being produced simultaneously (e.g., wheezes) [47].

Smaller airways have been shown to produce mid-to-late inspiratory and occasionally early expiratory crackles of short duration (<10 ms) and high frequencies (fine crackles). This type of crackles is rarely transmitted to the mouth; is unaffected by forced expiratory maneuvers, such as cough or huff; and is gravity-dependent. Restrictive pulmonary diseases have been associated with the production of fine crackles [50]. Larger, more proximal airways, such as trachea and main bronchi, are thought to produce longer (>10 ms) and low-frequency crackles (coarse crackles) in early inspiration and throughout expiration. This type of crackles is scanty, usually audible at the mouth, and gravity-independent and is more associated with obstructive pulmonary disease and secretions [16, 19, 51]. Due to their characteristics, coarse crackles may change or disappear during auscultation, forced expiratory maneuvers, or even during pulmonary function tests, possibly due to the effect of lung expansion [48]. Considering crackles' different characteristics and clinical interpretation, it seems essential to consider their timing within the respiratory cycle, as it allows direct estimation of the sound origin [52].

Besides crackles' frequency, duration, gravity (in)dependence, (non)response to forced expiratory maneuvers, and timing within the respiratory cycle, their number and the anatomical place from where they are being auscultated should also be considered. As the disease progresses, crackles tend to increase in number and occur first in the basal areas and later in the upper zones of the lungs [2]. In addition to the described crackles' characteristics, some investigations have also used crackles' initial deflection width (IDW), largest deflection width (LDW), and two-cycle duration (2CD) for diagnostic and monitoring purposes [47].

10.2.1.1 In Healthy People

The appearance of crackles has been interpreted as an early sign of respiratory disease [19]; however some studies have reported that crackles are present in healthy people [11, 29, 53–55]. In this population, the number of crackles have been found to vary between 1 and 4 per respiratory cycle and have been heard mainly in the upper and lateral right chest, especially during inspiration [29, 55–57]. Studies have reported the presence of both fine [54, 55] and coarse [56] crackles in healthy people, with frequencies ranging from 148.1 to 387 Hz in inspiration, from 144.2 to 404 Hz in expiration [29, 56], and from 259 to 864 Hz in all respiratory cycle [54]. A synthesis of crackle features in healthy people can be found in Table 10.2.

10.2.1.2 In the Presence of a Respiratory Condition

The use of crackles for diagnostic purposes has been recently revised [62]. Crackles have been associated with the process and severity of the disease in patients with interstitial lung disorders [19, 47], pneumonia [56, 63, 64], and COPD [58, 65]. Additionally, a number of inspiratory crackles recorded at anterior/upper regions have been shown to differ between healthy smokers and nonsmokers (2.2 [1.8–3.7] vs. 1.5 [1.2–2.2], $p = 0.0081$) [29]. These findings further point toward the possible use of crackles as first indicators of respiratory disease. However, these results have only been reported by one study and require investigation.

Some studies have also explored crackle's different features among diseases, e.g., COPD [30, 55, 57, 59, 66], fibrosis alveolitis, bronchiectasis, heart failure [30], asbestosis [67, 68], pulmonary edema [68], pneumonia, asthma, and interstitial pulmonary fibrosis [49, 57, 66], and between different phases of the same disease, e.g., stable versus exacerbated COPD [58, 63, 65]. A synthesis of crackle features in healthy people can be found in Table 10.2.

Crackles are also commonly used to monitor patients' responses to respiratory interventions, and yet few studies [60, 64, 69] have been conducted assessing their use as an outcome measure [70]. From the limited evidence available, LDW seemed to be the most valuable parameter to be used as an outcome measure due to its high effect sizes found in patients with pneumonia following medical intervention (1 and 1.25) [64]. This is supported by what has already been proposed by Hoevers and Loudon [71]. However, LDW has been the variable less explored among studies. Conflicting information has been found for the number of crackles and 2CD [60, 64, 69]. Timing of crackles has also showed to be sensitive to the clinical course of pneumonia [64] and has been described as a sensitive parameter to discriminate between respiratory diseases and heart failure [47]. However, similar to LDW limited research has been conducted considering this parameter as an outcome measure. Thus, it can be concluded that despite all available information, and the clear potential of crackles to contribute for the diagnosis and monitoring of respiratory conditions and interventions, much research is still needed to recommend auscultation of crackles as diagnostic and outcome measure for respiratory interventions. As described by Pasterkamp et al. [2], what seems well established is the presence or absence of crackles to distinguish pulmonary fibrosis from sarcoidosis (crackles usually absent) [50], fine and late inspiratory crackles indicating fibrotic lung disease and early coarse crackles indicating obstructive lung disease [58, 72, 73], crackles as an early sign of asbestos [67, 74, 75], and crackles indicating heart failure [30, 76, 77].

Table 10.2 Synthesis of crackle features in healthy people and in people with respiratory conditions

	No of crackles	IDW (ms)	2CD (ms)	LDW (ms)	Frequency (Hz)	Direction of the first deflection
Healthy [29, 55–57]	Respiratory cycle 1–4	Inspiration 3.2 Expiration 3–3.1	Inspiration 12.5–12.6 Expiration 12.3–12.8	Inspiration 3–3.1 Expiration 3–3.2	Inspiration 148.1–387 Expiration 144.2–404 Respiratory cycle 259–864	
COPD [30, 55, 57–59]	Inspiration 1.20–5 Expiration 0.73–8	Inspiration 1.88–2.1 Respiratory cycle 0.91 ± 0.43	Inspiration 7.74–11.6 Respiratory cycle 5.4 ± 2.4	Inspiration 2.69	Inspiration 233–311 Expiration 309	INP 90% ENP 53%
Asthma [57]	Inspiration 3 ± 3 Expiration 3 ± 3				Inspiration 329 ± 63 Expiration 309 ± 98	
Bronchiectasis [30, 60]	Inspiration 8.5 ± 5.1 Respiratory cycle 4.14 ± 2.31	Inspiration 1.8 ± 0.2	Inspiration 10.6 ± 1.0 Respiratory cycle 11.8 ± 1.50	Inspiration 2.45 ± 0.28		
Fibrosing alveolitis [30]	Inspiration 7.6 ± 3.7	Inspiration 1.3 ± 0.2	Inspiration 7.7 ± 1.3	Inspiration 1.83 ± 0.30		
Interstitial pulmonary fibrosis [49, 55, 57]	Inspiration 24–25 Expiration 8–9	Inspiration 0.65 ± 0.18	Inspiration 4.6 ± 1.2		Inspiration 441–448 Expiration 405–42	INP 76 ± 9% ENP 4 ± 14%
Heart failure [30, 49, 55, 57, 61]	Inspiration 5.3–13 Expiration 2–6	Inspiration 2.1 ± 0.3 Respiratory cycle 1.09 ± 0.20	Inspiration 11.8 ± 1.3 Respiratory cycle 6.59–6.6	Inspiration 2.86 ± 0.32	Inspiration 310–326 Expiration 285–303	INP 76 ± 10% ENP 38 ± 18%
Pneumonia [49, 55–57, 61]	Inspiration 7–9 Expiration 5–6	Respiratory cycle 0.85 ± 0.40	Respiratory cycle 5–6.61		Inspiration 302–316 Expiration 278–289	INP 75 ± 14% ENP 29 ± 18%

Values are presented as mean or as mean ± standard deviation per breathing phase
No number, *IDW* initial deflection width, *INP* inspiratory negative polarity, *ENP* expiratory negative polarity, *2CD* two-cycle deflection, *LDW* largest deflection width

10.2.1.3 Wheezes

Wheezes are continuous and musical adventitious respiratory sounds usually longer than 80–100 ms and with frequencies from less than 100 Hz to 1 kHz or even higher if measured inside the airways [78]. The mechanisms underlying wheeze production appear to involve an interaction between the airway wall and the gas moving through the airway and causing its oscillation [79]. These oscillations start when the airflow velocity reaches a critical value, called flutter velocity, due to narrowed airways [19, 79, 80]. The flutter mechanisms mainly explain expiratory wheezes, but inspiratory wheezes, which are normally associated with more severe and upper airway obstruction, are not yet well understood [19, 79].

It has been proposed that wheezes always occur when there is a flow limitation, but flow limitation is not necessarily accompanied by wheezes [81–83]. They can therefore be produced by all the mechanisms that reduce airway caliber such as bronchospasm, mucosal edema, intraluminal tumor, secretions, foreign bodies, or external compression. The frequency of a wheeze is dependent on the mass and elasticity of the airway walls and on the flow velocity. It is, however, not influenced by the length or the size of the airway [79]. Wheezes, which are usually louder than the underlying normal respiratory sounds, are often audible at the patient's mouth or by auscultation over the larynx [2].

Clinically, wheezes can be defined by their frequency (complexity—mono- or polyphonic), intensity, number, duration and position in the respiratory cycle, gravity influence, and respiratory maneuvers. Duration, complexity, and position in the respiratory cycle have been mostly used in the clinical setting to quantify the severity of an airway obstruction and to monitor its progression. Duration in the respiratory cycle, or wheeze occupation rate, has been indicated do be directly related to the degree of bronchial obstruction [19]. Regarding the complexity and position in the respiratory cycle, it is generally accepted that polyphonic wheezes and presence of wheezes in both inspiratory and expiratory phases indicate a more serious obstruction stage than monophonic wheezes and presence in expiration only [79, 84, 85].

To facilitate wheeze interpretation, a classification based on complexity and position in the respiratory cycle has been adopted. Wheezes have been classified as fixed monophonic, random monophonic, and sequential inspiratory or expiratory polyphonic [86]. Fixed monophonic wheezes imply hearing only one frequency and are usually indicative of an incomplete occlusion of the bronchus (e.g., tumor). Random monophonic wheezes occur when there is widespread airflow obstruction (e.g., asthma) [86]. This specific type of wheeze occurs randomly across the respiratory cycles, during inspiration or expiration, and is usually a result of bronchial spasm or swelling of the mucous membrane [86]. Sequential inspiratory wheezes are typically generated when peripheral airways open and oscillate, late in inspiration. They are characterized as sequences of short, monophonic wheezes, each with a different pitch and sound intensity [86]. Pulmonary diseases associated with sequential inspiratory wheezes include fibrosing alveolitis, asbestosis, and other diffuse interstitial pulmonary diseases [86]. Expiratory polyphonic wheezes are produced by the passage of air through several bronchial airways simultaneously obstructed [19], creating harmonic unrelated musical sounds. This type of wheezing is often associated with COPD [86].

In Healthy People

A literature review on respiratory sounds has synthetized the studies that analyzed wheezes in healthy people [11]. The presence of wheezes in healthy people has been studied [29, 56, 57]; however only two studies have reported the characteristics of these sounds [29, 57]. The average wheeze occupation rate in healthy people seems to vary between 0 and 51.6% both in inspiration and expiration [29, 57]. Mean frequencies of wheezes have been found to be higher in expiration (309–526.8 Hz) than in inspiration (283–300 Hz) [29, 57]. A synthesis of wheeze features in healthy people can be found in Table 10.3.

In the Presence of a Respiratory Condition

Wheezes have been used for diagnostic purposes [62] and widely reported in several respiratory conditions in children (i.e., cystic fibrosis [89], asthma [88, 90] with prolonged cough [91], and bronchiolitis [69]) and in adults (i.e., asthma [87, 92–94], pneumonia [56], COPD [87, 95, 96], lower respiratory tract infections [97, 98]). Table 10.3 provides a synthesis of wheeze features in several respiratory conditions.

Wheezes have also been used as an outcome measure in respiratory interventions [70]. Wheeze occupation rate seemed to be the most promising parameter to be used as an outcome measure in children and adults [70, 92, 98]. In a systematic review on respiratory sounds in COPD [95], it was found that during forced expiratory maneuvers, only 13.7% of the time was not occupied by wheezes; most were polyphonic (53.6% vs. 32.6% monophonic) [87] and were more frequent during expiration than in inspiration (inspiratory wheeze rate 2% vs. expiratory wheeze rate 12%) [57]. A strong association between the proportion of the respiratory cycle occupied by wheezes and the degree of bronchial obstruction has been widely demonstrated [87, 88, 90, 91]. This wheeze parameter, even when identified with conventional auscultation, has shown to be sensitive to assess the effectiveness of respiratory interventions in children [99, 100]. The wheeze complexity may also be a variable of interest as the presence of polyphonic wheeze indicates a more serious obstruction than monophonic wheeze [94]; however, this has been vaguely explored [94]. Wheeze monitoring has been found to provide more information on the changes of airway obstruction than measurements of pulmonary function [92], such as the percentage predicted of FEV_1 in people with asthma [93]. Thus, wheezes and their variables seem to be a promising objective measure for all populations with a special emphasis on non-collaborative populations such as children, people with cognitive deficit, and people in the intensive care.

There are three other sounds within the wheeze classification that, due to their specific characteristics and relationship with a disease process, are normally described apart, i.e., squawks, stridor, and rhonchus.

Table 10.3 Synthesis of wheeze features in healthy people and in people with respiratory conditions

	No. of wheeze	Wz%	Wz% monophonic wheeze	Wz% polyphonic wheeze	Frequency (Hz)	Rhonchus (%)	Frequency (Hz)
Healthy [48, 58, 65]		Inspiration 0–36.3 Expiration 0–51.6	Inspiration 3 ± 13 Expiration 7 ± 16		Inspiration 283–300 Expiration 309–526.8		
COPD [57, 58, 87]	Expiration (forced maneuvers) 10.4 ± 6.1	Inspiration 1.12–2 Expiration 1.77–12	Expiration (forced maneuvers) 32.6 ± 19	Expiration (forced maneuvers) 53.6 ± 25.5	Inspiration 232 ± 58 Expiration 301 ± 119 Expiration (forced maneuvers) 669.4 ± 250.1	Inspiration 3 ± 11 Expiration 7 ± 19	Inspiration 129 ± 29 Expiration 132 ± 30
Asthma [57, 87, 88]	Expiration (forced maneuvers) 8.4 ± 6.4	Inspiration 10 ± 16 Expiration 25 ± 32 Expiration (forced maneuvers) 58 ± 20	Inspiration 55.9 ± 17.7	Inspiration 21.9 ± 15.3	Inspiration 340 ± 142 Expiration 259 ± 67 Expiration (forced maneuvers) 440–560.9	Inspiration 5 ± 15 Expiration 7 ± 20	Inspiration 142 ± 34 Expiration 142 ± 37
Interstitial pulmonary disease [57]		Inspiration 0 Expiration 2 ± 4			Inspiration 0 Expiration 346 ± 124	Inspiration 0 Expiration 0	Inspiration 0 Expiration 0
Heart failure [56, 57]		Inspiration 3 ± 13 Expiration 6 ± 16			Inspiration 320 ± 129 Expiration 297 ± 83	Inspiration 3 ± 12 Expiration 4 ± 12	Inspiration 117–127 Expiration 11 ± 45
Pneumonia [56, 57]		Inspiration 3 ± 13 Expiration 7 ± 16			Inspiration 248 ± 61 Expiration 304 ± 89	Inspiration 5–30 Expiration 6–35	Inspiration 138–140 Expiration 126–127

Values are presented as mean or as mean ± standard deviation per respiratory phase
No. number, *Wz%* wheeze occupation rate

Squawks

Squawks can be considered a subgroup of wheezes and are characterized by specific parameters. A squawk is a high-frequency inspiratory short wheeze caused by airway wall oscillation as airways open, generally accompanied by crackles. Normally, the duration of a squawk is between 50 and 400 ms [1, 47, 57], and their frequency rarely exceeds 300 Hz [1, 2]. The term "squawk" should only be used to describe inspiratory short wheezes in patients with interstitial lung diseases or in acute patients with pneumonia, where small airways are involved, or they should be called simply "short wheezes." Although relatively common, little attention has been paid to this adventitious respiratory sound [101], and further education on its identification and interpretation has been recommended [102].

Stridor

Stridor is a very loud wheeze, resulting from a morphologic or dynamic obstruction in the larynx or trachea [1]. It occurs during inspiration when the obstruction is extra-thoracic and during expiration when it is intra-thoracic, unless the obstruction is fixed, in which case, stridor may appear in both phases of respiration [1, 79]. The frequency of stridor is between 500 Hz [16] and 1000 Hz, and it is common in infants and babies due to their small airway dimensions or supraglottic inflammation (laryngitis) [1]. In adults the frequency of stridor is usually much lower <200 Hz [103].

Rhonchus

Rhonchus should be placed between musical and nonmusical sounds [102]. They are low-pitch sounds, generated in the central/larger airways (associated with the presence of secretions, narrowing of large airways, or abnormal airway collapsibility) that can be heard during inspiration, expiration, or both and can disappear with forced expiratory maneuvers such as cough or huffing. The main frequency of rhonchus is below 300 Hz, and their duration is above 80–100 ms [1, 2, 16].

Table 10.4 Summary table of normal and adventitious respiratory sounds, from their mechanisms to clinical interpretation

Respiratory sounds	Mechanism	Origin	Acoustics	Clinical characteristics	Clinical interpretation	Sound wave
Normal (basic) respiratory sounds						
Normal or basic tracheal/mouth sound	Turbulent airflow, flow impinging in the bronchi and trachea	Pharynx, larynx, trachea, upper airways	Continuous Noise with resonances—range < 100—>1500 Hz	Loud and tubular (hollow) sound, nonmusical, heard in both phases of respiratory cycle	Transports intrapulmonary sounds; can become more noisy or musical if upper airway patency is altered Used to monitor sleep apnea	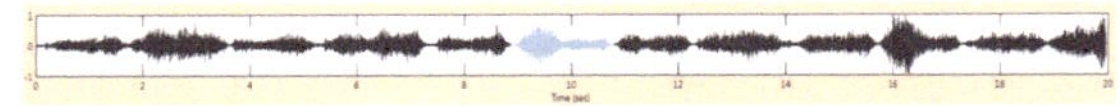 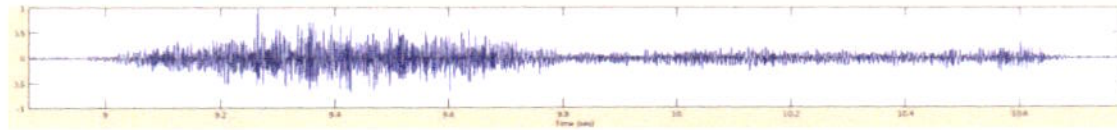 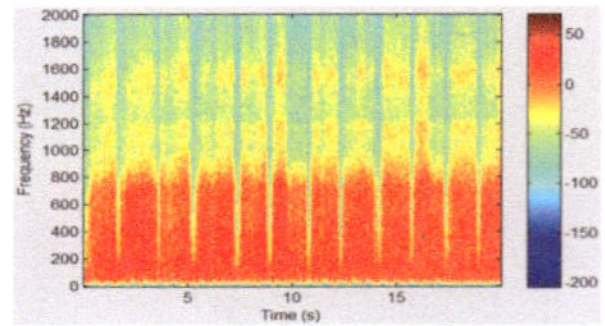

Normal or basic lung sound	Turbulent flow vortices along bronchi, outside alveoli	Central airways (expiration), lobar to segmental airway (inspiration)	Continuous Low-pass filter noise—<100–1000 Hz	Soft, nonmusical, heard only in inspiration and early expiration Expiration is clearly audible if closer to trachea, i.e., right upper lung areas and posterior upper zones in children	Diminished or enhanced due to sound generation and sound transmission factors. If heard in both respiratory cycles implies bronchial breathing Diminished—sound generation (e.g., hypoventilation, airway narrowing); sound transmission (e.g., lung destruction, pleural effusion, pneumothorax) Enhanced—sound generation (e.g., airway patency surrounded by consolidated lung tissue); sound transmission (e.g., pneumonia, atelectasis, fibrosis)	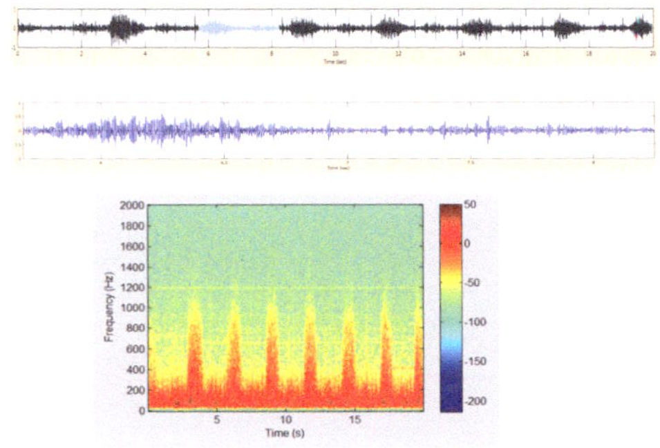

(continued)

Table 10.4 (continued)

Respiratory sounds	Mechanism	Origin	Acoustics	Clinical characteristics	Clinical interpretation	Sound wave
Bronchial breathing	Turbulent flow vortices along airways	Central airways, lobar to segmental airway	Continuous Frequency band up to 600–1000 Hz	Soft, nonmusical, heard on inspiration and expiration (mimics tracheal sound) An intermediate sound between tracheal and normal respiratory sound	Normal in infants and children (heart sounds can be superimposed) In adults indicates patent airway surrounded by consolidated lung tissue (e.g., pneumonia) or fibrosis	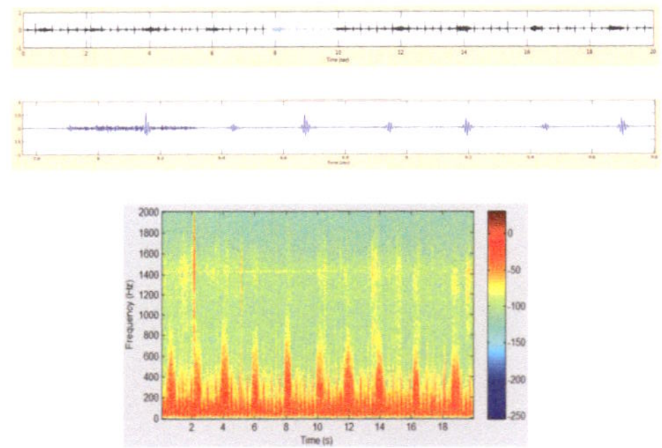
Adventitious respiratory sounds						
Fine crackles	Airway wall stress relaxation	Central and lower airways	Discontinuous Rapidly dampened wave deflection; duration <10 ms	Nonmusical, short, explosive, heard on mid-to-late inspiration and occasionally on expiration Unaffected by forced expiratory maneuvers such as cough, gravity-dependent, not transmitted to mouth	Related with sudden airway closing during expiration and sudden airway reopening during inspiration and not to secretions. Frequently present is some conditions of the lower airways, e.g., congestive heart failure, idiopathic pulmonary fibrosis, pneumonia, asbestosis	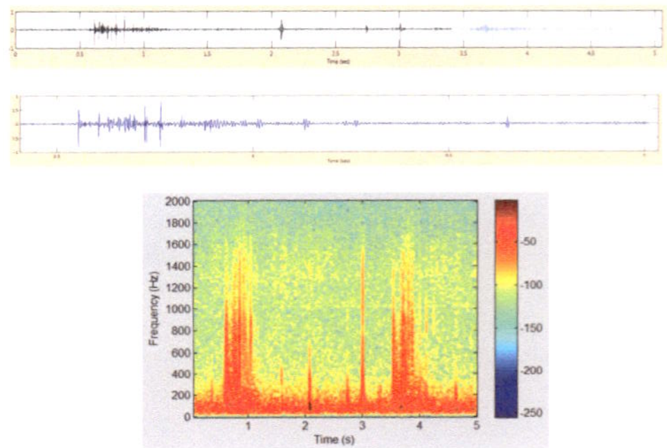

Coarse crackles	Rupture of fluid menisci and mucus bubbles	Central and lower airways	Discontinuous Rapidly dampened wave deflection; duration >10 ms	Nonmusical, short, explosive, heard on early inspiration and all expiration Affected by forced expiratory maneuvers such as cough, non-gravity-dependent, transmitted to the mouth	May be related to secretions and indicates intermittent airway opening (e.g., COPD)	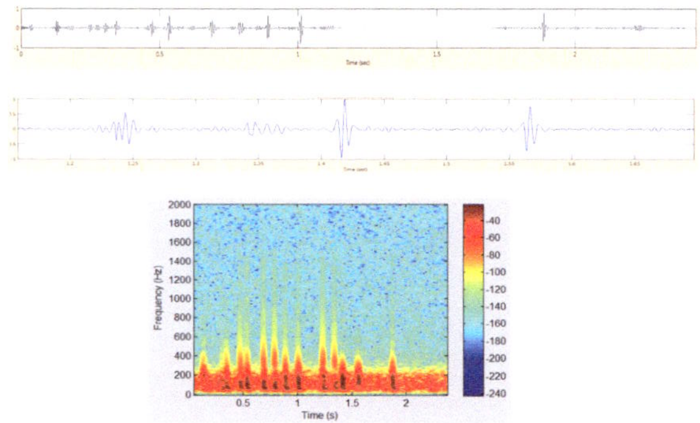
Monophonic wheeze	Airway wall flutter, vortex shedding	Central and upper airways	Continuous Sinusoid—range ≈100—>1000 Hz; duration >80 ms	Musical, continuum of flutter frequency from low to high, heard on inspiration, expiration or both Contains one frequency component.	Airway obstruction (e.g., foreign body, tumor), airflow limitation (e.g., asthma, COPD). The severity of the disease can be indicated by the percentage of the respiratory cycle occupied by wheezes. May be absent if airflow is too low or if the airway wall is too massive (e.g., thickened like in cystic fibrosis) to get into flutter at flow limitation	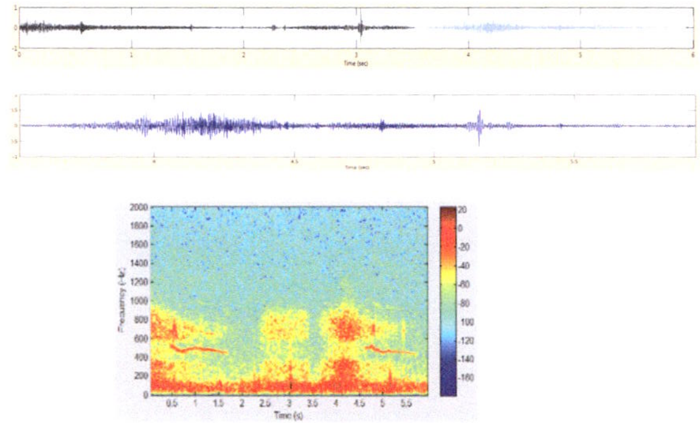

(continued)

Table 10.4 (continued)

Respiratory sounds	Mechanism	Origin	Acoustics	Clinical characteristics	Clinical interpretation	Sound wave
Polyphonic wheeze	Airway wall flutter, vortex shedding	Larger and central airways	Continuous Sinusoid—Range ≈100—>1000 Hz; duration >80 ms	Multiple musical notes starting and ending at the same time, continuum of flutter frequency from low to high, heard on expiration Contains two or more frequency components	Severe airway obstruction and airflow limitation (e.g., asthma, COPD)	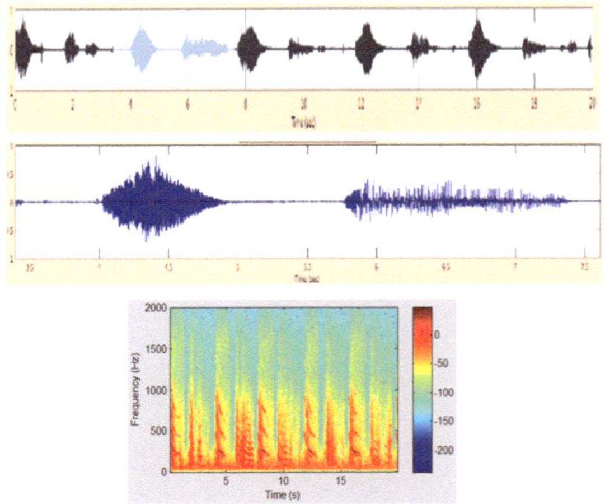
Squawk	Oscillation of peripheral airways (in deflated lung zones) whose walls remain in apposition long enough to oscillate under the action of the inspiratory airflow	Lower airways	Continuous Sinusoid – range ≈100 to >1000 Hz; duration 50–400 ms	Mixed sound (prolonged whistle, dull sound, or musical), high pitched, short, heard exclusively on inspiration and often preceded by crackles	Can be heard in chronic conditions when a patient is clinically stable, e.g., hypersensitivity pneumonia or other interstitial lung diseases or in acute ill patients, e.g., pneumonia	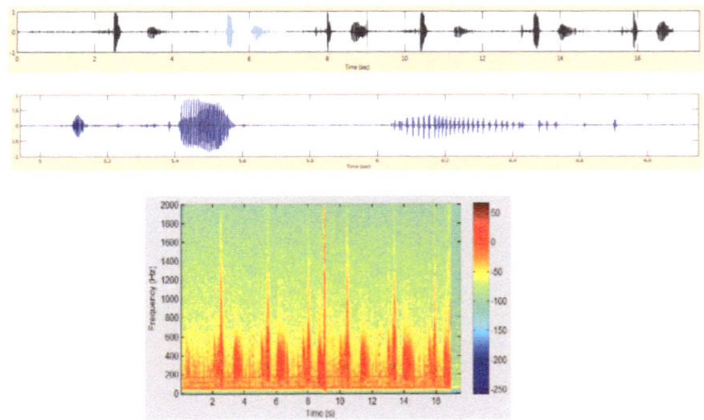

Rhonchus	Rupture of fluid films, airway wall vibrations, and collapsibility	Central airways	Continuous, Series of rapidly dampened sinusoids—<300 Hz; duration >100 ms	Quasi-musical, low pitched; may be heard on inspiration, expiration, or both Often disappears with forced expiratory maneuvers such as cough	Is common with airway narrowing caused by mucosal thickening or edema or bronchospasm (e.g., bronchiolitis in infants or bronchitis in older children and adults or COPD)	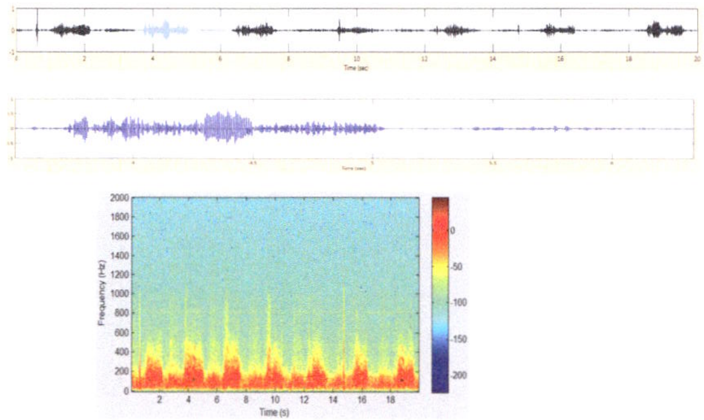

Conclusion

This chapter summarizes the main characteristics of respiratory sounds in healthy people and in some of the most representative respiratory diseases worldwide. Respiratory sounds exhibit different acoustic properties depending on the person's characteristics (e.g., age, gender, height, position, and airflow), local of sound acquisition, and position in the respiratory phase. The definition of such characteristics and the mastering of the pulmonary auscultation technique, by health professionals, will allow objective interpretations of respiratory sound alterations and, potentially, enhance the early detection, treatment, and monitoring of respiratory diseases.

Most of the evidence in respiratory sounds is now gathered through computerized acoustic devises, such as electronic stethoscopes and microphones. However, the methods for recording, analyzing, and reporting respiratory sounds still differ significantly among studies, which impair our understanding of the clinical meaning of each respiratory sound and the changes in their acoustics. Thus, the development of up-to-date international standard guidelines in the recording, analysis, and storage of respiratory sounds is immediately warranted. This standardization will enable comparisons of results among research and clinical centers and will facilitate the integration of the information provided by respiratory sounds in the clinical processes of patients along with other clinical measures. These developments are essential to further enhance the utility of auscultation at patients' bedside.

References

1. Sovijärvi A, Dalmasso F, Vanderschoot J, Malmberg L, Righini G, Stoneman S (2000) Definition of terms for applications of respiratory sounds. Eur Respir Rev 10:597–610
2. Pasterkamp H, Kraman SS, Wodicka GR (1997) Respiratory sounds: advances beyond the stethoscope. Am J Resp Crit Care 156:974–987
3. Gavriely N, Nissan M, Rubin A-H, Cugell DW (1995) Spectral characteristics of chest wall breath sounds in normal subjects. Thorax 50:1292–1300
4. Lessard CS, Wong WC (1986) Correlation of constant flow rate with frequency spectrum of respiratory sounds when measured at the trachea. IEEE Trans Biomed Eng 33(4):461–463
5. Krumpe PE, Cummiskey JM (1980) Use of laryngeal sound recordings to monitor apnea. Am Rev Respir Dis 122(5):797–801
6. East KA, East TD (1985) Computerized acoustic detection of obstructive apnea. Comput Methods Prog Biomed 21(3):213–220
7. Sanna A, Lorimier P, Dachy B, D'Hondt A, Sergysels R (1991) Value of monitoring of tracheal respiratory sounds in the diagnosis of nocturnal respiratory dysrhythmias. Acta Clin Belg 46(3):159–164
8. Pasterkamp H, Schafer J, Wodicka GR (1996) Posture-dependent change of tracheal sounds at standardized flows in patients with obstructive sleep apnea. Chest 110(6):1493–1498
9. Beckerman RC, Wegmann MJ, Waring WW (1982) Tracheal breath sounds for detection of apnea in infants and children. Crit Care Med 10(6):363–366
10. Beckerman RC, Wegmann MJ (1985) A comparison of tracheal breath sounds, airflow, and impedance pneumography in the detection of childhood apnea. Sleep 8(4):342–346

11. Oliveira A, Marques A (2014) Respiratory sounds in healthy people: a systematic review. Respir Med 108(4):550–570
12. Pasterkamp H, Sanchez I (1996) Effect of gas density on respiratory sounds. Am J Respir Crit Care Med 153(3):1087–1092
13. Leblanc P, Macklem PT, Ross WR (1970) Breath sounds and distribution of pulmonary ventilation. Am Rev Respir Dis 102(1):10–16
14. Forgacs P (1978) The functional basis of pulmonary sounds. Chest 73(3):399–405
15. Bohadana AB, Kanga JF, Kraman SS (1988) Does airway closure affect lung sound generation? Clin Physiol 8(4):341–349
16. Bohadana A, Izbicki G, Kraman SS (2014) Fundamentals of lung auscultation. N Engl J Med 370(8):744–751. https://doi.org/10.1056/NEJMra1302901
17. Pasterkamp H, Powell RE, Sanchez I (1996) Lung sound spectra at standardized air flow in normal infants, children, and adults. Am J Resp Crit Care 154(2):424–430. https://doi.org/10.1164/ajrccm.154.2.8756817
18. Dalmay F, Antonini MT, Marquet P, Menier R (1995) Acoustic properties of the normal chest. Eur Respir J 8:1761–1769
19. Sovijärvi A, Malmberg L, Charbonneau G, Vanderschoot J, Dalmasso F, Sacco C, Rossi M, Earis J (2000) Characteristics of breath sounds and adventitious respiratory sounds. Eur Respir Rev 10(77):591–596
20. Malmberg LP, Pesu L, Sovijarvi ARA (1995) Significant differences in flow standardised breath sound spectra in patients with chronic obstructive pulmonary disease, stable asthma and health lungs. Thorax 50:1285–1291
21. Malmberg LP, Sovijarvi ARA, Paajanen E, Piirila P, Haahtela T, Katila T (1994) Changes in frequency spectra of breath sounds during histaminic challenge test in adult asthmatics and healthy control subjects. Chest 105(1):122–132
22. Gavriely N, Cugell DW (1996) Airflow effects on amplitude and spectral content of normal breath sounds. J Appl Physiol 80(1):5–13
23. Hidalgo HA, Wegmann MJ, Waring WW (1991) Frequency spectra of normal breath sounds in childhood. Chest 100(4):999–1002
24. Jones A, Jones RD, Kwong K, Burns Y (1999) Effect of positioning on recorded lung sound intensities in subjects without pulmonary dysfunction. Phys Ther 79(7):682–690
25. Kraman SS (1984) The relationship between airflow and lung sound amplitude in normal subjects. Chest 86(2):225–229
26. Kompis M, Pasterkamp H, Oh Y, Wodicka GR (1997) Distribution of inspiratory and expiratory respiratory sound intensity on the surface of the human thorax. Engineering in Medicine and Biology Society, 1997 Proceedings of the 19th Annual International Conference of the IEEE 5:2047-2050
27. Kiyokawa H, Pasterkamp H (2002) Volume-dependent variations of regional lung sound, amplitude and phase. J Appl Physiol 93:1030–1038
28. Mineshita M, Kida H, Handa H, Nishine H, Furuya N, Nobuyama S, Inoue T, Matsuoka S, Miyazawa T (2014) The correlation between lung sound distribution and pulmonary function in COPD patients. PLoS One 9(9):e107506
29. Oliveira A, Sen I, Kahya YP, Afreixo V, Marques A (2016) Computerised respiratory sounds can differentiate smokers and non-smokers. J Clin Monit Comput:1–10
30. Piirila P, Sovijarvi ARA, Kaisla T, Rajala H-M, Katila T (1991) Crackles in patients with fibrosing alveolitis, bronchiectasis, COPD, and heart failure. Chest 99(5):1076–1083
31. Schreur HJ, Diamant Z, Vanderschoot J, Zwinderman AH, Dijkman JH, Sterk PJ (1996) Lung sounds during allergen-induced asthmatic responses in patients with asthma. Am J Respir Crit Care Med 153(5):1474–1480
32. Ono H, Taniguchi Y, Shinoda K, Sakamoto T, Kudoh S, Gemma A (2009) Evaluation of the usefulness of spectral analysis of inspiratory lung sounds recorded with phonopneumography in patients with interstitial pneumonia. J Nippon Med Sch 76(2):67–75
33. Piirila P, Lehtola H, Zitting A, Kivisaari L, Koskinen H, Luukkonen R, Salo SP, Vehmas T, Nordman H, Sovijarvi ARA (2000) Lung sounds in asbestos induced pulmonary disorders. Eur Respir J 16(5):901–908

34. Fiz JA, Jane R, Salvatella D, Izquierdo J, Lores L, Caminal P, Morera J (1999) Analysis of tracheal sounds during forced exhalation in asthma patients and normal subjects: bronchodilator response effect. Chest 116(3):633–638
35. Dosani R, Kraman SS (1983) Lung sound intensity variability in normal men. A contour phonopneumographic study. Chest 83(4):628–631
36. O'Donnell DM, Kraman SS (1982) Vesicular lung sound amplitude mapping by automated flow-gated phonopneumography. J Appl Physiol Respir Environ Exerc Physiol 53(3):603–609
37. Ploysongsang Y, Martin RR, Ross WRD, Loudon RG, Macklem PT (1977) Breath sounds and regional ventilation. Am Rev Respir Dis 116:187–199
38. Kraman SS (1983) Lung sounds - relative sites of origin and comparative amplitudes in normal subjects. Lung 161(1):57–64
39. Schreur HJ, Vanderschoot J, Zwinderman AH, Dijkman JH, Sterk PJ (1995) The effect of methacholine-induced acute airway narrowing on lung sounds in normal and asthmatic subjects. Eur Respir J 8(2):257–265
40. Schreur HJW, Vanderschoot J, Zwinderman AH, Dijkman JH, Sterk PJ (1994) Abnormal lung sounds in patients with asthma during episodes with normal lung function. Chest 106(1):91–99
41. Ishimatsu A, Nakano H, Nogami H, Yoshida M, Iwanaga T, Hoshino T (2015) Breath sound intensity during tidal breathing in COPD patients. Internal medicine (Tokyo, Japan) 54(10):1183–1191
42. Schreur H, Sterk P, Vanderschoot J, Klink H, Vollenhoven E, Dijkman J (1992) Lung sound intensity in patients with emphysema and in normal subjects at standardised airflows. Thorax 47(9):674–679
43. Nath AR, Capel LH (1974) Inspiratory crackles and mechanical events of breathing. Thorax 29(6):695–698
44. Forgacs P (1967) Crackles and wheezes. Lancet 2(7508):203–205
45. Forgacs P (1978) Lung Sounds. Bailliere Tindall, London
46. Fredberg JJ, Holford SK (1983) Discrete lung sounds: crackles (rales) as stress-relaxation quadrupoles. J Acoust Soc Am 73(3):1036–1046
47. Piirila P, Sovijarvi ARA (1995) Crackles: recording, analysis and clinical significance. Eur Respir J 8(12):2139–2148
48. Kiyokawa H, Geenberg M, Shirota K, Pasterkamp H (2001) Auditory detection of simulated crackles in breath sounds. Chest 119:1886–1892
49. Vyshedskiy A, Alhashem RM, Paciej R, Ebril M, Rudman I, Fredberg JJ, Murphy R (2009) Mechanism of inspiratory and expiratory crackles. Chest 135(1):156–164
50. Baughman RP, Shipley RT, Loudon RG, Lower EE (1991) Crackles in interstitial lung disease. Comparison of sarcoidosis and fibrosing alveolitis. Chest 100(1):96–101
51. Nath AR, Capel LH (1974) Inspiratory crackles - early and late. Thorax 29(2):223–227
52. Kompis M, Pasterkamp H, Wodicka GR (2001) Acoustic imaging of the human chest. Chest 120(4):1309–1321
53. Workum P, Holford SK, Delbono EA, Murphy RL (1982) The prevalence and character of crackles (rales) in young women without significant lung disease. Am Rev Respir Dis 126(5):921–923
54. Thacker RE, Kraman SS (1982) The prevalence of auscultatory crackles in subjects without lung disease. Chest 81(6):672–674
55. Bettencourt PE, Del Bono EA, Spiegelman D, Hertzmark E, Murphy RL Jr (1994) Clinical utility of chest auscultation in common pulmonary diseases. Am J Respir Crit Care Med 150(5 Pt 1):1291–1297
56. Murphy RLH, Vyshedskiy A, Power-Charnitsky V-A, Bana DS, Marinelli PM, Wong-Tse A, Paciej R (2004) Automated lung sound analysis in patients with pneumonia. Respir Care 49(12):1490–1497
57. Murphy RLH (2008) In defense of the stethoscope. Respir Care 53(3):355–369
58. Jacome C, Oliveira A, Marques A (2015) Computerized respiratory sounds: a comparison between patients with stable and exacerbated COPD. Clin Respir J. https://doi.org/10.1111/crj.12392

59. Munakata M, Ukita H, Doi I, Ohtsuka Y, Masaki Y, Homma Y, Kawakami Y (1991) Spectral and waveform characteristics of fine and coarse crackles. Thorax 46(9):651–657
60. Marques A, Bruton A, Barney A, Hall A (2012) Are crackles an appropriate outcome measure for airway clearance therapy? Respir Care 57(9):1468–1475
61. Ponte DF, Moraes R, Hizume DC, Alencar AM (2013) Characterization of crackles from patients with fibrosis, heart failure and pneumonia. Med Eng Phys 35(4):448–456
62. Gurung A, Scrafford CG, Tielsch JM, Levine OS, Check W (2011) Computerized lung sound analysis as diagnostic aid for the detection of abnormal lung sounds: a systematic review and meta-analysis. Respir Med 105(9):1396–1403
63. Morillo DS, Leon Jimenez A, Moreno SA (2013) Computer-aided diagnosis of pneumonia in patients with chronic obstructive pulmonary disease. J Am Med Inform Assoc 20(e1):2012–001171
64. Piirila P (1992) Changes in crackle characteristics during the clinical course of pneumonia. Chest 102(1):176–183
65. Sánchez Morillo D, Astorga Moreno S, Fernández Granero MÁ, León Jiménez A (2013) Computerized analysis of respiratory sounds during COPD exacerbations. Comput Biol Med 43(7):914–921
66. Wang Z, Xiong YX (2012) Lung sound patterns help to distinguish congestive heart failure, chronic obstructive pulmonary disease, and asthma exacerbations. Acad Emerg Med 19(1):79–84
67. Shirai F, Kudoh S, Shibuya A, Sada K, Mikami R (1981) Crackles in asbestos workers: auscultation and lung sound analysis. Br J Dis Chest 75(4):386–396
68. Urquhart RB, McGhee J, Macleod JES, Banham SW, Moran F (1981) The diagnostic value of pulmonary sounds: a preliminary study by computer-aided analysis. Comput Biol Med 11(3):129–139
69. Beck R, Elias N, Shoval S, Tov N, Talmon G, Godfrey S, Bentur L (2007) Computerized acoustic assessment of treatment efficacy of nebulized epinephrine and albuterol in RSV bronchiolitis. BMC Pediatr 7(22):1–6
70. Marques A, Oliveira A, Jacome C (2014) Computerized adventitious respiratory sounds as outcome measures for respiratory therapy: a systematic review. Respir Care 59(5):765–776. https://doi.org/10.4187/respcare.02765
71. Hoevers J, Loudon RG (1990) Measuring crackles. Chest 98(5):1240–1243
72. Epler GR, Carrington CB, Gaensler EA (1978) Crackles (rales) in the interstitial pulmonary diseases. Chest 73(3):333–339
73. Sovijarvi AR, Piirila P, Luukkonen R (1996) Separation of pulmonary disorders with two-dimensional discriminant analysis of crackles. Clin Physiol 16(2):171–181
74. Workum P, DelBono EA, Holford SK, Murphy RLH Jr (1986) Observer agreement, chest auscultation, and crackles in asbestos-exposed workers. Chest 89(1):27–29
75. Murphy RL Jr, Gaensler EA, Holford SK, Del Bono EA, Epler G (1984) Crackles in the early detection of asbestosis. Am Rev Respir Dis 129(3):375–379
76. Al Jarad N, Davies SW, Logan-Sinclair R, Rudd RM (1994) Lung crackle characteristics in patients with asbestosis, asbestos-related pleural disease and left ventricular failure using a time-expanded waveform analysisDOUBLEHYPHENa comparative study. Respir Med 88(1):37–46
77. Deguchi F, Hirakawa S, Gotoh K, Yagi Y, Ohshima S (1993) Prognostic significance of posturally induced crackles. Long-term follow-up of patients after recovery from acute myocardial infarction. Chest 103(5):1457–1462
78. Akasaka K, Konno K, Ono Y, Mue S, Abe C (1975) Acoustical studies on respiratory sounds in asthmatic patients. Tohoku J Exp Med 117(4):323–333
79. Meslier N, Charbonneau G, Racineux JL (1995) Wheezes. Eur Respir J 8(11):1942–1948
80. Beck R, Gavriely N (1990) The reproducibility of forced expiratory wheezes. Am Rev Respir Dis 141(6):1418–1422
81. Grotberg JB, Gavriely N (1989) Flutter in collapsible tubes: a theoretical model of wheezes. J Appl Physiol 66(5):2262–2273

82. Gavriely N, Kelly KB, Grotberg JB, Loring SH (1985) Forced expiratory wheezes are a manifestation of airway flow limitation. J Appl Physiol 62(6):2398–2403
83. Gavriely N, Shee TR, Cugell DW, Grotberg JB (1985) Flutter in flow-limited collapsible tubes: a mechanism for generation of wheezes. J Appl Physiol 66(5):2251–2261
84. Baughman RP, Loudon RG (1985) Lung sound analysis for continuous evaluation of airflow obstruction in asthma. Chest 88(3):364–368
85. Oud M, Dooijes EH, van der Zee JS (2000) Asthmatic airways obstruction assessment based on detailed analysis of respiratory sound spectra. IEEE 47(11):1450–1455
86. Yi GA (2004) A software toolkit for acoustic respiratory analysis. Massachusetts Institute of Technology, Massachusetts
87. Fiz J, Jané R, Homs A, Izquierdo J, García M, Morera J (2002) Detection of wheezing during maximal forced exhalation in patients with obstructed airways. Chest 122(1):186–191
88. Baughman RP, Loudon RG (1984) Quantitation of wheezing in acute asthma. Chest 86(5):718–722
89. Sanchez I, Powell RE, Pasterkamp H (1993) Wheezing and airflow obstruction during methacholine challenge in children with cystic fibrosis and in normal children. Am Rev Respir Dis 147(3):705–709
90. Bentur L, Beck R, Shinawi M, Naveh T, Gavriely N (2003) Wheeze monitoring in children for assessment of nocturnal asthma and response to therapy. Eur Respir J 21(4):621–626
91. Bentur L, Beck R, Berkowitz D, Hasanin J, Berger I, Elias N, Gavriely N (2004) Adenosine bronchial provocation with computerized wheeze detection in young infants with prolonged cough: correlation with long-term follow-up. Chest 126(4):1060–1065
92. Baughman RP, Loudon RG (1988) The utility of the estimated Tw/Ttot in evaluating a long acting sympathomimetic agent used for nocturnal asthma. Ann R Chron 5:157–160
93. Cortes S, Jane R, Fiz JA, Morera J (2005) Monitoring of wheeze duration during spontaneous respiration in asthmatic patients. Conf Proc IEEE Eng Med Biol Soc 6:6141–6144
94. Fiz JA, Jane R, Izquierdo J, Homs A, Garcia MA, Gomez R, Monso E, Morera J (2006) Analysis of forced wheezes in asthma patients. Respiration 73(1):55–60
95. Jacome C, Marques A (2015) Computerized respiratory sounds in patients with COPD: a systematic review. COPD 12(1):104–112. https://doi.org/10.3109/15412555.2014.908832
96. Seemungal TA, Donaldson GC, Bhowmik A, Jeffries DJ, Wedzicha JA (2000) Time course and recovery of exacerbations in patients with chronic obstructive pulmonary disease. Am J Respir Crit Care Med 161(5):1608–1613
97. Oliveira A, Pinho C, Dinis J, Oliveira D, Marques A (2013) Automatic wheeze detection and lung function evaluation: a preliminary study. In: Stacey D, Solé-Casals J, Fred A, Gamboa H (eds) Healthinf - 6th International Conference on Health Informatics, Barcelona, pp 323–326
98. Dinis J, Oliveira A, Pinho C, Campos G, Rodrigues J, Marques A (2013) Automatic wheeze and respiratory phase detectors to evaluate respiratory physiotherapy in LRTI: a preliminary study. In: Stacey D, Solé-Casals J, Fred A, Gamboa H (eds) Healthinf - 6th International Conference on Health Informatics, Barcelona, pp 233–238
99. Postiaux G, Louis J, Labasse HC, Gerroldt J, Kotik AC, Lemuhot A, Patte C (2011) Evaluation of an alternative chest physiotherapy method in infants with respiratory syncytial virus bronchiolitis. Respir Care 56(7):989–994
100. Gomes EL, Postiaux G, Medeiros DR, Monteiro KK, Sampaio LM, Costa D (2012) Chest physical therapy is effective in reducing the clinical score in bronchiolitis: randomized controlled trial. Rev Bras Fisioter 16(3):241–247
101. Paciej R, Vyshedskiy A, Bana D, Murphy R (2004) Squawks in pneumonia. Thorax 59(2):177–178
102. Pasterkamp H, Brand PL, Everard M, Garcia-Marcos L, Melbye H, Priftis KN (2016) Towards the standardisation of lung sound nomenclature. Eur Respir J 47(3):724–732
103. Charbonneau G, Ademovic E, Cheetham B, Malmberg L, Vanderschoot J, Sovijärvi A (2000) Basic techniques for respiratory sound analysis. Eur Respir Rev 10(77):625–635

11 Wheezing as a Respiratory Sound

Grigorios Chatziparasidis, Kostas N. Priftis, and Andrew Bush

The auscultation of breathing sounds dates back to the years of Hippocrates and was revolutionized after the invention of the stethoscope by Läennec in 1816. Wheezing was amongst the five different types of respiratory sounds described by Läennec. His original description was "the whistling of little birds". Interestingly, whereas the roentgenogram when discovered verified the accuracy of the stethoscopic findings in many cases, this was not the case for wheeze. Subsequently the value of wheezing as a clinical finding was confirmed by lung function studies, in particular spirometry. It was more a physics-based approach that allowed the understanding of how wheeze is produced and clinical meaning of the noise.

In this chapter, we present an overview of the wheezing as a respiratory sound in the light of lung acoustics, sound analysis, its pathogenesis and clinical importance.

11.1 Wheezing Defined

Wheezing is usually referred to as a musical sound. It is considered to be a high-pitched, continuous noise, often associated with a prolonged expiratory phase [1–3].

"Continuous" in the context of respiratory sound nomenclature means that a sound has a minimum duration of 250 ms [4]. As far as the respiratory phase is concerned, wheezing is usually expiratory, but may also be inspiratory if airway

G. Chatziparasidis · K. N. Priftis (✉)
Children's Respiratory and Allergy Unit, Third Department of Paediatrics, "Attikon" Hospital, National and Kapodistrian University of Athens, Athens, Greece
e-mail: kpriftis@otenet.gr

A. Bush
Imperial College, London, UK

National Heart and Lung Institute, London, UK

Royal Brompton Harefield NHS Foundation Trust, London, UK
e-mail: A.Bush@rbht.nhs.uk

K. N. Priftis et al. (eds.), *Breath Sounds*, https://doi.org/10.1007/978-3-319-71824-8_11

obstruction is severe [5]. In 1977, the American Thoracic Society (ATS) [6] and the Tenth International Conference on Lung Sounds [7] added a new definition to the then nomenclature. According to this, "wheezes" are high-pitched continuous sounds, and low-pitched continuous sounds are to be called "rhonchi". Other investigators have proposed that the term rhonchus should be abandoned and only the term wheeze to be used, further divided into high-pitched or low-pitched wheezes [6, 8].

Despite the efforts to clearly define wheezing over the years, the intra-observer agreement on lung sound terminology is still not good [9, 10].

11.2 Production of Wheeze

11.2.1 A Physics-Based Approach to Wheeze Production

To understand the generation of wheeze, one has to understand basic physiology. Centuries ago, Poiseuille determined the pressure drop of a constant viscosity fluid exhibiting laminar flow through a rigid pipe. Although his work was on moving liquids, the results can also be applied in the gaseous phase.

All moving fluids (liquids and gases) exhibit viscosity, which is a measure of the resistance of a fluid to flow. Knowledge of viscosity is a basic necessity for fluid flow analysis. Fluid friction describes a fluid's internal resistance to movement. The greater the viscosity, the "thicker" the fluid and the more the fluid will resist movement.

When a fluid (e.g. air) flows past a stationary wall, the fluid closer to the wall does not move (Fig. 11.1). A velocity gradient exists, due to adhesive, cohesive and frictional forces. The magnitude of this gradient is characteristic of the fluid. Viscosity is a proportionality constant relating an applied shear stress to the resulting shear

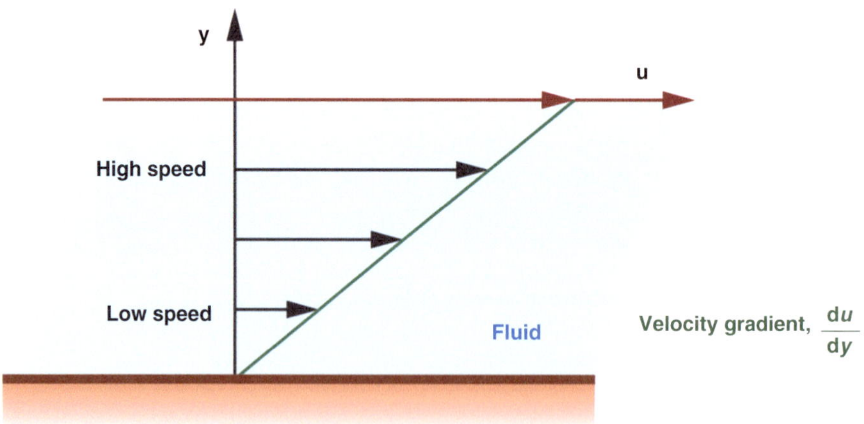

Fig. 11.1 A fluid flows between two plates. A velocity gradient exists, due to adhesive, cohesive and frictional forces. The magnitude of this gradient is characteristic of the fluid (du = flow velocity difference between the layers; dy = instance between the layers)

velocity. When a force is applied to a fluid, creating a shear stress, the fluid will undergo a certain displacement. The viscosity of the fluid is its resistance to this displacement.

In analysing the properties of moving fluids, it is necessary to determine the nature of flow of the fluid. This is generally split into three categories: laminar, turbulent and mixed tubular-laminar flow [11].

11.2.1.1 Laminar Flow

Laminar flow consists of a regular flow pattern with constant flow velocity throughout the fluid volume and is much easier to analyse than turbulent flow.

Laminar flow is often encountered in common hydraulic systems, such as where fluid flow is through an enclosed, rigid pipe; the fluid is Newtonian, namely, incompressible, and has constant viscosity, and the Reynolds number is below the lower critical threshold value.

The Reynolds number is a dimensionless quantity that is used to help predict similar flow patterns in different fluid flow situations. Arnold Sommerfeld named it in 1908 after Osborne Reynolds (1842–1912), who popularized its use in 1883. The Reynolds number [12] is defined as

$$\mathrm{Re} = \rho VL / \mu$$

where ρ is the density of the fluid (SI units, kg/m^3), V is the characteristic velocity of the fluid with respect to the object (m/s), L is a characteristic linear dimension (m), and μ is the dynamic viscosity of the fluid (kg/m s) [11].

Laminar flow is characterized by the flow of a fluid in parallel layers, in which there is no disruption or interaction between the different layers and in which each layer flows at a different velocity along the same direction [13].

The variation in velocity between adjacent parallel layers is due to the viscosity of the fluid and resulting shear forces. Figure 11.2 gives a representation of the relative magnitudes of the velocity vectors of each of these layers for laminar fluid flow through a circular pipe, in a direction parallel to the pipe axis.

Considering laminar flow of a constant density, incompressible fluid travelling in a pipe, with a Reynolds number below the upper limit level for fully laminar flow, the pressure difference between two points along the pipe can be found from the volumetric flow rate, or vice versa. For such a system with a pipe radius of r, fluid viscosity η, distance between the two points along the pipe $\Delta x = x2 - x1$ and the volumetric flow rate Q of the fluid, the pressure difference between the two points along the pipe, Δp, is given by Poiseuille's equation as shown below:

$$\Delta p = 8\eta Q \Delta x / \pi r^4$$

This can be used to determine the pressure drop of a constant viscosity fluid exhibiting laminar flow through a rigid pipe.

This equation is valid for laminar flow of incompressible (Newtonian) fluids in an infinitely long tube only and may be used to determine a number of properties in the hydraulic system, if the others are known or can be measured. In practice,

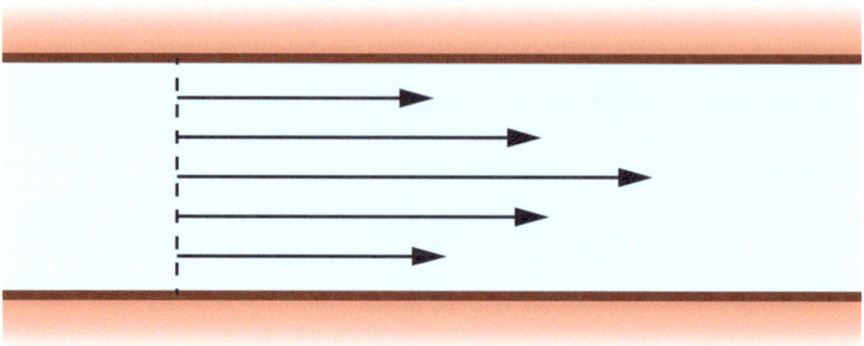

Fig. 11.2 Relative magnitudes of velocity vectors. Laminar fluid flow in a circular pipe at the same direction

Poiseuille's equation holds for most systems involving laminar flow of a fluid, except at regions where features disrupting laminar flow, such as the ends of a pipe or bifurcations are present [14].

11.2.1.2 Turbulent Flow

Turbulent flow is characterized by irregular flow of a fluid in which there are both inconsistent flow patterns and velocity variations throughout the volume of the fluid in motion [11].

Analysis of turbulent flow can be very complex and often requires advanced mathematical analysis to simulate flow in systems on a near case-by-case basis. It occurs when the Reynolds number is above a certain critical threshold (numerically 2000).

11.2.1.3 Mixed Tubular-Laminar Flow

This is the type of flow that is mostly encountered in human airways. It is a combination of laminar and localized turbulent fluid movements referred as *eddies*. Eddies occur where the tube either narrows or branches or where there are irregularities in the tube surface. Its predominance in the bronchial tree is explained by the rapidity with which the airway tree bifurcates [13].

At the lower limit of this mixed turbulent-laminar flow Reynolds number region, there is another critical threshold value, below which only laminar flow is possible (see below).

11.2.1.4 Application of Poiseuille's Equation to the Airflow Along the Tracheobronchial Tree

The production of a respiratory sound necessitates airflow along the airways; despite this fact, it is only turbulent airflow which is capable of producing sounds [15].

The mechanism of sound production in turbulent airflow involves the collision of the air molecules with each other and with the airway walls. This mechanism is in accordance with the Flutter theory initially described by Gavriely [16]. He concluded that the fluttering of both fluid and airway walls produces wheezes, and the flutter velocity depends on the mechanical and physical characteristics of the airway and the gas. The mechanism of flutter can be explained by Bernoulli's principle, which states that when gas flows through a narrow tube at high velocity, it causes a fall in pressure within the airway. This low pressure causes the airway to vibrate.

Turbulence occurs when the Reynolds number exceeds 2000. So, when gas travels through a large-diameter airway at a high velocity, and even more considering the irregular walls of bronchi and trachea, or in a system which branches rapidly, then turbulent flow occurs. This type of flow is completely disorganized and chaotic without a high axial flow velocity.

It is the gas density and not the viscosity that affects the flow properties. Based on this principle, mixing of oxygen with helium generates a lighter gas mixture, reducing turbulent airflow, and may convert turbulent flow to laminar.

The air layers are travelling parallel to the bronchial walls with the central layers moving faster than the peripheral, with little or no transverse flow, as Poiseuille's equation implies.

According to this equation, $Q = \Delta P \cdot n \cdot r^4/8\eta l$, where Q is the volume of flow rate, ΔP is the driving pressure, n is the viscosity, r the radius and l the length of the tube. Since Q is directly proportional to the driving pressure ΔP and the tube radius r, it is obvious that small airways (<2 mm) are not the site of wheeze production [17].

The clinical importance of the result of this equation is that since in the small airways the airflow is laminar (low Reynolds number), it is thus silent. Furthermore, the very low flow rates contribute to the absence of sound production as the total cross-sectional generational airway area is greatly increased.

11.2.2 An "Instrumental" Approach of Wheeze Production

As a general rule, wheeze is produced by the oscillation of opposing airway walls narrowed nearly to the point of closure [18, 19].

Airway oscillation leading to wheeze production requires sufficient airflow; thus, the absence of wheeze in an acute asthma patient represents an ominous sign. This of course is the mechanism underlying the "silent chest" in acute really severe asthma, where impending exhaustion means that very low flows are being generated.

The underlying mechanism of wheeze production involves a constant interaction between the gas moving through the airways and the airway wall. The wheeze is by definition a musical sound, and this has inevitably led to its comparison with wind musical instruments. The sound production in these instruments relates to the oscillations of an air jet (flute) or to the vibration of a reed (clarinet). Furthermore, the pitch of the sound depends upon the length of the air column coupled to the sound source and upon the gas mixture density in the resonating column. In a toy trumpet, a vibrating reed produces the sound [18–20].

Forgacs used the toy trumpet to try to clarify the mechanism of wheeze production. He demonstrated that the pitch of a toy trumpet sound is dependent upon the mass and the elasticity of the reed and independent of the attached horn. He further discovered that high-pitched musical sounds are only produced when the airway calibre is narrowed to the point that the opposite walls are almost in contact. He assumed that it is the acceleration of the gas flow through the narrowed lumen which is responsible for the airway wall oscillation. Thus, three parameters affected the pitch of the wheeze: the flow velocity, the mass and the elasticity of the airway wall. The length and the calibre of the airway have no influence on the sound pitch [20]. So, he contradicted Läennec's suggestion, demonstrating that high-pitched wheezes are not solely produced by peripheral airways and also those low-pitched wheezes not necessarily produced by the more central airways.

In 1980, Grotberg and Davis [21] proposed a new model of wheeze production, analysing mathematically the stability of the airflow as it moves through a collapsible tube. They suggested that the origin of the wheeze production is the fluttering of the fluid and the airway walls together. When the airflow velocity reaches a critical level, called *flutter velocity*, the oscillation begins. This critical level depends on the physical and mechanical features not only of the tube but also of the gas travelling through this tube.

By the late 1980s, this model was perfected by Grotberg and other researchers and is the basis of today's understanding of wheeze production. The new model could predict both the critical flow velocity for the airway wall oscillations and also the oscillation frequency. Furthermore, the model made clear that wheeze is always accompanied by limitation of flow but that flow limitation is not necessarily accompanied by wheezing.

Gavriely and co-workers focused on time and frequency features of breath sounds in ten wheezing patients. The results of their study were in agreement with the Grotberg model [16, 17]. Though revolutionary, the above model could only explain expiratory wheezing, leaving the mechanism of inspiratory wheezes (often associated with more severe obstruction) unclarified.

The Grotberg model of flutter or flattened tube can cast light on the mechanism of wheeze production in diseases like asthma where there is a reduction in the airway calibre or pulmonary oedema where there is a reduction in pulmonary elastance. The model could also be applied in some chronic obstructive lung diseases characterized by a reduction in bronchial stiffness. In all these cases, there is a lower critical flutter velocity, and thus, oscillations of the airway walls will start more easily.

It is worth mentioning that even healthy subjects can produce wheezes during forced expiration [22–24]. These are caused by airflow limitation, but they may also be produced by eddy-induced wall oscillation without underlying airflow limitation. This mechanism fits perfectly in cases of exercise-induced laryngeal obstruction (EILO, also named "vocal cord dysfunction"), where the pathology of the wheeze lies in the larynx and not the bronchial tree.

11.2.3 A Modern Understanding of Wheezing Production

The respiratory system integrates two anatomically different parts: the conducting and the respiratory airways. Trachea, bronchi and bronchioles, the constituents of the conducting airways, differ in architecture. Bronchioles lack the cartilaginous support which is present in the more central airways. As a result, the bronchiolar wall tends to collapse in response to changes in the pressure within the pleural cavity (intrapleural pressure, P_{pl}) or the airway pressure.

During expiration, a pressure is generated in the alveoli (P_{alv}) and transmitted along the airways. As a result of airflow resistance, there is a pressure drop as the air moves towards the mouth during expiration [25, 26]. This phenomenon is known as friction loss. When airway pressure drops to a level where it equals the intrapleural pressure during forced expiration, an equal pressure point (EPP) is reached [27]. If the EPP occurs in the distal airway (not supported by cartilages), the airway will collapse. In case of a healthy lung, the EPP will be reached in cartilaginous airways due to sufficient alveolar driving pressure and the gradual drop in pressure as the airway resistance is minimal [27]. In diseased lung, such as in cases of airway obstruction, resistance to airflow will be much greater and the pressure drop much steeper (Fig. 11.3). The EPP will be reached in the thin-walled bronchioles, causing airway collapse and the typical depression in the flow-volume curve [26, 28].

Being familiar with the EPP theory, researchers attempted to approach the mechanism of wheeze production from a different angle. They used bronchoprovocation and the forced expiratory wheeze manoeuvre to analyse and better clarify this mechanism.

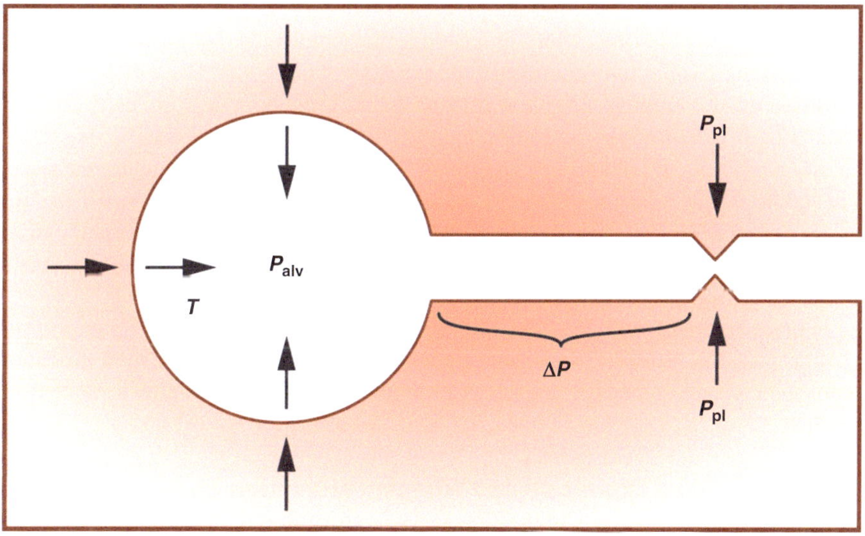

Fig. 11.3 Schematic representation of the respiratory system, enclosed by the intrapleural cavity. Alveolar pressure (P_{alv}) is generated as a result of elastic recoil due to wall tension (T) and intrapleural pressure (P_{pl}). Where the pressure drop (ΔP) over a certain distance from the alveoli equals recoil pressure, an equal pressure point will arise. Cartilaginous airways (on the right side) are barred

11.2.3.1 Bronchoprovocation Tests and Wheeze Production

Since 1990, different groups of investigators started using the computerized lung sound analysis (LSA) to delineate the effects of bronchoconstriction on lung sounds [29, 30].

They all concluded that wheeze was detected by LSA at a much lower PC_{20} or PC_{15} (the provocation concentration of a bronchoconstrictive agent that produces a 20% or 15%, respectively, fall in FEV_1) than that producing symptoms (e.g. cough, subjective wheeze). By analysing the correlation between FEV_1 drop from the baseline and clinically detected wheezing, they found cases where even though the FEV_1 dropped by 55%, wheeze was not detected. This implies that FEV_1 is dependent on the narrowing of many airways, though wheezing on the critical degree of narrowing in a solitary bronchus. In this study, Spence and co-workers tried to establish a relation between the presence of wheeze and the development of symptoms. They found that airflow limitation during tidal breathing preceded the onset of wheezing, and more interestingly, wheezing may not occur at all even though flow limitation patterns were present. The importance of this finding in clinical practice is more than obvious as it disconnects wheezes from symptoms. The researchers put this down to the higher degree of abdominal muscle activation in the wheeze group during the challenge protocol. They concluded that the increase in lung volume is associated with increased abdominal muscle activity and hence a greater force available to deform the airway wall. This could explain the interconnection between abdominal muscle fatigue and silent chest in case of a life-threatening asthma attack [31].

Furthermore, LSA was found to be reliable in wheeze detection even in small children as it requires minimal cooperation rendering the investigation clinically suitable in young children. More interesting, they confirmed that airway narrowing caused an increase in lung sound frequency [32].

Based on this finding, Shreur et al. studied the frequency and intensity of lung sounds both in asthmatics and normal subjects. They induced the same degree of airway narrowing in both groups and found that the asthmatic group wheezed more. This could not be attributed to the airway narrowing alone since that was the same in two groups (at least as judged by spirometry) but also to the morphological changes of the airway walls in asthma. It seems that increased wall thickness enhances airflow limitation even at a similar change of FEV_1 [33].

Is there any difference in the pathogenesis of inspiratory wheeze? Spence et al. [34] proposed that inspiratory wheezing happens when mid and maximal flow rate is reached. On the other hand, expiratory wheeze happens when flow limitation is reached.

11.2.3.2 Forced Expiration and Wheeze Production

Forced expiration is an easy to perform bedside procedure to detect airway narrowing in both asthmatics and normals. It has been used to compare the properties of the airway between stable asthmatics and normal subjects. By recording the lung sounds produced during forced expiration wheeze, researchers came to the conclusion that lung sounds were lower in intensity and higher in pitch in stable asthmatics [35]. When treated with a bronchodilator, there was a greater decrease in forced expiration wheeze in the asthmatic group [36].

Korenbaum and colleagues [37] added more to our understanding of wheeze pathogenesis. They suggested that a forced expiration wheeze duration of more than 1.8 s is a sensitive index of bronchial obstruction. Analysis of the forced expiration wheeze frequency at sequential time domains (time domain is the analysis of physical signals, with respect to time) led Korenbaum to the assumption that forced expiration wheeze may be fitted with a model of vortex shedding in the bronchial tree [38]. In fluid dynamics, vortex shedding is an oscillating flow that takes place when a fluid such as air or water flows past a bluff (as opposed to streamlined) body at certain velocities, depending on the size and shape of the body. In this flow, vortices are created at the back of the body and detach periodically from either side of the body. The fluid flow past the object creates alternating low-pressure vortices on the downstream side of the object. The object will tend to move towards the low-pressure zone. When they used different mixed gases, they found that the vortices inside the trachea or large bronchi were the source of forced expiration wheeze [39].

All previously mentioned studies using forced expiration wheeze as a means of uncovering the mechanism of wheeze production assumed that flow limitation is a prerequisite for generation of the wheeze. They also suggested vortex shedding and airway wall oscillation as possible mechanisms [22, 40, 41].

These suggestions were further supported by the study of Gavriely et al. He used the predictions of five theories of wheeze production and compared them with the spectral shape, mode of appearance and frequency range of wheezes. He concluded that theories of fluid dynamic flutter and vortex-induced wall resonator better matched the experimental observations [16, 17, 42].

He also used a theoretical model simulation based on transmural pressure (P_{tm}) calculations in conjunction with airway opening for four different tube laws (normal, constricted, stiff and floppy), to clarify the mechanism of inspiratory wheeze production. He concluded that intrathoracic wheeze is produced by the same flutter/flow limitation mechanisms as expiratory wheeze.

11.3 Acoustic Characteristics of Wheezes

Over the centuries, medical schools have trained doctors to largely rely on their auditory skills for interpretation of the sounds acquired using the stethoscope. So, the accuracy of the diagnosis goes hand in hand with the doctor's training and experience. Realisation of this fact immediately poses the question "What happens with the junior doctors?" Numerous attempts have been made to turn the "gap" between graduation from medical school and acquisition of experience in a manner that is safe for both doctors and patients. The roots of this effort can be found back in 1977 when Murphy and co-workers [43] managed to depict the acoustic characteristics of wheezing on a screen in the form of waves. By analysing them in the time and frequency domain using a computerized time-expanded waveform analysis, they represented wheezing as a continuous undulating sinusoidal deflection replacing the normal waveform of lung sounds. They used fast Fourier transform (FFT) to describe these sinusoidal deflections in the frequency domain by computing their power spectrum (Fig. 11.4) [16, 17, 44].

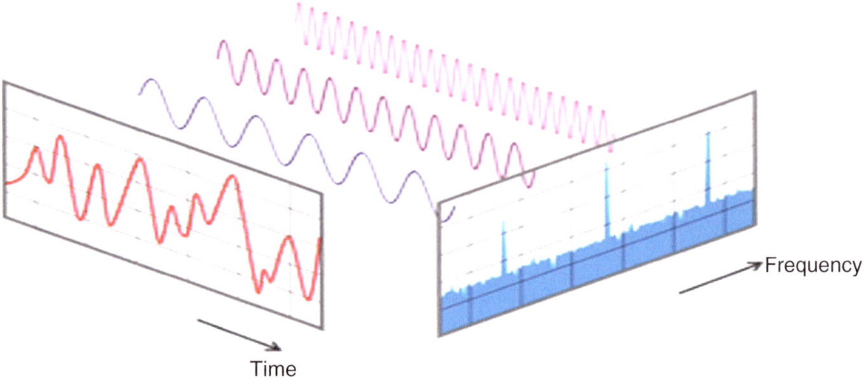

Fig. 11.4 View of a signal in the time and frequency domain (source: Wikipedia)

The fast Fourier transform is a mathematical method for transforming a function of time into a function of frequency. Sometimes it is described as transforming from the time domain to the frequency domain. It is very useful for analysis of time-dependent phenomena. One important application is for the analysis of sound.

Subsequently, Gavriely and Pasterkamp used the same technique and showed that wheezing produce a well-defined small number of peaks in the power spectrum with highly variable frequencies. Since then, the advancement in computer applications has brought a new era in lung sound analysis focusing on assisting doctors in more accurate diagnosis. New methods of spectral analysis facilitate the identification of the patterns of common normal and abnormal lung sounds. Power spectrum, spectrogram and time-expanded waveform analysis are the most popular tools amongst researchers for visual detection of these patterns.

The following sections will try to give a modern insight into the above-mentioned physical phenomena.

Pitch and duration are the main characteristics of wheezes. Their frequency lies between 400 and 1000 Hz. The power spectrum can depict the power distribution of a sound with respect to frequency [45].

Figure 11.4 represents the view of a signal in the time and frequency domain.

Spectrograms are a collective form of a sound power spectrum. They allow the visualization of the spectral information as depicted on an x–y axis system. The y-axis corresponds to frequency and the x-axis to time. This has two advantages; firstly, it provides information regarding the instant at which a frequency occurs. Secondly, it gives a colour representation of the sound amplitude which changes in colour depending on the intensity of the sound at a particular instant.

Figure 11.5 represents the spectrogram of normal breath sounds. It is characterized by a continuous magnitude decay from lower to higher frequencies, and higher spectral components lie in the region lower than 100 Hz [47].

Since wheezes are continuous high-pitched sounds with a frequency greater than 100 Hz and a duration greater than 100 ms, they give a different printout, characterized by harmonics of higher pitch [47].

In practice, there may be a collection of lung sounds and distinguishing between them is easier with the time-expanded waveform analysis (TEWA). In this

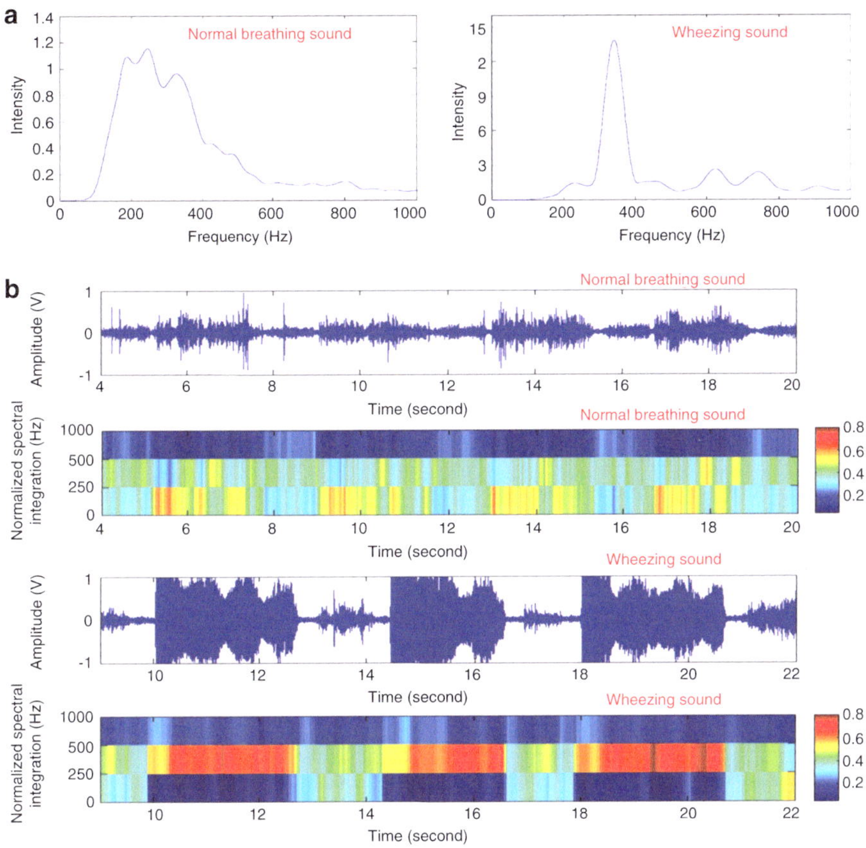

Fig. 11.5 (**a**) Spectrum of wheezing and healthy breathing sounds and (**b**) raw data and feature patterns for wheezy and healthy breathing sounds [46]

technique, the resolution of an acoustic signal is increased so it becomes more detailed by zooming in on the time axis of the waveform. Normal lung sounds present with an irregular shape without any repetitive pattern. In contrast, wheezes have a sinusoidal or more complex periodic waveform. Crackles have initially a sudden short deflection with secondary greater amplitude deflections.

11.4 Wheeze: From Lab to Clinical Application

11.4.1 Large Airway Obstruction and Wheezing

Theoretically, when a lesion affects the calibre of the intrathoracic trachea or main bronchi, the local airflow turns from laminar to turbulent at the point of the narrowing, and the emerging wheezing sound may be well localized over this point. This type of wheeze is classified as monophonic [48].

Monophonic wheezing consists of a single musical note. In terms of the underlying pathology, the obstruction may be from a tumour, an inflammation, a mucus plugging or an endobronchial foreign body. If the obstruction is fixed, the resultant wheezing will be heard in both inspiration and expiration, whereas if the obstruction is dynamic, the wheezing may be either inspiratory or expiratory. Variable obstruction located in the extrathoracic region (trachea) leads to inspiratory monophonic wheeze; variable intrathoracic large airway obstruction leads to expiratory monophonic wheeze. A further clue to the diagnosis is the intensity change with the change in posture, e.g. indicating the presence of a partially obstructing tumour.

11.4.2 Small Airway Obstruction and Wheezing

Pathologies that cause small airway obstruction lead to the generation of high pleural pressure swings in an attempt to maintain normal airway flow. The pitch of the wheeze increases at the end of the expiration as the equal point pressure moves towards the periphery [18, 19].

This causes expiratory compression (inward collapse) of the large airways and generalized expiratory wheezing. This is particularly the case in infants and neonates where the chest wall is more compliant and the large airways are relatively soft and thus very prone to collapse. Because the point of collapse is not fixed, the wheezing sounds consist of multiple musical notes that start and end at the same time. This type of wheeze is termed as polyphonic [48] and can be heard, for example, in cases of asthma and bronchiolitis. Tracheobronchomalacia can produce an identical noise due to dynamic collapse of the malacic airways.

11.5 Wheeze: From Theory to Clinical Practice

11.5.1 What Do Parents Understand by Wheeze?

The term wheeze is widely used by parents during an office/emergency department consultation to describe a diversity of respiratory symptoms in their child. In a hospital-based observational study [49, 50], children aged 4 months to 15 years were assessed in the ED. The aim of the study was to measure the agreement between parental report of wheeze and clinicians' report of the noise. The range of agreement was found to be less than 50%. In detail, when a child presented to ED with alleged wheeze or asthma and the attending physician confirmed the presence of wheeze, 39% of the accompanying parents used words other than wheeze during history taking (mainly difficulty in breathing and/or cough). Moreover, in 14% of cases, parents used the word wheeze to describe upper airway noises in wheeze-free children.

During the same study, clinicians focused on 160 parents attending the outpatient chest clinic due to wheeziness of their child.

Parents were asked: "What do you understand by wheeze, and how do you recognize wheeze in your child?" They answered with a variety of terms like squeaking, rasp, hissing and whistle. More interesting, 25% of the parents did not consider wheeze as a noise, and 49% used nonauditory cues. What does this study reveal? Nothing but the obvious. There are a significant proportion of parents that used wheezing with a very different meaning to that used by clinicians. This study gave rise to much controversy over the accuracy of a number of paediatric epidemiological studies reporting on answers to the question "Has your child wheezed in the past 12 months?" or "Has your child ever wheezed?" or "Has your child asthma symptoms?" It is difficult to believe such studies have any meaning whatever.

More sophisticated studies which involved other lung function tests (LFTs) such as sRaw [51] confirmed the gap between parent- and physician-reported wheeze with the latter being more accurate.

11.5.2 Do Parents Over-/Underestimate the Severity of Wheeze?

In 2004, Lowe and co-workers [51] conducted an observational study measuring the lung function of children with clinician-confirmed wheeze and unconfirmed parent-reported wheeze. The study was part of a large UK birth cohort (n = 1000) and focused on a subgroup of 454 children followed to the age of 3 years. Forty-one percent of these children had parent-reported wheeze, and 29% had their wheeze confirmed by a clinician. At the age of 3 years, the children had their specific airway resistance (sRaw) measured by plethysmography. sRaw was significantly higher in children with clinician-confirmed wheeze, compared with children who had never wheezed and those with parent-reported wheeze.

The use of video questionnaire (VQ) as a mean of better communication between parents and doctors has been evaluated over the previous decade. Saglani et al. used a VQ to present four clips (wheeze, stridor and two other upper respiratory noises) to the parents of preschool children with reported wheeze. The children underwent fibre-optic bronchoscopy for clinical investigation of troublesome noisy breathing. The VQ helped parents who previously thought their child has wheeze to identify a noise other than wheeze. The noise generated from an upper airway abnormality [52].

In another study, five clinicians agreed on ten video clips of children with audible breathing. These responses were the "gold standard". The clips were shown to parents of children (a) with asthma/wheeze, (b) with other respiratory complaints and (c) without respiratory complaints. Parents were asked what they called the sounds, where they originated, and whether their own child made similar sounds. The authors concluded that with the use of VQ, parents locate sounds better than describing them. At least 30% of all parents use other words for wheeze, and 30% labelled other sounds as "wheeze". This could have important clinical implications [50].

11.6 Wheeze in the Era of Modern Technology

Computerized respiratory sound analysis (CORSA) has brought a new approach to detection and analysis of normal and adventitious lung sounds in both children and adults with asthma-related wheeze [45, 53].

It has been also used to monitor their response to treatment [54–57].

CORSA has the advantage of better compliance with objective definition criteria of lung sounds [53], along with a reduced interobserver variability [56–59].

It has also been used to quantify nocturnal wheeze with success [60, 61]. Bentur et al. investigated the usefulness of nocturnal wheeze monitoring and quantification for assessment of asthma activity in symptomatic school-aged children before and during treatment. They concluded that wheeze monitoring provides quantitative and most of all noninvasive information about the extent of nocturnal wheezing, has a good correlation with conventional indices of asthma activity and assists in assessment of treatment efficacy [62].

For decades, physicians relied on lung function tests (LFTs) as a means to diagnose airway obstruction. This practice is only applicable in a research context in infants and neonates where more complicated techniques such as the raised volume rapid thoracoabdominal compression technique has to be applied. CORSA could overcome this obstacle as it can easily measure bronchial responsiveness [63] and monitor the progression of obstructive airway disease even from birth.

Until recently, there were no evidence-based studies to support the safe use of CORSA in daily practice in small infants. In 2016, Fischer et al. [64] used the "Pulmo Track" CORSA device as a means for recording LFTs in infants recovering in the neonatal intensive care unit. They found good correlation between automatically detected wheeze and increased resistance indices.

Their findings could change our approach to wheeze detection in uncooperative patients since CORSA is (a) more reliable than parental reported wheeze [65] and auscultation findings of experienced physicians [45, 56], (b) less time consuming and less costly than conventional infant LFTs, (c) does not require sedation [65–67] and can be performed outside a specialized LFT unit.

In this case, any concerns regarding the interference of ambient sounds with the CORSA recordings, successfully addressed by studies reporting of CORSA use in the noisy environment of a paediatric intensive care unit [56].

Computerized acoustic assessment of lung sounds has also been used for objectively differentiating between wheeze and ruttles [68] and also to assess treatment efficacy of nebulized epinephrine and albuterol in RSV bronchiolitis [69].

Jacome et al. studied 13 adult patients with COPD and 14 with an acute exacerbation of COPD. During the study, they used computerized respiratory sounds, crackles and wheezes for the diagnosis and monitoring of an acute exacerbation of COPD. The use of CORSA contributed to the objectiveness and accuracy of the clinical findings [70].

11.7 Summary

For centuries, medical professionals have tried to record, define, analyse and typify wheeze by all available means. They managed to expand their knowledge about several aspects of the wheezing sound, and this has helped them to provide better treatment. But there is more to achieve. Incorporation of modern technology into daily medical practice sounds really promising, and its implementation may simplify the accurate diagnosis of wheeze and lead to a faster symptom-oriented treatment.

References

1. Mellis C (2009) Respiratory noises: how useful are they clinically? Pediatr Clin N Am 56:1–17
2. Grigg J, Silverman M (2006) Wheezing disorders in young children: one disease or several phenotypes? In: Frey U, Gerritsen J (eds) Respiratory diseases in infants and children, vol 37. The European Respiratory Soceity, Sheffield, UK, pp 153–169
3. Brand PL, Baraldi E, Bisgaard H, Boner AL, Castro-Rodriguez JA, Custovic A et al (2008) Definition, assessment and treatment of wheezing disorders in preschool children: an evidence-based approach. Eur Respir J 32:1096–1110
4. Meslier N, Charbonneau G, Racineux J (1995) Wheezes. Eur Respir J 8:1942–1948
5. Hull J, Forton J, Thomson AH (2015) Pediatric respiratory medi cine, 2nd edn. Oxford University Press, New York
6. American Thoracic Society Ad Hoc Committee on Pulmonary Nomenclature (1977) Updated nomenclature for membership reaction. ATS News 3:5–6
7. Mikami R, Murao M, Cugell DW, Chretien J, Cole P, Meier-Sydow J et al (1987) International symposium on lung sounds. Synopsis of proceedings. Chest 92:342–345
8. Pasterkamp H, Brand PL, Everard M, Garcia-Marcos L, Melbye H, Priftis KN (2016) Towards the standardisation of lung sound nomenclature. Eur Respir J 47:724–732
9. Pasterkamp H, Montgomery M, Wiebicke W (1987) Nomenclature used by health-care professionals to describe breath sounds in asthma. Chest 92:346–352
10. Melbye H, Garcia-Marcos L, Brand P, Everard M, Priftis K, Pasterkamp H (2016) Wheezes, crackles and rhonchi: simplifying description of lung sounds increases the agreement on their classification: a study of 12 physicians' classification of lung sounds from video recordings. BMJ Open Respir Res 3(1):e000136
11. Sarkar M, Madabhavi I, Niranjan N, Dogra M (2015) Auscultation of the respiratory system. Ann Thorac Med 10:158–168
12. Rott N (1990) Note on the history of the Reynolds number. Annu Rev Fluid Mech 22:1–11
13. Osborne S (2006) Airways resistance and airflow through the tracheobronchial tree. In: Schwartzstein R, Parker MJ (eds) Respiratory physiology, a clinical approach. Lippincott Williams & Wilkins, Philadelphia, p 17–23, 8–168
14. Pfitzner J (1976) Poiseuille and his law. Anaesthesia 31:273–275
15. Forgacs P (1969) Lung sounds. Br J Dis Chest 63:1–12
16. Gavriely N, Palti Y, Alroy G, Grotberg JB (1984a) Measurement and theory of wheezing breath sounds. J Appl Physiol Respir Environ Exerc Physiol 57:481–492
17. Gavriely N, Palti Y, Alroy G, Grotberg JB (1984b) Measurement and theory of wheezing breath sound. J Appl Physiol 57:481–492
18. Forgacs P (1978a) The functional basis of pulmonary sounds. Chest 73:399–405
19. Forgacs P (1978b) Lung sounds. Bailliere Tindall, London
20. Forgacs P (1967) Crackles and wheezes. Lancet 2(7508):203–205
21. Grotberg JB, Davis SH (1980) Fluid-dynamic flapping of a collapsible channel: sound generation and flow limitation. J Biomech 13:219–230
22. Charbonneau G, Sudraud M, Racineux JL, Meslier N, Tuchais E (1987) Forced expirations in normal subjects. Is the shape of the flow rate curve related to existence of a wheeze? Chest 92:825–831
23. Gavriely N, Kelly KB, Grotberg JB, Loring SH (1987) Forced expiratory wheezes are a manifestation of airway flow limitation. J Appl Physiol 62:2398–2403
24. Gavrieli N (1987) Inspiratory wheezes and intrathoracic inspiratory flow limitation. J Appl Physiol 52:1988–1992
25. Boron WF, Boulpaep EL (2012) Mechanics of ventilation. In: Boron WF (ed) Medical physiology. Elsevier Saunders, Philadelphia, PA, pp 637–641
26. Jordanoglou J, Pride NB (1968) Factors determining maximum inspiratory flow and maximum expiratory flow of the lung. Thorax 23:33–37
27. Mead J, Turner JM, Macklem PT, Little JB (1967) Significance of the relationship between lung recoil and maximum expiratory flow. J Appl Physiol 22:95–108

28. Frew AJ, Holgate ST (2009) Respiratory diseases. In: Kumar P, Clark M (eds) Kumar & Clark clinical medicine. Elsevier Saunders, Edinburgh, pp 815–817
29. Anderson K, Aitken S, Carter R, Macleod JES, Moran F (1990) Variation of breath sound and airway caliber induced by histamine challenge. Am Rev Respir Dis 141:1147–1150
30. Beck R, Dickson U, Montgomery MD, Mitchell I (1992) Histamine challenge in young children using computerized lung sound analysis. Chest 102:759–763
31. Spence DPS, Bentley S, Evans DH, Morgan MDL (1992) Effect of methcholine induced bronchosconstriction on the spectral characteristics of breath sounds in asthma. Thorax 47:680–683
32. Malmberg LP, Sovijarvi ARA, Paajanen E, Piirila P, Haahtela T, Katila T (1994) Changes in frequency spectra of breath sounds during histamine challenge test in adult asthmatics and healthy control subjects. Chest 105:122–132
33. Shreur HJW, Vanderschoot J, Zwinderman AH, Dijkman JH, Sterk PJ (1995) The effect of methacholine induced acute airway narrowing on lung sounds in normal and asthmatic subjects. Eur Respir J 8:257–265
34. Spence DP, Graham DR, Jamieson G, Cheetham BM, Calverley PM, Earis JE (1996) The relationship between wheezing and lung mechanics during methacholine-induced bronchoconstriction in asthmatic subjects. Am J Respir Crit Care Med 154:290–294
35. Shreur HJW, Vanderschoot J, Zwinderman AH, Dijkman JH, Sterk PJ (1994) Abnormal lung sounds in patients with asthma during episodes with normal lung function. Chest 106:91–99
36. Fiz JA, Jane R, Salvatella D, Izquierdo J, Lores L, Caminal P et al (1999) Analysis of tracheal sounds during forced exhalation in asthma patients and normal subjects. Chest 116:633–638
37. Pochektova IA, Korenbaum VI (2009). Forced expiratory tracheal noise duration in bronchial obstruction among young men. Numerical description of vesicular and bronchial breath sounds [abstract]. The 34th annual conference of international lung sounds association, Haifa, Israel
38. Korenbaum VI (2009) Statistical simulation of vortex shedding on bronchial tree bifurcations as mechanism of tracheal forced expiratory wheezes origin healthy subjects [abstract]. The 34th annual conference of international lung sounds association, Haifa, Israel
39. Dyachenko A, Korenbaum VI, Tagiltsev A (2011) Measurements of forced expiratory noise over trachea and infrascapular region [abstract]. The 36th annual conference of international lung sounds association, Manchester, UK
40. Gavriely N, Kelly KB, Grotberg JB, Loring SH (1989a) Critical pressure required for generation of forced expiratory wheezes. J Appl Physiol 66:1136–1142
41. Beck R, Gavriely N (1990) The reproducibility of forced expiratory wheezes. Am Rev Respir Dis 141:1418–1422
42. Gavriely N, Shee TR, Cugell DW, Grotberg JB (1989b) Flutter in flow-limited collapsible tubes: a mechanism for generation of wheezes. J Appl Physiol 66:2251–2261
43. Murphy RLH, Holford SK, Knowler WC (1977) Visual lung sound characterization by time-expanded waveform analysis. N Engl J Med 296:968–971
44. Pasterkamp H, Tal A, Leahy F, Fenton R, Chernik V (1985) The effect of anticholinergic treatment on postexertional wheezing in asthma studied by phonopneumography and spirometry. Am Rev Respir Dis 132:16–21
45. Sovijara ARA, Dalmasso F, Vanderschoot J, Malmberg LP, Righini G, Stoneman SAT (2000) Definition of terms for application of respiratory sounds. Eur Respir Rev 10(77):597–610
46. Li S-H, Lin B-S, Tsai C-H, Yang C-T, Lin B-S (2017) Design of wearable breathing sound monitoring system for real-time wheeze detaction. Sensors 17(1):171
47. Riella RJ, Nohama P, Maia JM (2009) Method for automatic detection of wheezing inlung sounds. Braz J Med Biol Res 42:674–684
48. Fakhoury K, Seilheimer D, Hoppin A. Approach to wheezing in children. 2008. http://www.uptodate.com
49. Cane R, Ranganathan S, McKenzie S (2000) What do parents of wheezy children understand by "wheeze"? Arch Dis Child 82:327–332
50. Cane RS, SA MK (2001) Parents' interpretations of children's respiratory symptoms on video. Arch Dis Child 84:31–34

51. Lowe L, Murray C, Martin L et al (2004) Reported versus confirmed wheeze and lungfunction in early life. Arch Dis Child 89:540–543
52. Saglani S, McKenzie SA, Bush A, Payne DN (2005) A video questionnaire identifies upper airway abnormalities in preschool children with reported wheeze. Arch Dis Child 90:961–964
53. Kiyokawa H, Greenberg M, Shirota K, Pasterkamp H (2006) Auditory detection of simulated crackles in breath sounds. Chest 119:1886–1892
54. Bahoura M (1999) Analyse des signaux acoustiques respiratoires: contribution a'ladetection automatique des sibilants par paquets d'ondelettes. PhD thesis Univ, Univ. Rouen, France
55. Chuah JS, Moussavi ZK (2004) Automated respiratory phase detection by acoustic means. University of Manitoba Dept of Electrical and Computer Engineering
56. Earis JE, Cheetham BM (2000) Future perspectives for respiratory sound research. Techniques for respiratory sound analysis. Eur Respir Rev 10:636–640
57. Sestini P, Renzoni E, Rossi M, Beltrami V, Vagliasindi M (1995) Multimedia presentation of lung sounds as a learning aid for medical students. Eur Respir J 8:783–788
58. Pasterkamp H, Kraman SS, Wodicka GR (1997) Respiratory sounds, advances beyond the stethoscope. Am J Respir Crit Care Med 156(3 Pt 1):974–987
59. Elphick HE, Sherlock P, Foxall G, Simpson EJ, Shiell NA, Primhak RA et al (2001) Survey of respiratory sounds in infants. Arch Dis Child 84:35–39
60. Rossi M, Sovijarvi AR, Piirila P, Vannuccini L, Dalmasso F, Vanderschoot J (2000) Environmental and subject conditions and breathing manœuvres for respiratory sound recordings. Eur Respir Rev 10:611–615
61. Vanuccini L, Earis JE, Helisto P, Cheetham BM, Rossi M, Sovijarvi AR et al (2000) Capturing and preprocessing of respiratory sounds. Eur Respir Rev 10:616–620
62. Bentur L, Beck R, Shinawi M, Naveh T, Gavriely N (2003) Wheeze monitoring in children for assessment of nocturnal asthma and response to therapy. Eur Respir J 21:621–626
63. Welsby PD, Parry G, Smith D (2003) The stethoscope: some preliminary investigations. Postgrad Med J 79(938):695–698
64. Fischer HS, Puder LC, Wilitzki S, Usemann J, Bührer C, Godfrey S et al (2016) Relationship between computerized wheeze detection and lung function parameters in young infants. Pediatr Pulmonol 51:402–410
65. Kompis M, Pasterkamp H, Wodicka GR (2001) Acoustic imaging of the human chest. Chest 120:1309–1321
66. Mazic J, Sovilj S, Magjarevic R (2003) Analysis of respiratory sounds in asthmatic infants. Meas Sci Rev 3:11–21
67. Benedetto G, Dalmasso F, Spagnolo R (1988) Surface distribution of crackles sounds. IEEE Trans Biomed Eng 35:406–412
68. Elphick HE, Ritson S, Rodgers H, Everard ML (2000) When a "wheeze" is not a wheeze: acoustic analysis of breath sounds in infants. Eur Respir J 16:593–597
69. Beck R, Elias N, Shoval S, Tov N, Talmon G, Godfrey S, Bentur L (2007) Computerized acoustic assessment of treatment efficacy of nebulized epinephrine and albuterol in RSV bronchiolitis. BMC Pediatr 7:22
70. Jácome C, Oliveira A, Marques A (2017) Computerized respiratory sounds: a comparison between patients with stable and exacerbated COPD. Clin Respir J 11(5):612–620

Crackles and Other Lung Sounds

12

Konstantinos Douros, Vasilis Grammeniatis, and Ioanna Loukou

12.1 Introduction

The auscultation of the respiratory system is one of the oldest diagnostic techniques for bronchopulmonary ailments, going back to the time of Hippocrates who advocated the method of applying the ear directly to the chest in order to detect the accumulation of fluid within the pleural space [1]. However, it was the invention of stethoscope in 1816 by Rene Theophile Laënnec that made this technique comfortable for patients and physicians; auscultation has since remained an important part of medical culture. Effective chest auscultation is a skill that depends greatly on the training and experience of physicians; when efficiently mastered, it allows physicians to gain easily, quickly, and inexpensively a wealth of information on diagnosing and observing different types of pulmonary diseases. Nevertheless, with the advance of technology and the now widely available imaging and laboratory procedures that can detect lung diseases with an accuracy never dreamed before, the art of auscultation has started to fade and lose its primary importance and often is performed "as a bedside ritual, in deference to tradition" [2]. To make things worse, there is an actual difficulty to describe in words a sensory experience and convey its essence in a way conceivable by others. Indeed, trained physicians tend to disagree over the use of basic descriptors such as coarse, low pitched, etc. when they listen to recorded respiratory sounds [3, 4]. These semantic ambiguities become more evident when more than one language is involved and remain a major obstacle in developing an effective communication language between health professionals. Fortunately, modern automated computerized methods of signal processing and analysis of lung sounds have provided us with valuable tools to standardize

K. Douros (✉) · V. Grammeniatis
Pediatric Allergy and Respiratory Unit, Third Department of Pediatrics, "Attikon" Hospital, University of Athens School of Medicine, Athens, Greece

I. Loukou
Cystic Fibrosis Unit, "Aghia Sophia" Children's Hospital, Athens, Greece

K. N. Priftis et al. (eds.), *Breath Sounds*, https://doi.org/10.1007/978-3-319-71824-8_12

terminology and improve our knowledge on the correlations between lung sounds' physical characteristics and the underlying pathology.

In this review we will attempt to summarize what is known about crackles—which constitute one of the most frequently encountered type of adventitious lung sounds—and discuss some of the controversies and misunderstandings surrounding this term. In addition, we will also discuss in less detail some of the other less common adventitious lung sounds.

12.2 Crackles

12.2.1 Definition and Auscultation of Crackles

Crackles are discrete, discontinuous, short-lived, explosive, and nonmusical adventitious lung sounds emitted from lung parenchyma during inspiration and sometimes during expiration, in the course of various pathological situations [2]. They are classified as fine or coarse depending on their frequency and duration. Fine crackles have high frequency and short duration, whereas coarse crackles have lower frequency and longer duration. The timing of crackles in the respiratory cycle is another important characteristic; crackles may appear in early, mid-, or end-inspiration or end-expiration [5]. Fine crackles are usually heard during mid-to-late inspiration and repeat in similar patterns over subsequent breaths, are more easily recognized in dependent lung regions, remain uninfluenced by coughing, but may alter with body position change [6, 7]. Fine crackles have a characteristic sound that is similar to the sound produced when two Velcro strips are gently separated. It has been suggested that the detection of Velcro-like crackles should be considered as a meaningful option for the early diagnosis of IPF [8–10]. Coarse crackles are usually found in early inspiration and occasionally in expiration; they have a "popping" quality and tend to be less reproducible from breath to breath [6, 7].

The term "crepitations" is widely used in English and some other European languages to describe crackling sounds, and the two terms are often used interchangeably. Originally, Laënnec had used the term crepitations to describe the sounds felt to resemble those created by agitating a container of moderately heated salt. Both crepitations and crackles refer to brief, nonmusical, discontinuous sounds. Potential confusion may arise when the qualifier "coarse" is added, since "crepitations," at least in the English language, more typically refers to fine crackles, e.g., bone crepitus in fractures [11].

In the past, crackles were commonly—but quite speculatively—believed to be caused by the moving and bubbling of intraluminal secretions. The repetitive nature of crackles in consecutive inspirations and their persistence after coughing contradict this theory [2, 5, 12]. Occasionally however, low-pitched, interrupted, quasi-musical sounds (rhonchi), generated by the movement of air through secretions with successive rupture of fluid menisci, can be confused with crackles [11]. The confusion has to be attributed to human's ear imperfect ability to detect and discriminate between sounds with similar waveforms, especially if they are of low amplitude [13, 14].

Crackle frequency ranges between 60 Hz and 2 kHz with the major contribution being from the range of 60 Hz–1.2 kHz [15]. Crackle's pitch tends to progressively increase during inspiration and to progressively decrease during expiration [16]. It has to be mentioned that in frequencies below 1 kHz, and especially below 500 Hz, the sensitivity of the ear falls sharply [5].

By definition, continuous lung sounds last for 250 ms or more, whereas discontinuous sounds last for 25 ms or less. Crackles are typically less than 20 ms in duration [7]. Human's ear ability to detect crackles during auscultation depends on the relative loudness and the duration of the sound. In case of very short intervals interposed between two discrete sounds, there is difficulty in hearing them distinctively. The minimum time interval that should separate two sounds in order to be heard clearly is not constant but depends on the frequency composition and intensity of the two individual sounds. Moreover, after a sound of high intensity, the hearing sense may get fatigued and fail to realize a second sound that follows shortly after the first one [5].

Stethoscope is an invaluable piece of medical equipment for listening and recognizing lung sounds, but it has some disadvantages. Multiple brands are available, but their frequency responses vary greatly depending on the kind of stethoscope [17]. All types of stethoscopes considerably attenuate all sound frequencies in a nonuniform way (Piirila and Sovijarvi [5]). Attenuation is greater with higher-frequency sounds [18]. There is no clear evidence on which stethoscope is better, and selection mostly relies on price and popularity, though there is no clear correlation between higher pay and better performance [19]. Noise contamination is a pragmatic problem encountered by physicians when they auscultate patients in busy clinical settings. Lung sounds can be covered or heard corrupted by environmental sounds. Furthermore, when pediatric auscultation is considered, almost inevitable sources of noise, such as agitation, movement, and cry, add additional difficulty in correctly acquiring and interpreting auscultation findings [20].

12.2.2 Mechanism of Crackle Generation

Forgacs first proposed a legitimate theory on the genesis of crackles [2, 21]. According to his model, small airways collapsed by the lack of aeration during expiration and snap open during inspiration. This explosive sound arises from gas pressure gradient equalization following the sudden opening of the barrier that separates two compartments containing gas with highly different pressures. Opening is the result of the development of a critical pressure gradient at the two sides of the point of closure and/or by radial traction on the airway by the expanding lung. Pressure equalization results in a pressure wave that oscillates the gas column and produces the popping crackling sound. Forgacs likened the production of a crackle with the sound occurring when the cork is removed from a champagne bottle. Expiratory crackles are infrequent, and according to Forgacs' theory, they represent the closing sounds of small airways. In short, each crackle represents an abrupt opening or closing of a single airway. Forgacs' theory has received further support from the study of Nath and Capel, who showed that the individual crackles had a recurrent pattern in consecutive respiratory cycles and occurred at similar inspired volumes and transpulmonary pressures during successive inspirations [12] .

Fredberg and Holford [22] proposed the mathematical model of stress-relaxation quadrupoles, which is also based on the idea of explosive opening of airways. According to their theory, whenever an airway's state changes from close to open (and vice versa), its static elastic stress alters in order to approach a new static equilibrium corresponding to the new state. The transition from one state to another results in vibration of airways' walls. These alterations in airways are propagated via the elastic matrix of lung parenchyma and can be sensed at a distance with a stethoscope as crackles. Fredberg and Holford modeled the changes in elastic stress as point sources (quadrupoles) in an ideal medium (homogeneous, lossless, linearly elastic, nondispersive continuum of infinite extent). This new hypothesis focuses solely upon the dynamical events that occur in and near the airway wall and considers the vibration in the walls of small airways, and not the vibration of air column within the airways, as the source of crackles. This theory can account for the existence of crackles even in the presence of collateral channels that might prevent development of gas pressure differences across collapsed airways.

Each opening of the airways is followed by its closure during expiration. The transition from a patent to a close state is thought to be a more gradual process than the corresponding transition from close to open because of the presence of surfactant. This lipoprotein complex lowers surface tension at the air-liquid interface reducing attractive forces between hydrogen bonds of water and thus greatly decreasing lung elastic recoil. Given the assumption of less rapid close, the quadrupole model by Fredberg and Holford predicts that the magnitude of the stress anomaly will be smaller upon closure and the corresponding crackle intensities proportionally smaller. Furthermore, the polarity of expiratory crackle waveforms ought to be reversed compared with inspiratory crackles. However, Vyshedskiy et al. [23] showed that airway closure is not a gradual process. In their study, both the temporal and spectral characteristics of expiratory crackles were similar to those of inspiratory crackles. Thus, the events responsible for crackle generation must be as fast in expiration as they are in inspiration. The study also showed that, as it had been predicted in the quadrupole model, the energy of expiratory crackles is substantially smaller than the energy of inspiratory crackles, and hence far fewer expiratory crackles can be detected.

Another interesting theory on the formation of crackles has been based on the hypothesis of liquid bridge formation [24–26]. In some circumstances, when a quantity of liquid is interposed between two solid bodies or in a pipe, a minimized surface of liquid or membrane is created connecting and adding an attractive force between the two bodies or the walls of the pipe. Its formation is the result of the liquid's surface tension acting on the nearby surfaces. Surfactant minimizes surface tension; however, in certain lung diseases, surfactant's properties change allowing the formation of liquid bridges inside the small airways and the blocking of airflow to the alveoli. During a deep breath, the overexpansion of the lung may open these blocked airways by breaking the liquid bridges. The produced sound is perceived as crackles and is the result of acoustical release of the energy that had been stored in the surfaces of liquid bridges prior to their rupture. Correspondingly, the emission of expiratory crackles results from the energy released in the form of acoustic waves during the formation of the liquid bridge [25].

12.2.3 Recording and Analysis of Crackling Sounds

Chest auscultation is an easy and inexpensive method for the evaluation of the respiratory disorders. However, as it has already been mentioned, auscultation performance is affected by a series of factors, and its interpretation is inherently subjective. Computerized lung sound analysis is a means of overcoming many of these issues and enhances our ability to understand the underlying pathology. It involves recording, processing, analysis, and finally classification of lung sounds on the basis of specific signal characteristics. Scientific activity in this field has grown considerably in the last two decades, boosted by advancing technology.

Many different automated systems are nowadays available to identify adventitious sounds [27–29] and describe their morphological features in the time [30, 31] and frequency [32, 33] domain. Unfortunately, most of these techniques are used only for research purposes. Experimental and clinical studies are warranted to determine their potential role in clinical practice [34]. What follows is not a thorough review of the numerous techniques used in lung sound processing but instead is aimed at explaining some of the common acoustical properties of crackles that have been extensively studied with lung sound analysis.

Visually, the timing of crackles in relation to the respiratory cycle is illustrated with a condensed time domain phonopneumogram. Phonopneumographic recordings serve as the basic method in the analysis of crackle sound timing; sound intensity signal is displayed simultaneously with the airflow (or air volume) signal as a function of time. The crackling sounds can be seen as transient peaks in the sound signal. With this mode the amplitude, waveforms, temporal relation of crackles with respiratory cycle and airflow (or volume), number per breath cycle, and duration can all be accurately measured [35]. However, in order to extract detailed information of sound waveforms, a slower playback mode is used where sounds are processed at the desired time-based resolution. The latter technique is called time-expanded waveform analysis (TEWA) and is considered a key tool in characterizing waveforms of crackles. A resolution of 3000 mm/sec is usually recommended [35]. Usually, lung sounds are recorded with high-pass filters in order to attenuate low-frequency components which are generated by muscles, large blood vessels, and the heart [5]. The characteristics of high-pass filtration have long been standardized [36].

The typical appearance of crackles in TEWA is a sudden short deflection followed by deflections of greater amplitude. Crackle amplitude is measured in arbitrary units. Measurable characteristics that are used as criteria in classifying crackles as coarse or fine are the duration of the initial deflection width (IDW), namely, the duration of the first deflection of the crackle and the two-cycle duration (2CD) which is defined as the time from the beginning of IDW up to the completion of two cycles. In each of these two parameters, low or large values correspond to the clinical concept of fine or coarse crackles, respectively. American Thoracic Society's (ATS) classifying criteria are the mean durations of IDW and 2CD for fine crackles 0.7 and 5 ms and for coarse crackles

1.5 and 10 ms, respectively [37]. However, ATS did not provide in the published article a detailed description of the method(s) these recommendations were based on. Computerized respiratory sound analysis (CORSA) project, a European initiative toward standardization of recording, processing, and analysis of lung sounds, proposed its own recommendations for characterizing crackles on the grounds of a standardized technique [38]; authors used only the 2CD duration and defined fine crackles as those having 2CD <10 ms and coarse crackles those with 2CD >10 ms [39].

The initial deflection of a crackle was originally used to characterize its polarity, and the typical pattern for inspiratory and expiratory crackles is to have opposite polarities [33]. In a more recent study, polarity was determined by the highest wave deflection and defined as positive or negative if the highest peak was upward or downward, respectively. Authors maintained that the definition of crackle polarity by the initial wave deflection was highly subjective because the latter is usually very small and sometimes not discernible from the noise floor [23]. In their study, crackles of both positive and negative polarity were observed during inspiration and expiration; however, in the vast majority of cases, there was predominantly negative polarity of inspiratory crackles and predominantly positive polarity of expiratory crackles [23].

Another way to visualize and study crackles is through spectrograms (or sonograms) where time is represented in x-axis and frequency in y-axis, and the intensity of signal is illustrated by a palette of colors. Many methods have been invented to automatically recognize crackles based on spectrogram analysis and extract mathematical information corresponding to specific features of the sounds [40].

There is considerable evidence that crackle rate remains stable and reproducible in a given examining session, but it decreases or increases in accordance with the improvement or deterioration of the disease. Therefore, serially measuring crackles could aid in following the course of illness [41]. Unfortunately, counting crackles with a stethoscope is associated with substantial inter- and intra-observer variability and cannot be used per se. In order to compensate for this limitation, there have been devised computer-based methods that can accurately count crackles and allow longitudinal monitoring of patients [41–43].

Many mathematical tools have been created to analyze lung sounds in general and crackles in particular. Methods, like Fourier transform, short-time Fourier transform, artificial neural network, k-nearest neighbor algorithm, fuzzy logic, wavelet, etc. [27, 44–50], have all been adapted to the special needs of sound analysis. A lot of mathematical algorithms have been designed based on the above methods, for the automatic recognition of crackles. Despite these methods having a substantial contribution in lung sound analysis, their understanding requires a robust mathematical background, and they will not be discussed further in this review.

12.2.4 Clinical Significance of Crackles in Lung Disorders

Clinical history and examination are still the cornerstones of clinical diagnosis, and lung auscultation is an integral part of this procedure. The ease and convenience of auscultation and the value of information it provides make it an indispensable everyday clinical tool. However, one should always bear in mind that failure to detect crackles and poor agreement among observers is not unusual, especially when the auscultation is not performed under ideal conditions [3, 13, 51].

The characteristics of pulmonary crackles, such as timing, number, regional distribution, and especially the distinction between fine and coarse, can all be used in the diagnosis and follow-up of various types of pulmonary diseases such as pneumonia, bronchiectasis, COPD, fibrosing alveolitis, asbestosis, sarcoidosis, etc. [5, 6]. In idiopathic pulmonary fibrosis, fine crackles appear first in the basal areas of the lungs and gradually extend to the upper zones, as the disease progresses. Fine crackles are also found in other interstitial disorders such as asbestosis, nonspecific interstitial pneumonitis, and interstitial fibrosis associated with collagen vascular disorders [6]. Sarcoidosis causes granulomatous lesions, most often in the upper zones of the lungs, but usually no auscultatory findings are present; fine crackles may appear only when the disease has progressed to the point of fibrosis, but even then they tend to be far fewer compared with other fibrotic disorders [5, 52]. In bronchiectasis crackles are coarse, appear early in inspiration, continue to mid-inspiration, and usually fade by the end of inspiration [53]. They have a relatively longer duration because the time required to open bronchiectatic segments is longer. In COPD, there are also rather coarse crackles, but they tend to occur earlier, and their crackling period is shorter compared to bronchiectasis [54].

Crackles are the most commonly found clinical sign in patients with clinically identified—and later radiographically confirmed—pneumonia [55]. In pneumonia, the characteristics of crackles may vary markedly and are associated with the stage of the disease. Some authors argue that crackles tend to change gradually from fine to coarse as the disease progresses from acute stage to resolution [5]. However, a computerized objective sound analysis showed that in the early phase of pneumonia, crackles are coarse and mid-inspiratory, and as the disease improves, they progressively become shorter and end-inspiratory [56].

Acute bronchiolitis is an infectious disease of the lower respiratory tract that occurs primarily in young infants; it is the most common cause of hospitalization and acute respiratory failure at this age [57]. It is characterized by the presence of diffuse fine crackles (especially in the youngest children) and/or wheeze on auscultation [58]. In the United Kingdom, crackles are regarded as the hallmark of bronchiolitis [59].

12.3 Other Lung Sounds

12.3.1 Squawks

Squawks (or squeaks) are short, late inspiratory, musical, wheeze-like sounds that were first described by Laënnec ("cry of a small bird"). Many years later Forgacs observed this auscultatory sign in patients with cryptogenic fibrosing alveolitis [60], and Earis et al. found squawks to be present in the majority of patients with different kinds of interstitial lung disorders [61]. However, squawks are not pathognomonic of these conditions, as they have also been documented in diseases with different pathologies such as bronchiectasis and pneumonia [62]. Usually, squawks occur along with crackles and often are preceded with a crackle. Their duration ranges from 40 ms to 400 ms [14, 47]. Although the mechanism underlying production of squawks is not known, it is believed that they are produced by the oscillation of small airway walls and surrounding tissues in deflated lung zones, as the inspired air rushes in to open them [61] .

12.3.2 Rhonchi

Of all the terms used to describe adventitious lung sounds, and despite being widely used across European languages, rhonchi appear to be the most difficult and ambiguous term resulting in poor observer agreement [11, 51]. Rhonchi denote continuous, low-pitched, snoring-type sounds with a rattling, rumbling, or bubbling quality [4, 37]. They may provide a more liquid acoustic perception compared with either wheezes or crackles, but they could also sound dry [47]. Rhonchi contain rapidly damping periodic waveforms with a duration of >100 ms and frequency of <300 Hz; however, the dominant frequency is below 200 Hz [14, 66]. Occasionally, they may sound similar to wheezes, and therefore may be difficult to distinguish from them. Rhonchi are often considered to be a variant of wheeze, and many physicians prefer to use the term low-pitched wheezes instead of rhonchi [6, 51]. The mechanism of rhonchi generation probably shares some common elements with that of wheeze, but the rhonchi, unlike the wheeze, may disappear after coughing, suggesting that secretions play a role. Simply defining rhonchus as a low-pitched wheeze does not take into account conspicuous differences in their waveforms, namely, the pure sinusoidal wave of a low-pitched wheeze in contrast to complex repetitive waves of similar tonal pitch but with rougher and snoring character of rhonchus [11].

12.3.3 Pleural Rub

The pleural friction rub is probably produced when the inflamed facing surfaces of the parietal and visceral pleurae rub against each other during breathing. It is a nonmusical, short, explosive sound, with a creaky or leathery quality. Typically, it is a biphasic sound, with the expiratory component mirroring the inspiratory [63]. It is a highly specific but moderately sensitive sign for the diagnosis of pleural effusion [64, 65]. It has been observed that this sound is more noticeable on auscultation of the basal regions than of the upper regions of the lung, probably because basal regions undergo greater expansion for a given change in transpulmonary pressure [6]. It has a waveform similar to that of crackles but with longer duration and lower frequency [6].

12.4 Concluding Remarks

Considerable research effort has been invested in the last years in the study of adventitious lung sounds. A substantial part of the progress made should be attributed to the advances of technology which provided researchers with a host of very sophisticated methods for digital recording, processing, and analysis of lung sound signals. The waveform characteristics of crackles and other lung sounds can help distinguish one from the other and constitute a useful tool in the diagnosis and follow-up of many pulmonary diseases. However, the use in current clinical practice of such computerized methods of lung sound analysis is not realistic. On the other hand, stethoscope is a handy medical instrument. However, its ease and simplicity of use and the wealth of information it provides make us overlook its technical shortcomings, as well as the limited abilities of human ear in sound perception. In general, we have not yet found the ideal means in terms of ease and accuracy to get the maximum of information from lung sounds. Maybe in the future, as the technology evolves, we will be able to combine the ease of auscultation with advanced high-end digital features to enhance the acquisition of clinically useful information to maximum.

References

1. Hajar R (2012) The art of listening. Heart views: the official journal of the Gulf Heart Association 13(1):24–25. Epub 2012/07/04
2. Forgacs P (1978) The functional basis of pulmonary sounds. Chest 73(3):399–405. Epub 1978/03/01
3. Elphick HE, Lancaster GA, Solis A, Majumdar A, Gupta R, Smyth RL (2004) Validity and reliability of acoustic analysis of respiratory sounds in infants. Arch Dis Child 89(11):1059–1063. Epub 2004/10/23
4. Mikami R, Murao M, Cugell DW, Chretien J, Cole P, Meier-Sydow J et al (1987) International symposium on lung sounds. Synopsis of proceedings Chest 92(2):342–345. Epub 1987/08/01
5. Piirila P, Sovijarvi AR (1995) Crackles: recording, analysis and clinical significance. Eur Respir J 8(12):2139–2148. Epub 1995/12/01
6. Bohadana A, Izbicki G, Kraman SS (2014) Fundamentals of lung auscultation. N Engl J Med 370(8):744–751. Epub 2014/02/21
7. Sarkar M, Madabhavi I, Niranjan N, Dogra M (2015) Auscultation of the respiratory system. Annals of thoracic medicine 10(3):158–168. Epub 2015/08/01
8. Cottin V, Cordier JF (2012) Velcro crackles: the key for early diagnosis of idiopathic pulmonary fibrosis? Eur Respir J 40(3):519–521. Epub 2012/09/04
9. Cottin V, Richeldi L (2014) Neglected evidence in idiopathic pulmonary fibrosis and the importance of early diagnosis and treatment. European respiratory review : an official journal of the European Respiratory Society 23(131):106–110. Epub 2014/03/05
10. Sellares J, Hernandez-Gonzalez F, Lucena CM, Paradela M, Brito-Zeron P, Prieto-Gonzalez S et al (2016) Auscultation of Velcro crackles is associated with usual interstitial pneumonia. Medicine 95(5):e2573. Epub 2016/02/06
11. Pasterkamp H, Brand PL, Everard M, Garcia-Marcos L, Melbye H, Priftis KN (2016) Towards the standardisation of lung sound nomenclature. Eur Respir J 47(3):724–732. Epub 2015/12/10
12. Nath AR, Capel LH (1974) Inspiratory crackles and mechanical events of breathing. Thorax 29(6):695–698. Epub 1974/11/01
13. Kiyokawa H, Greenberg M, Shirota K, Pasterkamp H (2001) Auditory detection of simulated crackles in breath sounds. Chest 119(6):1886–1892. Epub 2001/06/16
14. Reichert S, Gass R, Brandt C, Andres E (2008) Analysis of respiratory sounds: state of the art. Clin Med Circ Respirat Pulm Med 2:45–58. Epub 2008/01/01
15. Abbas A, Fahim A (2010) An automated computerized auscultation and diagnostic system for pulmonary diseases. J Med Syst 34(6):1149–1155. Epub 2009/06/26

16. Vyshedskiy A, Murphy R (2012) Crackle pitch rises progressively during inspiration in pneumonia, CHF, and IPF patients. Pulmonary medicine 2012:240160. Epub 2012/04/25
17. Callahan D, Waugh J, Mathew GA, Granger WM (2007) Stethoscopes: what are we hearing? Biomedical instrumentation & technology / Association for the Advancement of Medical Instrumentation 41(4):318–323. Epub 2007/09/14
18. Grenier MC, Gagnon K, Genest J Jr, Durand J, Durand LG (1998) Clinical comparison of acoustic and electronic stethoscopes and design of a new electronic stethoscope. Am J Cardiol 81(5):653–656. Epub 1998/03/26
19. Mehmood M, Abu Grara HL, Stewart JS, Khasawneh FA (2014) Comparing the auscultatory accuracy of health care professionals using three different brands of stethoscopes on a simulator. Medical devices (Auckland, NZ) 7:273–281. Epub 2014/08/26
20. Emmanouilidou D, Elhilal M 2013 Characterization of noise contaminations in lung sound recordings. In: Conference proceedings: Annual International Conference of the IEEE Engineering in Medicine and Biology Society IEEE Engineering in Medicine and Biology Society Annual Conference, vol 2013. P 2551–4. Epub 2013/10/11
21. Forgacs P (1969) Lung sounds. Br J Dis Chest 63(1):1–12. Epub 1969/01/01
22. Fredberg JJ, Holford SK (1983) Discrete lung sounds: crackles (rales) as stress-relaxation quadrupoles. J Acoust Soc Am 73(3):1036–1046. Epub 1983/03/01
23. Vyshedskiy A, Alhashem RM, Paciej R, Ebril M, Rudman I, Fredberg JJ et al (2009) Mechanism of inspiratory and expiratory crackles. Chest 135(1):156–164. Epub 2008/08/12
24. Alencar AM, Wolfe E Fau - Buldyrev SV, Buldyrev SV Monte Carlo simulation of liquid bridge rupture: application to lung physiology: (1539–3755 (Print))
25. Almeida AB, Buldyrev SV, Alencar AM (2013) Crackling sound generation during the formation of liquid bridges: a lattice gas model. Physica A: Statistical Mechanics and its Applications 392(16):3409–3416
26. Majumdar A, Alencar AM, Buldyrev SV, Hantos Z, Stanley HE, Suki B (2003) Fluid transport in branched structures with temporary closures: a model for quasistatic lung inflation. Physical review E, Statistical, nonlinear, and soft matter physics 67(3 Pt 1):031912. Epub 2003/04/12
27. Mastorocostas PA, Theocharis JB (2007) A dynamic fuzzy neural filter for separation of discontinuous adventitious sounds from vesicular sounds. Comput Biol Med 37(1):60–69. Epub 2005/12/13
28. Tolias YA, Hadjileontiadis LJ, Panas SM (1998) Real-time separation of discontinuous adventitious sounds from vesicular sounds using a fuzzy rule-based filter. IEEE transactions on information technology in biomedicine : a publication of the IEEE Engineering in Medicine and Biology Society 2(3):204–215. Epub 2000/03/17
29. Mastorocostas PA, Tolias YA, Theocharis JB, Hadjileontiadis LJ, Panas SM (2000) An orthogonal least squares-based fuzzy filter for real-time analysis of lung sounds. IEEE Trans Biomed Eng 47(9):1165–1176. Epub 2000/09/29
30. Murphy RL Jr, Holford SK, Knowler WC (1977) Visual lung-sound characterization by time-expanded wave-form analysis. N Engl J Med 296(17):968–971. Epub 1977/04/28
31. al Jarad N, Strickland B, Bothamley G, Lock S, Logan-Sinclair R, Rudd RM (1993) Diagnosis of asbestosis by a time expanded wave form analysis, auscultation and high resolution computed tomography: a comparative study. Thorax 48(4):347–353. Epub 1993/04/01
32. Mori M, Kinoshita K, Morinari H, Shiraishi T, Koike S, Murao S (1980) Waveform and spectral analysis of crackles. Thorax 35(11):843–850. Epub 1980/11/01
33. Munakata M, Ukita H, Doi I, Ohtsuka Y, Masaki Y, Homma Y et al (1991) Spectral and waveform characteristics of fine and coarse crackles. Thorax 46(9):651–657. Epub 1991/09/01
34. Spieth PM, Zhang H (2011) Analyzing lung crackle sounds: stethoscopes and beyond. Intensive Care Med 37(8):1238–1239. Epub 2011/06/30
35. Charbonneau G, Ademovic E, Cheetham B, Malmberg L, Vanderschoot J, Sovijarvi A (2000) Basic techniques for respiratory sound analysis. European Respiatory Review 10:625–635
36. Sovijärvi ARA, Vanderschoot J, Earis J (2000) Computerized respiratory sound analysis (CORSA) recommended standards for terms and techniques. European Respiatory Review 10:585–649

37. ATS (1977) Updated nomenclature for membership reaction. Reports of the ATS-ACCP ad hoc committee. Am Thorac Soc News:5–6
38. Vannuccini L, Earis J, Helistö P, Cheetham B, Rossi M, Sovijärvi A et al (2000) Capturing and preprocessing of respiratory sounds. European Respiatory Review 10(77):616–620
39. Sovijärvi A, Dalmasso F, Vanderschoot J, Malmberg L, Righini G, Stoneman S (2000) Definition of terms for applications of respiratory sounds. European Respiatory Review 10(77):597–610
40. Zhang K, Wang X, Han F, Zhao H (2015) The detection of crackles based on mathematical morphology in spectrogram analysis. Technology and health care : official journal of the European Society for Engineering and Medicine 23(Suppl 2):S489–S494. Epub 2015/09/28
41. Vyshedskiy A, Ishikawa S, Murphy RL Jr (2011) Crackle pitch and rate do not vary significantly during a single automated-auscultation session in patients with pneumonia, congestive heart failure, or interstitial pulmonary fibrosis. Respir Care 56(6):806–817. Epub 2011/02/22
42. Kaisla T, Sovijarvi A, Piirila P, Rajala HM, Haltsonen S, Rosqvist T (1991) Validated method for automatic detection of lung sound crackles. Med Biol Eng Comput 29(5):517–521. Epub 1991/09/01
43. Murphy RL Jr, Del Bono EA, Davidson F (1989) Validation of an automatic crackle (rale) counter. Am Rev Respir Dis 140(4):1017–1020. Epub 1989/10/01
44. Charleston-Villalobos S, Gonzalez-Camarena R, Chi-Lem G, Aljama-Corrales T (2007) Crackle sounds analysis by empirical mode decomposition. Nonlinear and nonstationary signal analysis for distinction of crackles in lung sounds. IEEE engineering in medicine and biology magazine : the quarterly magazine of the Engineering in Medicine & Biology Society 26(1):40–47. Epub 2007/02/07
45. Guler I, Polat H, Ergun U (2005) Combining neural network and genetic algorithm for prediction of lung sounds. J Med Syst 29(3):217–231. Epub 2005/07/30
46. Hadjileontiadis LJ (2005) Wavelet-based enhancement of lung and bowel sounds using fractal dimension thresholding--part II: application results. IEEE Trans Biomed Eng 52(6):1050–1064. Epub 2005/06/28
47. Kandaswamy A, Kumar CS, Ramanathan RP, Jayaraman S, Malmurugan N (2004) Neural classification of lung sounds using wavelet coefficients. Comput Biol Med 34(6):523–537. Epub 2004/07/22
48. Mastorocostas PA, Theocharis JB (2006) A stable learning algorithm for block-diagonal recurrent neural networks: application to the analysis of lung sounds. IEEE Trans Syst Man Cybern B Cybern 36(2):242–254. Epub 2006/04/11
49. Serbes G, Sakar CO, Kahya YP, Aydin N (2011) Feature extraction using time-frequency/scale analysis and ensemble of feature sets for crackle detection. Conference proceedings : Annual International Conference of the IEEE Engineering in Medicine and Biology Society IEEE Engineering in Medicine and Biology Society Annual Conference 2011:3314–3317. Epub 2012/01/19
50. Chen CH, Huang WT, Tan TH, Chang CC, Chang YJ (2015) Using K-Nearest Neighbor Classification to Diagnose Abnormal Lung Sounds. Sensors (Basel, Switzerland) 15(6):13132–13158. Epub 2015/06/09
51. Melbye H, Garcia-Marcos L, Brand P, Everard M, Priftis K, Pasterkamp H (2016) Wheezes, crackles and rhonchi: simplifying description of lung sounds increases the agreement on their classification: a study of 12 physicians' classification of lung sounds from video recordings. BMJ Open Respir Res 3(1):e000136. Epub 2016/05/10
52. Baughman RP, Shipley RT, Loudon RG, Lower EE (1991) Crackles in interstitial lung disease. Comparison of sarcoidosis and fibrosing alveolitis. Chest 100(1):96–101. Epub 1991/07/01
53. Nath AR, Capel LH (1980) Lung crackles in bronchiectasis. Thorax 35(9):694–699. Epub 1980/09/01
54. Piirila P, Sovijarvi AR, Kaisla T, Rajala HM, Katila T (1991) Crackles in patients with fibrosing alveolitis, bronchiectasis, COPD, and heart failure. Chest 99(5):1076–1083. Epub 1991/05/01

55. van Vugt SF, Verheij TJ, de Jong PA, Butler CC, Hood K, Coenen S et al (2013) Diagnosing pneumonia in patients with acute cough: clinical judgment compared to chest radiography. Eur Respir J 42(4):1076–1082. Epub 2013/01/26
56. Piirila P (1992) Changes in crackle characteristics during the clinical course of pneumonia. Chest 102(1):176–183. Epub 1992/07/01
57. Yanney M, Vyas H (2008) The treatment of bronchiolitis. Arch Dis Child 93(9):793–798. Epub 2008/06/10
58. Zorc JJ, Hall CB (2010) Bronchiolitis: recent evidence on diagnosis and management. Pediatrics 125(2):342–349. Epub 2010/01/27
59. Baumer JH (2007) SIGN guideline on bronchiolitis in infants. Archives of disease in childhood Education and practice edition 92(5):ep149–ep151. Epub 2007/09/27
60. Forgacs P (1967) Crackles and wheezes. Lancet (London, England) 2(7508):203–205. Epub 1967/07/22
61. Earis JE, Marsh K, Pearson MG, Ogilvie CM (1982) The inspiratory "squawk" in extrinsic allergic alveolitis and other pulmonary fibroses. Thorax 37(12):923–926. Epub 1982/12/01
62. Paciej R, Vyshedskiy A, Bana D, Murphy R (2004) Squawks in pneumonia. Thorax 59(2):177–178. Epub 2004/02/05
63. Forgacs P (1978) Lung sounds. Baillière Tindall, London
64. Wong CL, Holroyd-Leduc J, Straus SE (2009) Does this patient have a pleural effusion? JAMA 301(3):309–317. Epub 2009/01/22
65. Kalantri S, Joshi R, Lokhande T, Singh A, Morgan M, Colford JM Jr et al (2007) Accuracy and reliability of physical signs in the diagnosis of pleural effusion. Respir Med 101(3):431–438. Epub 2006/09/13
66. Meslier N, Charbonneau G, Racineux JL (1995) Wheezes. Eur Respir J 8(11):1942–1948. Epub 1995/11/01

Suggested Sites with Recordings of Lung Sounds

European Respiratory Society - Reference Database of Respiratory Sounds http://www.ers-education.org/e-learning/reference-database-of-respiratory-sounds/

The R.A.L.E.® Repository – http://www.rale.ca

Respiratory Sounds: Laryngeal Origin Sounds

13

Nicola Barker and Heather Elphick

13.1 Normal Laryngeal Sounds

Laryngeal sounds are primarily generated by turbulent airflow in upper airways, including the pharynx, glottis and trachea. The anatomy of the laryngeal area can be subdivided into the supraglottic, glottic and subglottic regions (Fig. 13.1).

Turbulent flow and jet formation cause pressure fluctuations within the airway lumen. Sound pressure waves within the airway gas and airway wall motion cause vibrations that reach the neck surface and are heard as laryngeal sounds [1]. A linear relationship between tracheal sound and flow has been demonstrated [2, 3], and models for calculation of flow based on sound data have been proposed [4]. Normal laryngeal sounds are characterised as harsh, loud, high-pitched sounds heard over the trachea or lateral neck [5]. The sounds can be generated through both phases of the respiratory cycle. The sound originating from the laryngeal and tracheal areas is broad spectrum, covering a frequency range from less than 100 Hz to 1500 Hz, and can reach up to 4000 Hz [6, 7], compared with the frequency of lung sounds which rarely exceed 2500 Hz. A sharp drop in power above a frequency of approximately 800 Hz (the cut-off frequency) has been described [8]. Pasterkamp and Sanchez analysed tracheal sounds at standardised airflows in children and adults and found a close relationship between the cut-off frequency and body height. Children with shorter tracheal lengths had higher cut-off frequencies than adults [9]. The spectral shape of tracheal sounds is highly variable between subjects but quite reproducible within the same person, reflecting the strong influence of individual airway anatomy [10].

N. Barker · H. Elphick (✉)
Department of Paediatric Respiratory Medicine, Sheffield Children's Hospital, Sheffield, UK
e-mail: Heather.Elphick@sch.nhs.uk

K. N. Priftis et al. (eds.), *Breath Sounds*, https://doi.org/10.1007/978-3-319-71824-8_13

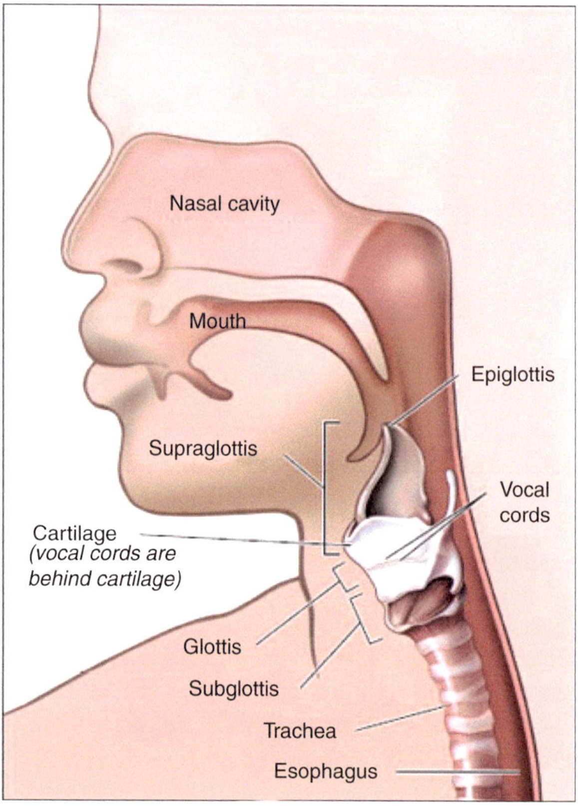

Fig. 13.1 Anatomy of the larynx

Measurements of tracheal sounds provide valuable and in some cases unique information about respiratory health. Apnoea monitoring by simple acoustical detection of tracheal sounds is an obvious application and has been successfully applied in adults and children [11]. Tracheal sound microphones have become incorporated into commercial apnoea monitoring devices. Pasterkamp measured normal tracheal sounds at standardised airflow in awake patients with obstructive sleep apnoea (OSA) and in snorers without OSA. Pharyngeal dynamics appeared to be different in the patients with OSA who showed a significantly greater increase of tracheal sound intensity in the supine position reflecting presumed structural and functional abnormalities in OSA.

Abnormal sounds heard over the neck and trachea can indicate pathologies associated with upper airway obstruction (UAO) in children. Extrathoracic UAO produces an inspiratory stridor, whereas intrathoracic UAO is associated with biphasic or expiratory wheezing sounds. In some cases the anatomical origin of the sound can be identified from the sound, providing diagnostic information. Figure 13.1 provides a reference for identification of pathological causes of the different laryngeal sounds.

13.2 Pathological Laryngeal Sounds

13.2.1 Stridor

13.2.1.1 Acoustic Properties of Stridor

The term stridor is derived from the Latin verb *stridere*, meaning to creak or make a harsh grating noise. The sound results from turbulent airflow passing through a narrowed segment of the airway at the level of the supraglottis, glottis, subglottis or trachea [12]. Its presence suggests significant obstruction of the large airway. Stridor should not to be confused with stertor, which is a lower-pitched, snoring-type sound generated at the level of the nasopharynx, oropharynx and, occasionally, supraglottis.

Stridor is a high-pitched, continuous, musical sound that can be heard near the patient without a stethoscope [13]. Terms have been used to compare it to known noises, for example, "like a little pig", "whistle of snake" and "foghorn" [14, 15]. Using a stethoscope, unlike wheeze, it is louder over the neck than chest wall. The stridor usually occurs during inspiration, indicating extrathoracic supraglottic lesions such as laryngomalacia or a vocal cord lesion, although can be heard during expiration when the underlying cause is an intrathoracic tracheobronchial lesion, for example, tracheomalacia, bronchomalacia and extrinsic compression of the airway. If the obstruction is fixed, for example, tracheal stenosis, the stridor may be biphasic, appearing in both phases of respiration [13, 16].

The sinusoidal waveform and spectrum patterns characteristic of stridor are similar to those of a wheeze. Stridor is usually characterised by a prominent peak at about 1000 Hz in its frequency spectrum. The frequency of the peak and the number of peaks or harmonics in the spectrum are highly variable and depend on the underlying disease, the site of obstruction, the airflow and the volume as well as the elasticity of the obstruction and the surrounding tissues. A fixed obstruction will generate a constant pitch, and a dynamic obstruction such as with laryngomalacia will modulate the pitch in frequency. Its tonal characteristics may be harsh, musical or breathy; however, when combined with the phase of respiration, volume, duration, rate of onset and associated symptoms, the tonal characteristics of the sound may be used as an indication of the location and size of the airway obstruction.

Zwartenkot et al. attempted to use sounds recorded with a high-quality digital recorder to diagnose the location of the underlying pathology in 19 infants in whom a diagnosis was confirmed by endoscopy. The sounds were presented to 38 experienced healthcare professionals. The participants were requested to score the sounds as pharyngeal, supraglottic, glottic, subglottic or tracheal. Even though the two most common diagnoses, laryngomalacia and tracheomalacia, were localised more correctly, the general performance was not significantly higher than random [17]. Studies of the cry of infants with infectious or congenital disorders of the larynx including infectious laryngitis, laryngomalacia, paresis of the recurrent nerve and subglottic stricture have revealed no clear parameters except for the presence of inspiratory stridor [18].

The use of flow, acoustic and structural airway models to study the relationship between the acoustic characteristics of stridor and localisation of the obstructive lesion has the potential to reduce the need to invasive procedures such as laryngoscopy for diagnosis of obstructive airway lesions [19]. The relationship is complex however, and normative data would be needed in order to understand the significance of changes in acoustic parameters that would indicate any specific pathology [20].

Figure 13.2 shows an acoustic recording of an infant with a diagnosis of subglottic stenosis. The sound recording and analysis were performed using the R.A.L.E. (respiration acoustics laboratory environment), developed by PixSoft Inc. [21]. This infant was born at 28 weeks gestation with intrauterine growth retardation and

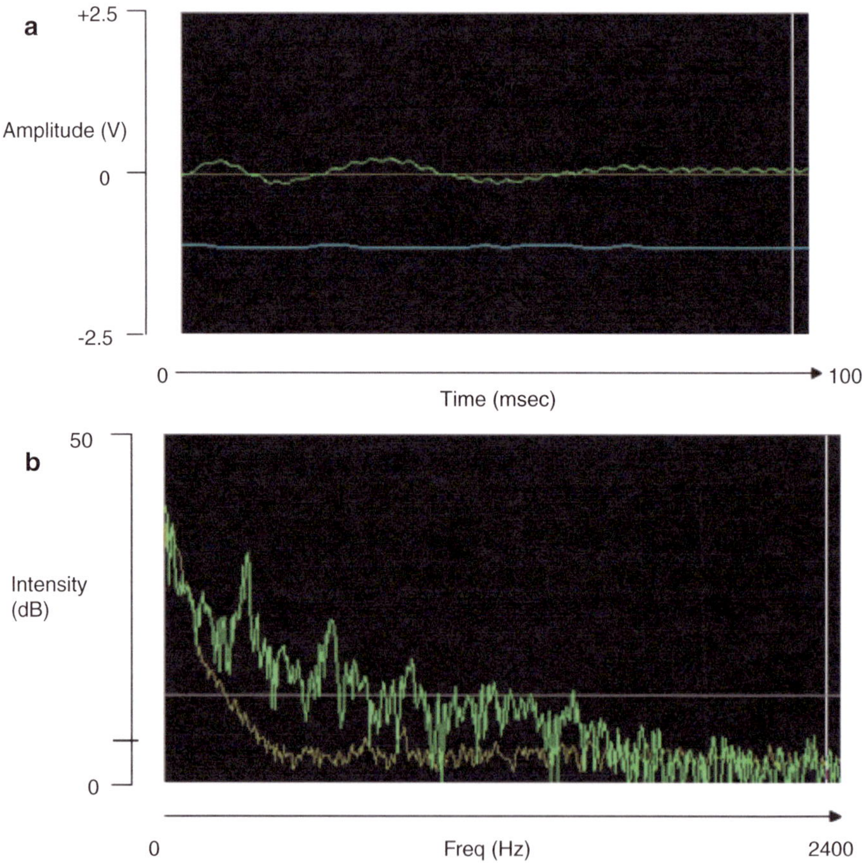

Fig. 13.2 (**a**) Waveform pattern from infant with soft stridor. The characteristic sinusoidal pattern of wheeze is also present in stridor but takes place during inspiration. The green line is the sound pattern; the blue or paler line is the corresponding flow trace. (**b**) Power spectrum with individual the same 100 ms interval as 21a, after fast Fourier transformation. The brighter line represents the respiratory noise; the lower line is the background noise. (**c**) Waveform pattern during harsh stridor. The sinusoidal characteristic is more marked. The green line is the sound pattern; the blue line is the corresponding flow trace. (**d**) Corresponding power spectrum. The brighter line represents the respiratory noise; the lower line is the background noise

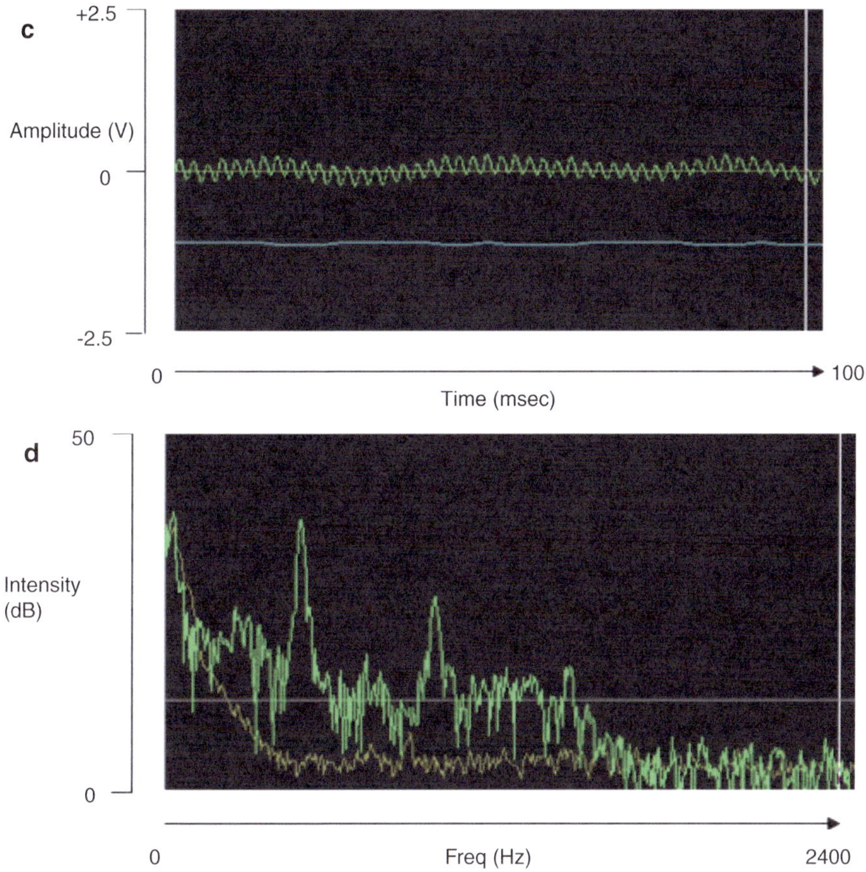

Fig. 13.2 (continued)

was recorded at the age of 1 year, post-gestation. The recording took place over the trachea for a duration of 1 min, and a stridor was audible throughout, the character of which varied according to the activity of the infant. At rest a baseline soft stridor was present (Fig. 13.2a, b); when the infant became excited, the stridor was coarser (Fig. 13.2c, d).

13.2.1.2 Causes of Stridor

Stridor is a symptom, not a diagnosis or a disease, and further investigation is needed in order to identify the underlying cause. Stridor may be inspiratory (most common), expiratory or biphasic, depending on its timing in the respiratory cycle, and the three forms each suggest different causes, as follows:

- Inspiratory stridor suggests a laryngeal obstruction.
- Expiratory stridor implies tracheobronchial obstruction.
- Biphasic stridor suggests a subglottic or glottic anomaly.

Common causes of stridor are airway oedema, aspiration and airway infections. For clinical purposes, the causes of stridor may be divided into acute and chronic causes.

13.2.1.3 Acute Stridor

Laryngotracheobronchitis, commonly known as croup, is the most common cause of acute stridor in children aged 6 months to 2 years. The patient has a barking cough that is worse at night and may have low-grade fever. Pasterkamp and Sanchez [22] observed that tracheal sound levels reflected the degree of inspiratory flow obstruction in a child with subglottic narrowing secondary to infectious laryngotracheitis who presented with noisy breathing. Acoustic measurements of the boy's tracheal sounds at standardised airflows correlated well with the clinical course and with spirometric assessments indicating the potential value of respiratory sound characterisation in patients with upper airway obstruction.

Other infectious causes can cause obstruction at different anatomical levels. Bacterial tracheitis is relatively uncommon and mainly affects children younger than 3 years. It is a secondary infection (most commonly due to *Staphylococcus aureus*) that follows a viral process (commonly croup or influenza). Retropharyngeal abscess is a complication of bacterial pharyngitis that is observed in children younger than 6 years. The patient presents with abrupt onset of high fevers, difficulty swallowing, refusal to feed, sore throat, hyperextension of the neck and respiratory distress. Peritonsillar abscess is an infection in the potential space between the superior constrictor muscles and the tonsil. It is common in adolescents and preadolescents. The patient develops severe throat pain, trismus and trouble with swallowing or speaking. Epiglottitis is a medical emergency that occurs most commonly in children aged 2–7 years. Clinically, the patient experiences an abrupt onset of high-grade fever, sore throat, dysphagia and drooling. The introduction of the Hib vaccine in 1989 has almost eliminated this diagnosis, but it is still a cause of death if treated inappropriately.

Aspiration of foreign body is common in children aged 1–2 years. Often, foreign bodies are food (e.g. nuts) or a small toy that is inhaled. A history of coughing and choking that precedes development of respiratory symptoms may be present. Allergic reaction (i.e. anaphylaxis) occurs within 30 min of an adverse exposure. Hoarseness and inspiratory stridor may be accompanied by symptoms (e.g. dysphagia, nasal congestion, itching eyes, sneezing and wheezing) that indicate the involvement of other organs.

13.2.1.4 Chronic Stridor

Laryngomalacia is the most common cause of inspiratory stridor in the neonatal period and early infancy [23]. Stridor in this condition may be exacerbated by crying or feeding. Placing the patient in a prone position with the head up alleviates the stridor; a supine position exacerbates the stridor. Long-time average spectral (LTAS) characteristics of crying episodes in babies with laryngomalacia differ from normal with a longer overall duration of the crying episode, proportionately fewer expiratory phonations and more inspiratory phonations compared to normal infants [24]. Laryngomalacia is usually benign and self-limiting and improves as the child reaches age 1 year [25]. In cases where significant obstruction or lack of weight gain is present, surgical correction or supraglottoplasty may be considered. Tracheomalacia is caused either by a defect on the cartilage, resulting in loss of the rigidity necessary to keep the tracheal lumen patent, or by an extrinsic compression of the trachea. If present in the proximal (extrathoracic) trachea, tracheomalacia can be associated with inspiratory stridor. If it is present in the distal (intrathoracic) trachea, it is associated more with expiratory or biphasic noise.

Vocal cord paralysis is probably the second most common cause of stridor in infants. Unilateral vocal cord paralysis can be either congenital or secondary to birth or surgical trauma (e.g. from cardiothoracic procedures). Patients with a unilateral vocal cord paralysis present with a weak cry and biphasic stridor that is louder when awake and improves when lying with the affected side down. Bilateral vocal cord paralysis is a more serious entity. Patients usually present with aphonia and a high-pitched biphasic stridor that may progress to severe respiratory distress. This condition is often associated with CNS abnormalities, such as Arnold-Chiari malformation or increased intracranial pressure. In some cases, the airway obstruction is severe enough to require tracheostomy [26].

Congenital stenoses of the airway include tracheal and subglottic stenosis. Patients with significant tracheal stenosis demonstrate an increase in the peak spectral power at 1 kHz, and there is also an increase in the mean spectral power from 600 to 1300 Hz, compared to control subjects [27]. Subglottic stenosis occurs when an incomplete canalization of the subglottis and cricoid rings causes a narrowing of the subglottic lumen. Acquired stenosis is most commonly caused by prolonged intubation. Patients with subglottic stenosis can present with inspiratory or biphasic stridor. Symptoms can be evident at any time during the first few years of life. If symptoms are not present in the neonatal period, this condition may be misdiagnosed as asthma. Common extrinsic causes of stenosis include vascular rings, pulmonary artery slings and double aortic arch that encircles the trachea and oesophagus. Pulmonary artery slings are also associated with complete tracheal rings. Patients usually present during the first year of life with noisy breathing, intercostal retractions and a prolonged expiratory phase.

Other congenital laryngeal malformations include webs, cysts and haemangiomas. Webs are caused by an incomplete recanalization of the laryngeal lumen during embryogenesis. Most are in the glottic area. Infants with laryngeal webs have a weak cry and biphasic stridor. Surgical intervention is recommended in the setting of significant obstruction. Shah et al. described unique acoustic and aerodynamic voice features of a 5-year-old girl with chronic dysphonia and high-pitched voice since birth. Endoscopic division of an anterior glottic web was performed with significant improvement in vocal quality and quality of life [28]. Laryngeal cysts are a less frequent cause of stridor. They are usually found in the supraglottic region in the epiglottic folds. Patients may present with stridor, hoarse voice or aphonia. Cysts may cause obstruction of the airway lumen if they are very large. Laryngeal haemangiomas are rare, and around 50% are accompanied by cutaneous haemangiomas in the head and neck. Typically, haemangiomas present in the first 3–6 months of life during the proliferative phase and regress by age 12–18 months.

Patients usually present with inspiratory or biphasic stridor that may worsen as the haemangioma enlarges. Treatment options consist of oral steroids, intralesional steroids, laser therapy and surgical resection. Oral propranolol has proved to be an effective medical treatment in the appropriate population [29, 30]. Vocal nodules are acquired and may cause stridor and changes in voice quality. In a group of 26 age- and size-matched male children, 13 with vocal nodules and 13 without vocal nodules, the fundamental frequencies, obtained from narrow-band sonograms that were magnified to expand the spectrum from 0 to 1300 Hz, were significantly higher in the group with vocal nodules than the normal group [31]. The acoustic properties before and after treatment significantly change such that the parameters following treatment approach normal values, suggesting that the evaluation of acoustic parameters may be useful in monitoring response to surgical treatment [32].

13.2.1.5 Vocal Cord Dysfunction

Paradoxical vocal cord dysfunction (pVCD) is a condition which occurs in both children and adults. It presents as disproportionate shortness of breath along with other symptoms such as stridor and throat tightness [33, 34] and is characterised by incorrect vocal cord adduction, primarily during inspiration [35].

Paradoxical vocal cord dysfunction (pVCD) forms one element of a group of conditions increasingly referred to as inducible laryngeal obstruction (ILO), where ILO is defined as a transient obstruction of the larynx associated with breathlessness in the presence of a definite "inducer" or triggering factor [36]. The most common form of trigger, particularly in young people, is exercise, but other examples include perfumes, smoke and various chemicals [37]. The primary traits observed in ILO are (1) the "attack-like" or varying nature of condition, (2) the upper airway location of the airflow limitation and (3) the primary symptom being breathing problems [36]. Other conditions encompassed by ILO include exercise-induced laryngomalacia and exercise-induced paradoxical arytenoid motion (EPAM) [38–44], but pVCD is the more heavily researched to date.

pVCD is also one of a number of conditions where diagnosis is difficult due to similar clinical presentations to other conditions, for example, asthma [45]. The underlying mechanism of these conditions is very different; asthma classically presents with an expiratory wheeze, whereas pVCD presents with inspiratory stridor. As the acoustic properties of these sounds are distinguishable, acoustic analysis offers a means of differential diagnosis. This is however complicated by the concurrent presentation of these conditions in some cases. In a cohort of 370 elite athletes, Rundell and Spiering demonstrated that, whilst 5% of this group presented with inspiratory stridor indicative of pVCD, 53% of those with stridor also demonstrated exercise-induced bronchospasm [46]. The different acoustic profiles (with distinct patterns displayed in different parts of the breathing cycle) should however mean that both the pVCD- and asthma-related sounds remain identifiable. The situation may be further complicated however by the potential presence of structural causes of symptoms including unilateral cord palsy and subglottic stenosis [47].

Preliminary pilot data comparing children with and without nasendoscopically proven pVCD demonstrated that at least 67% of participants with pVCD presented with abnormal respiratory sounds compared to 24% of the healthy control group during exercise [48]. This pilot data indicates that acoustic analysis offers a potentially viable, non-invasive alternative to the diagnosis of pVCD.

Conclusion

Laryngeal sounds reflect turbulence of air in the upper airway and are harsher and higher in pitch than normal lung sounds. Stridor is characterised by a high-pitched musical sound and reflects underlying pathology in the airway. Inspiratory stridor indicates an obstruction in the extrathoracic airway, and obstruction in the intrathoracic airway results in an expiratory or biphasic sound.

Acute and chronic stridor indicates a range of underlying pathologies, some of which have been characterised further using digital sound analysis. Many studies are descriptive rather than quantitative, and there is little specific research that uses prospective and formal outcome measures before and after interventions. Acoustic analysis may have useful applications in treatment monitoring, surgical planning, voice quality analysis after laryngeal reconstruction, speech development, voice training, therapy and rehabilitation, and these potential applications require further evaluation.

The gold standard diagnostic tool for upper airway lesions in children is upper airway endoscopy, often requiring general anaesthesia. Paradoxical vocal cord dysfunction is a form of inducible laryngeal obstruction which can co-exist with asthma and is currently diagnosed using laryngoscopy during exercise. The use of acoustic analysis to study the relationship between the acoustic characteristics of stridor and localisation of the obstructive lesion has the potential to reduce the need for invasive procedures; however normative data are needed in order to understand the significance of changes in acoustic parameters that would indicate any specific pathology.

References

1. Pasterkamp H, Kraman SS, Wodicka GR (1997) Respiratory sounds advances beyond the stethoscope. Am J Respir Crit Care Med 156:974–987
2. Yadollahi A, Moussavi Z (2008) Comparison of flow-sound relationship for different features of tracheal sound. In: Annual international conference of the IEEE engineering in medicine and biology society. IEEE Engineering in Medicine and Biology Society, pp 805–808
3. Soufflet G, Charbonneau G, Polit M, Attal P, Denjean A, Escourrou P, Gaultier C (1990) Interaction between tracheal sound and flow rate: a comparison of some different flow evaluations from lung sounds. IEEE Transactions on Bio-medical Engineering 37(4):384–391. 0018–9294 (April 1990)
4. Yadollahi A, Moussavi Z (2006) A robust method for estimating respiratory flow using tracheal sounds entropy. IEEE Transactions on Bio-medical Engineering 53(4):662–668. 0018–9294 (April 2006)
5. Sarkar M, Madabhavi I, Niranjan N, Dogra M (2015) Auscultation of the respiratory system. Ann Thorac Med 10(3):158–168
6. Reichert S, Gass R, Brandt C, Andrès E (2008) Analysis of respiratory sounds: state of the art. Clin Med Circ Respirat Pulm Med 2:45–58

7. Andrès E, Brandt C, Gass R, Reichert S (2010) New developments in the field of human auscultation. Rev Pneumol Clin 66:209–213
8. Gavriely N, Palti Y, Alroy G (1981) Spectral characteristics of normal breath sounds. J Appl Physiol Respir Environ Exerc Physiol 50:307–314
9. Sanchez I, Pasterkamp H (1993) Tracheal sound spectra depend on body height. Am Rev Respir Dis 148:1083–1087
10. Pasterkamp H, Schafer J, Wodicka GR (1996) Posture-dependent change of tracheal sounds at standardised flows in patients with obstructive sleep apnea. Chest 110:1493–1498
11. Nakano H, Hayashi M, Ohshima E, Nishikata N, Shinohara T (2004) Validation of a new system of tracheal sound analysis for the diagnosis of sleep apnea-hypopnea syndrome. Sleep 27:951–957
12. Cotton R, Reilly JS (1983) Stridor and airway obstruction. In: Bluestone CD, Stool SE (eds) Pediatric otolaryngology. Saunders, Philadelphia PA, pp 1190–1204
13. Bohadana A, Izbicki G, Kraman SS (2014) Fundamentals of lung auscultation. N Engl J Med 370:744–751
14. Elphick HE, Sherlock P, Foxall G, Simpson EJ, Shiell NA, Primhak RA, Everard ML (2001) Survey of respiratory sounds in infants. Arch Dis Child 84:35–39
15. Sovijarvi ARA, Malmberg LP, Charbonneau G, Vanderschoot J, Dalmasso F, Sacco C, Rossi M, Earis JE (2000) Characteristics of breath sounds and adventitious respiratory sounds. Eur Respir Rev 10:591–596
16. Ida JB, Thompson DM (2014) Pediatric stridor. Otolaryngol Clin N Am 47:795–819
17. Zwartenkot JW, Hoeve HLJ, Borgstein J (2010) Inter-observer reliability of localization of recorded stridor sounds in children. Int J Pediatr Otorhinolaryngol 74(10):1184–1188. 0165–5876
18. Raes J, Michelsson K, Dehaen F, Despontin M (1982) Cry analysis in infants with infectious and congenital disorders of the larynx. Int J Pediatr Otorhinolaryngol 4(2):157–169
19. van der Velden WC, van Zuijlen AH, de Jong AT, Lynch CT, Hoeve LJ, Bijl H (2016) Acoustic simulation of a patient's obstructed airway. Comput Methods Biomech Biomed Engin 19(2):144–158. https://doi.org/10.1080/10255842.2014.996877. Epub 2015 Jan 8
20. Koike Y, Takahashi H, Calcaterra TC (1977) Acoustic measures for detecting laryngeal pathology. Acta Otolaryngol 84(1–2):105–117
21. Pasterkamp H, Carson C, Daien D, Oh Y (1989) Digital respirosonography: new images of lung sounds. Chest 96:1405–1412
22. Pasterkamp H, Sanchez I (1992) Tracheal sounds in upper airway obstruction. Chest 102(3):963–965
23. Thorne MC, Garetz SL (2016) Laryngomalacia: review and summary of current clinical practice in 2015. Paediatr Respir Rev 17:3–8. https://doi.org/10.1016/j.prrv.2015.02.002. Epub 2015 Feb 28
24. Goberman AM, Robb MP (2005) Acoustic characteristics of crying in infantile laryngomalacia. Logoped Phoniatr Vocol 30(2):79–84
25. Isaac A, Zhang H, Soon SR, Campbell S, El-Hakim H (2016) A systematic review of the evidence on spontaneous resolution of laryngomalacia and its symptoms. Int J Pediatr Otorhinolaryngol 83:78–83. https://doi.org/10.1016/j.ijporl.2016.01.028. Review
26. Kaushal M, Upadhyay A, Aggarwal R, Deorari AK (2005) Congenital stridor due to bilateral vocal cord palsy. Indian J Pediatr 72(5):443–444
27. Yonemaru M, Kikuchi K, Mori M, Kawai A, Abe T, Kawashiro T et al (1993) Detection of tracheal stenosis by frequency analysis of tracheal sounds. J Appl Physiol 75(2):605–612
28. Shah J, White K, Dohar J (2015) Vocal characteristics of congenital anterior glottic webs in children: a case report. Int J Pediatr Otorhinolaryngol 79(6):941–945
29. Wang CF, Wang YS, Sun YF (2016) Treatment of infantile subglottic hemangioma with oral propranolol. Pediatr Int 58(5):385–388. https://doi.org/10.1111/ped.12813
30. Broeks IJ, Hermans DJ, Dassel AC, van der Vleuten CJ, van Beynum IM (2013) Propranolol treatment in life-threatening airway hemangiomas: a case series and review of literature. Int J Pediatr Otorhinolaryngol 77(11):1791–1800. https://doi.org/10.1016/j.ijporl.2013.08.011. Review

31. Hufnagle J (1982) Acoustic analysis of fundamental frequencies of voices of children with and without vocal nodules. Percept Mot Skills 55(2):427–432
32. Niedzielska G, Glijer E, Niedzielski A (2001) Acoustic analysis of voice in children with noduli vocales. Int J Pediatr Otorhinolaryngol 60(2):119–122
33. de Groot EP (2011) Breathing abnormalities in children with breathlessness. Paediatr Respir Rev 12(1):83–87
34. Noyes BE, Kemp JS (2007) Vocal cord dysfunction in children. Paediatr Respir Rev 8(2):155–163
35. Kenn K, Balkissoon R (2011) Vocal cord dysfunction: what do we know? Eur Respir J 37(1): 194–200
36. Halvorsen T, Walsted ES, Bucca C et al (2017) Inducible laryngeal obstruction: an official joint European Respiratory Society and European Laryngological Society statement. Eur Respir J 50:1602221. https://doi.org/10.1183/13993003.02221-2016
37. Shusterman D (2002) Review of the upper airway, including olfaction, as mediator of symptoms. Environ Health Perspect 110(Suppl 4):649–653
38. Tilles SA, Inglis AF (2009) Masqueraders of exercise-induced vocal cord dysfunction. J Allergy Clin Immunol 124(2):377–378
39. Bent JP, Miller DA, Kim JW, Bauman NM, Wilson JS, Smith RJ (1996) Pediatric exercise-induced laryngomalacia. Ann Otol Rhinol Laryngol 105(3):169–175
40. Fahey JT, Bryant NJ, Karas D, Goldberg B, DeStefano R, Gracco LC (2005) Exercise-induced stridor due to abnormal movement of the arytenoid area: Videoendoscopic diagnosis and characterization of the "at risk" group. Pediatr Pulmonol 39(1):51–55
41. Heimdal J-H, Roksund OD, Halvorsen T, Skadberg BT, Olofsson J (2006) Continuous laryngoscopy exercise test: a method for visualizing laryngeal dysfunction during exercise. Laryngoscope 116(1):52–57
42. Maat R, Roksund O, Olofsson J, Halvorsen T, Skadberg B, Heimdal J-H (2007) Surgical treatment of exercise-induced laryngeal dysfunction. Eur Arch Otorhinolaryngol 264(4):401–407
43. Røksund OD, Maat RC, Heimdal JH, Olofsson J, Skadberg BT, Halvorsen T (2009) Exercise induced dyspnea in the young. Larynx as the bottleneck of the airways. Respir Med 103(12):1911–1918
44. Maat R, Røksund O, Halvorsen T, Skadberg B, Olofsson J, Ellingsen T et al (2009) Audiovisual assessment of exercise-induced laryngeal obstruction: reliability and validity of observations. Eur Arch Otorhinolaryngol 266(12):1929–1936
45. Christensen P, Thomsen S, Rasmussen N, Backer V (2010) Exercise-induced laryngeal obstructions objectively assessed using EILOMEA. Eur Arch Otorhinolaryngol 267(3):401–407
46. Morris MJ, Allan PF, Perkins PJ (2006) Vocal cord dysfunction: etiologies and treatment. Clin Pulm Med 13(2):73–86
47. Rundell KW, Spiering BA (2003) Inspiratory stridor in elite athletes. Chest 123(2):468–474
48. Barker N, Thevasagayam R, Ugonna K, Smith L (2015) Paediatric paradoxical vocal cord dysfunction: Diagnosis and treatment in a multidisciplinary clinic. European Respiratory Journal Sep 46(Suppl 59):PA2809. https://doi.org/10.1183/13993003.congress-2015.PA2809

Sleep Evaluation Using Audio Signal Processing

14

Yaniv Zigel, Ariel Tarasiuk, and Eliran Dafna

14.1 Introduction

Millions of people worldwide experience sleep disorders, and unrecognized or ignored sleep problems can lead to poor health, accidents, and even death [1–10]. Early diagnosis and treatment can improve quality of life and health [10, 11]. However, due to the high cost of diagnostic technology and diagnostic procedures and the need for highly qualified personnel, many people are left undiagnosed and untreated [9, 12]. Moreover, despite the consistently increasing number of sleep studies worldwide each year [9, 10], many people are unaware of their sleep disorders and treatment. Polysomnography (PSG) is the gold standard sleep diagnostic study that requires a full-night laboratory stay [13]. PSG employs numerous collections of surface electrodes, each measuring physiologic parameters of sleep, including electroencephalography (EEG), electrooculography (EOG), electromyography (EMG), electrocardiography (ECG), and respiratory activity [13–16]. Time series data are aggregated, processed, and visually examined epoch-by-epoch (at 30 s resolution) by qualified personnel in order to evaluate sleep stages, respiratory activity during sleep, and other parameters. This study is labor intense and very costly [17].

Currently, the biomedical engineering field of sleep disorders evaluation is on a "fast track" toward home-based testing [17–28]. In recent years, extensive

Y. Zigel (✉) · E. Dafna
Department of Biomedical Engineering, Faculty of Engineering, Ben-Gurion University of the Negev, Beer-sheva, Israel
e-mail: yaniv@bgu.ac.il

A. Tarasiuk
Sleep-Wake Disorders Unit, Soroka University Medical Center, Beersheba, Israel

Department of Physiology, Faculty of Health Sciences, Ben-Gurion University of the Negev, Beersheba, Israel
e-mail: tarasiuk@bgu.ac.il

K. N. Priftis et al. (eds.), *Breath Sounds*, https://doi.org/10.1007/978-3-319-71824-8_14

efforts have been devoted to seeking alternative simple cost-effective technologies for objective home-based testing to increase accessibility to sleep disorders diagnosis. These new technologies are based on reduced channels and sensors and often involve algorithms that simplify diagnostic procedures and increase accessibility [17, 20, 23, 28–32]. Body-contact-based sensor technology may lead to poor data acquisition and often disturbs sleep; therefore, recently, new non-contact approaches were suggested for simple respiratory and sleep evaluation [19, 21, 33–37].

One of the approaches is audio analysis; the basic idea is that respiratory activity, which contains information regarding sleep stages and sleep breathing disorders, generates breathing (and snoring) sounds that can be acquired by a sensitive non-contact microphone and a digital audio recording device. The advantage of audio is the simplicity and safety of acquisition; a non-contact microphone will not disturb sleep.

There are several common sleep disorders that can be reliably analyzed using audio signals without the need of contact microphones, such as snoring, obstructive sleep apnea (OSA), and insomnia. *Snoring* is the resulting sound due to obstructed air movement during *breathing* while sleeping [38]. Snore sounds vary significantly; in some cases the snore sound may be soft, but in others it can be very loud [36]. It was concluded that to a large extent, snoring is "in the ear of the beholder" [38]. Snoring is a symptom of OSA. *OSA* is a prevalent disease in which upper airways are collapsed during sleep [6]. OSA causes breath cessation, frequent arousals, and can lead to sleepiness, accidents, cardiovascular morbidity, and even death. Generally, *insomnia* is having trouble sleeping; it is a sleep disorder in which there is an inability to fall asleep or to stay asleep as long as desired [13].

Currently, an audio signal is usually analyzed only for snoring intensity [dB] using a sound level meter during PSG study [39] or without a sound level meter in at-home testing [40]. This snoring intensity analysis is usually performed together with the analysis of respiratory activity to determine OSA severity. It has been assumed that greater loudness is correlated with OSA severity. Recently, we have shown that this is not very accurate [41], since sound level meters acquire all the sound signals in the room including movements.

We have shown that with higher sampling frequency and suitable signal processing algorithms, additional sleep information can be extracted from audio signals during sleep [21, 35, 36, 42–45] and even during wakefulness [46–49].

In this chapter, several audio-based signal processing algorithms for sleep evaluation are reviewed. These algorithms, developed in the Biomedical Signal Processing Lab. of Ben-Gurion University of the Negev in collaboration with the Sleep-Wake Disorder Unit, Soroka University Medical Center, evaluate snoring and breathing, sleep-wake stages, sleep quality parameters (such as total sleep time), and obstructive sleep apnea.

Our findings show that sleep can be evaluated by analysis of audio signals, using non-contact sensors such as microphones.

14.2 Sleep Evaluation Using Audio Signals

14.2.1 Breathing and Snoring Sound Detection

Breathing sounds during sleep vary significantly between soft and very loud; the definition of snore is unclear and is more "in the ear of the beholder" [38]. In the absence of a conclusive definition, the snoring is sometimes defined [41] as relatively loud breathing sounds (>50 dB) during sleep.

Figure 14.1 shows an example of snoring pattern during 30 s (epoch) of sleep. A study was performed on whole-night audio signals collected from subjects who were referred to sleep diagnosis [36]. In this work [36], we defined all audible inhale sounds during sleep as snores. We demonstrated that breathing sounds can be acquired and detected using a non-contact microphone.

The breathing and snoring sound detection can be an important step before estimating breathing and snoring statistics [41, 43] and OSA severity [42, 44, 45]. It can also be an important step before determining sleep-wake states and estimating sleep-wake parameters from audio signals [21, 22, 35].

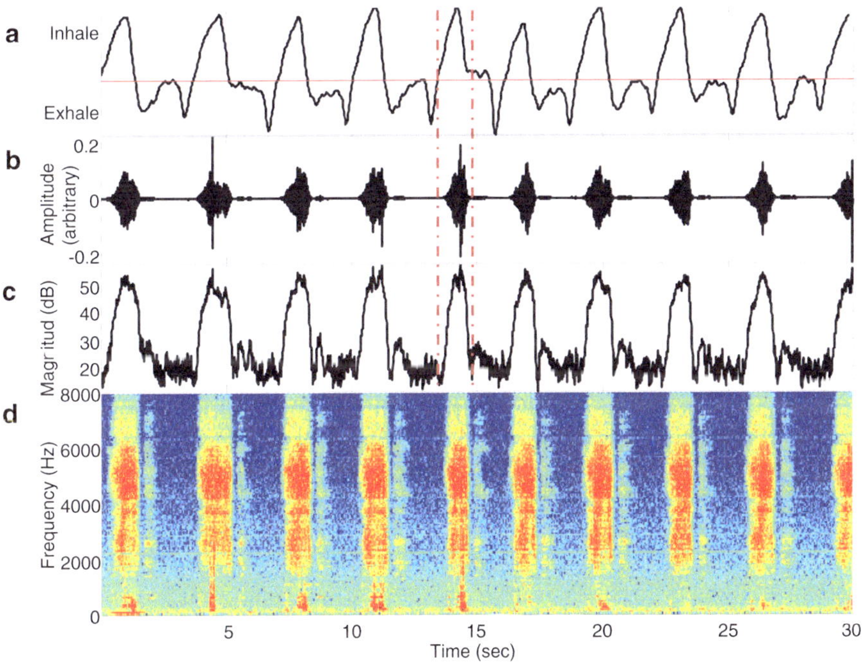

Fig. 14.1 Example of snoring pattern during 30 s epoch. (**a**) Air flow, (**b**) audio signal, (**c**) energy signal, (**d**) spectrogram. Dashed vertical lines highlight one inspiratory event. Note that snore events are predominantly apparent during the inspiratory phase of the respiratory cycle. Data was collected from a 57-year-old man (BMI = 31, AHI = 16, during sleep stage 2) [36]

14.2.1.1 Method

A breathing sound (snore) detection algorithm (system) was developed; this system can emphasize sound events (suspected snore events) from the background noise using an adaptive noise reduction algorithm and distinguish snore and non-snore events (such as movement of bed linen, cars, and barking dogs) [36]. For system design, snore and non-snore events were manually labeled and used to train an AdaBoost model fed by acoustic features from time and spectral domains. Using a feature selection algorithm on the design dataset, the best features were selected and used in the validation (testing) phase as well. After system design, the system was blindly tested using an additional audio dataset. Each sound event was processed and assigned a snore likelihood score (SLS); the higher the score, the greater its probability to be a snore event.

14.2.1.2 Experimental Setup and Results

A study was performed on whole-night audio signals collected from 67 subjects who were referred to sleep diagnosis in the Sleep-Wake Disorder Unit. A total detection rate of >98% was achieved on detection of snore vs. non-snore (noise) [36].

Recently, in a pilot study, we developed and validated an inspiratory (inhale) and expiratory (exhale) sounds detection system [50]. Random forests classifier (3-class) was trained and tested using inspiratory/expiratory/noise events, acquired from 84 subjects in sleep laboratory and at-home environments. More than 560,000 events were analyzed, including a variety of recording devices and different environments. The system's overall accuracy rates were 91.2% and 83.6% in in-laboratory and at-home environments, respectively, when classifying between inspiratory, expiratory, and noise classes.

Figure 14.2 shows how breathing pattern can be determined from audio signal using a non-contact microphone. Even in the case of a very quiet (faint) breathing sound signal (Fig. 14.2e), an emphasized signal of interest can be calculated (Fig. 14.2f). Using a 3-class breathing classifier, breathing pattern can be estimated (Fig. 14.2g) that is similar to the respiratory inductance plethysmography (RIP) signal (Fig. 14.2h).

In a recent study [41], breathing/snoring sounds were examined to see whether breathing properties are different between gender, sleep stages, and obstructive sleep apnea severity. In this study, we showed that snoring intensity was similar in both genders in all sleep stages and independent of OSA severity.

14.2.2 Extracting Sleep-Wake States from Breathing Sounds

The most commonly used technology to detect sleep and wake states in home-based testing is actigraphy [51]. In this approach movement is considered a wake state, and lack of movement implies a sleep state [24, 25, 52]. This is true most of the time, but fails when the subject is awake but lying still or has movement disorders while sleeping [6, 24]. This technology was validated versus PSG using in-laboratory data collection and showed an agreement (accuracy) ranging between 80% and 86% [24, 53, 54]. Currently, most sleep diagnosis technologies are based on body-contact-sensors that often affect natural sleep and may bias medical interpretation [24].

We provided evidence [21, 22] that sleep-wake states can be estimated using non-contact microphones. The idea is that during sleep, there is a considerable

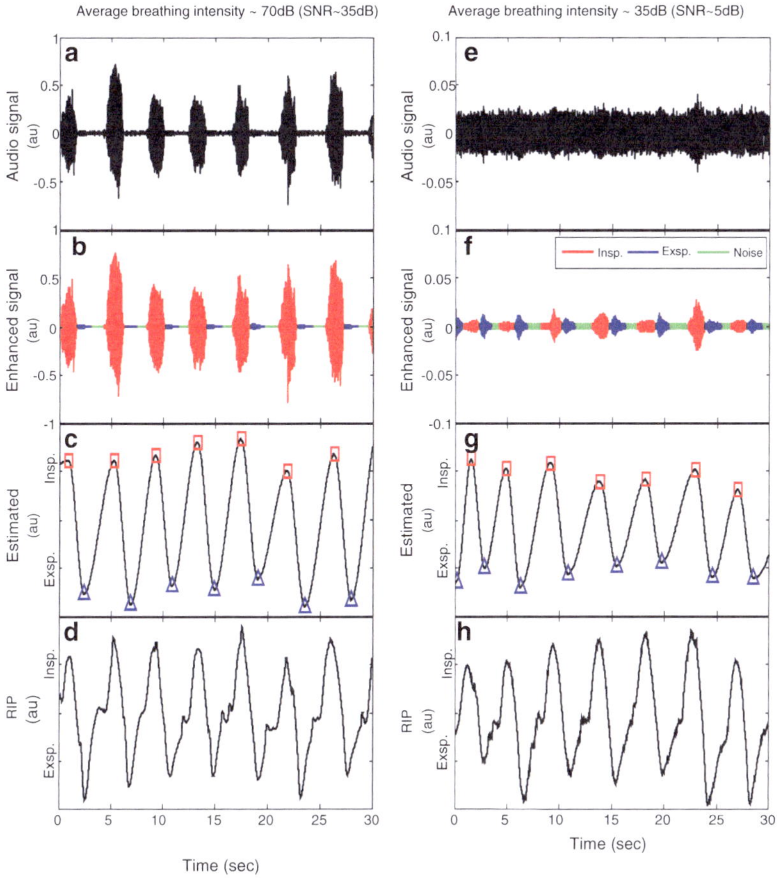

Fig. 14.2 Breathing activity detection from audio signal. Subject: male, age 61, BMI = 28, AHI 17, was recorded using an ambient microphone placed 1 m above the subject's head. Left and right columns present 30 s of loud and faint breathing, respectively. (**a** and **e**) The recorded audio signal. (**b** and **f**) The corresponding audio signal after enhancement (noise reduction). Colors represent segments after 3-class breathing sound detection: inspiration (red), expiration (blue), and non-breathing/noise (green). (**c** and **g**) Estimated breathing activity score. (**d** and **h**) Breathing activity measured by PSG's respiratory inductance plethysmography (RIP). Please notice that the left column presents loud breathing of about 70 dB (each) and the right column presents faint breathing of about 35 dB. For convenience, panels **e** and **f** are zoomed ×10 relative to **a** and **b** since the breathing signal's amplitude is relatively low and almost hidden within the background noise

increase of upper airway resistance [20, 55–58]; this elevated resistance is reflected by amplification of air-pressure oscillations in the upper airways during breathing. These air-pressure oscillations are perceived as typical breathing sounds during sleep [38]. In contrast, during wakefulness, there is an increase in activity of the upper airway dilating muscles [59, 60] and hence decreased upper airway resistance and airway oscillations. Our study [21, 22] was the first to illustrate that sleep can be reliably estimated using non-contact technology that can model sleep-wake breathing characteristics from audio signals.

14.2.2.1 Method

We formulated several acoustic features of sleep-wake breathing characteristics that were proven to be very beneficial: (1) *breathing pattern features* (such as breathing cycle period and cycle intensity) and (2) *snore likelihood score (SLS) features*.

Breathing pattern features evaluate the rhythmic pattern of the respiratory action. When sleeping, the respiratory action is more periodic. The idea of SLS features is that when someone is snoring, he is probably sleeping.

The *breathing pattern features* were calculated using the autocorrelation function. However, since the audio signal may contain noises in different frequencies, the autocorrelation was calculated selectively from the part of the spectrum in order to emphasize the periodicity of the interval. For this, a spectrogram, $X(k,n)$, was calculated for each signal interval (Fig. 14.3b), where k is the frequency component index and n is the time frame index. In order to find repeating breathing patterns, we kept the most periodic information in the spectrogram using the autocorrelation function. Therefore, the autocorrelation is calculated separately for each frequency component:

$$R(k,t) = \frac{1}{N-t} \sum_{n=1}^{N-t} X(k,n) \times X(k,n+t),$$

where t is the time frame-lag index and N represents the total number of frames in the interval.

The frequency components were sorted according to the first peak amplitude value as criterion $J(k)$ (see Fig. 14.3c):

$$J(k) = \max_{t} \left(R(k,t)_{t>2\text{s}} \right),$$

and it summed the top 50% ($\{J(k)\}_{50}$) frequency components. In this stage, the interval is represented with a single function of emphasized autocorrelation.

$$R(t) = \frac{1}{K} \sum_{k \in \{J(k)\}_{50}}^{K} R(k,t)$$

Then, the breathing pattern features can be extracted: for example, *breathing cycle intensity* is calculated as the autocorrelation value of the first peak, and *cycle period* is the time lag of the first peak. Figure 14.3 shows an example of sleep vs. wake.

The snores features are based on SLS parameter. SLS [21] is assigned to every detectable energetic audio event; the more positive this score is, the greater its probability to be a snore event. In a sleep interval of 30 s (epoch), the percentage of high positive values is much higher than in a wake interval of the same duration. We formulated two sets of SLS features: (1) *MaxSLS*, which is the maximum SLS in the epoch, and (2) *snoring index*, which is the estimation of number of snores (SLS > Threshold) per hour, calculated over an epoch interval.

Using the extracted features, sleep-wake likelihood (SWL) curve was estimated for each subject at 30 s epoch resolution. AdaBoost classifier was used as a time-series model in which each feature was fed along with two previous epochs. Figure 14.4 shows a typical example of an SWL curve estimated from whole-night audio recording of a subject from the validation design set. Higher values of SWL indicate increased likelihood toward wake state. Note the similarity between the hypnogram

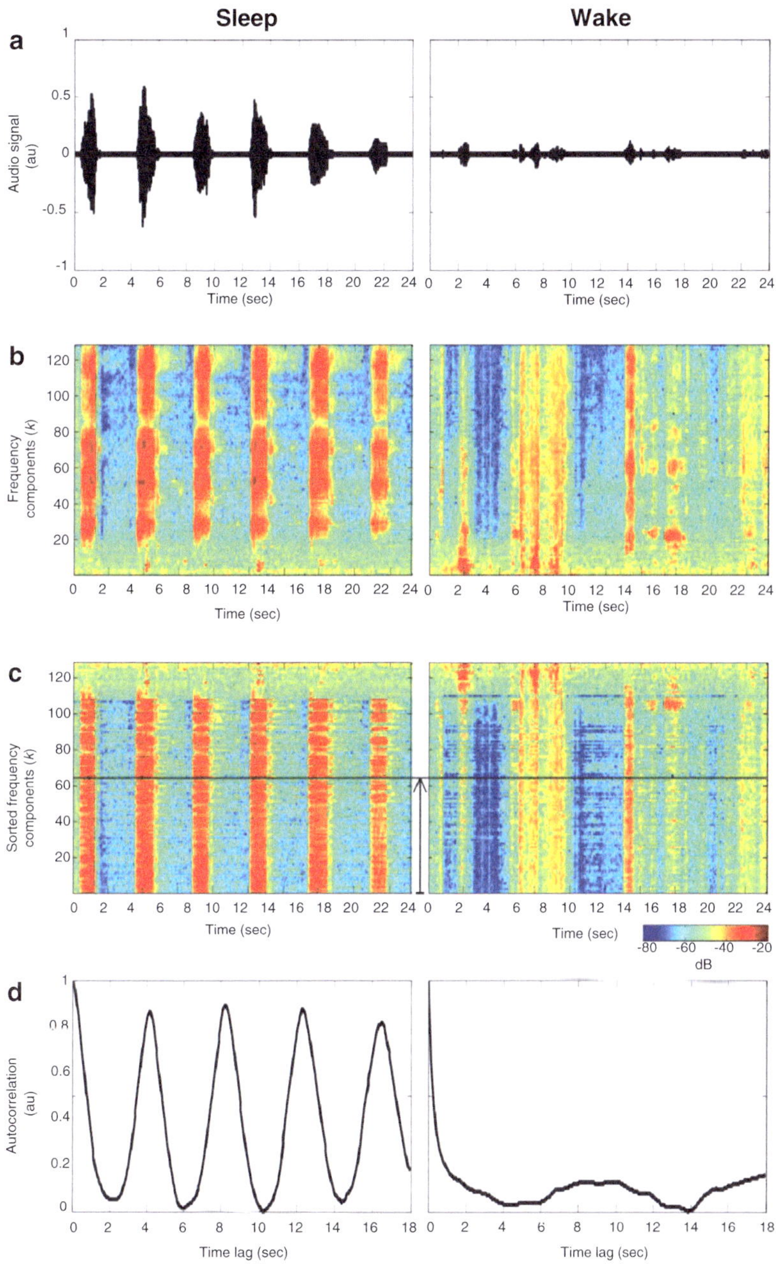

Fig. 14.3 An example of a 24 s interval of audio signal collected from 65-year-old female, BMI 36, AHI 12. Left column illustrates data collected during sleep; right column illustrates data collected during wake. (**a**) Audio signal following noise suppression. (**b**) The corresponding spectrogram (frequency components) of the audio signal in (**a**). (**c**) The sorted frequency components according to periodicity measure. (**d**) The enhanced autocorrelation of the interval calculated from the lower half of the sorted frequency components (**c**), visualized by the vertical solid line [22]

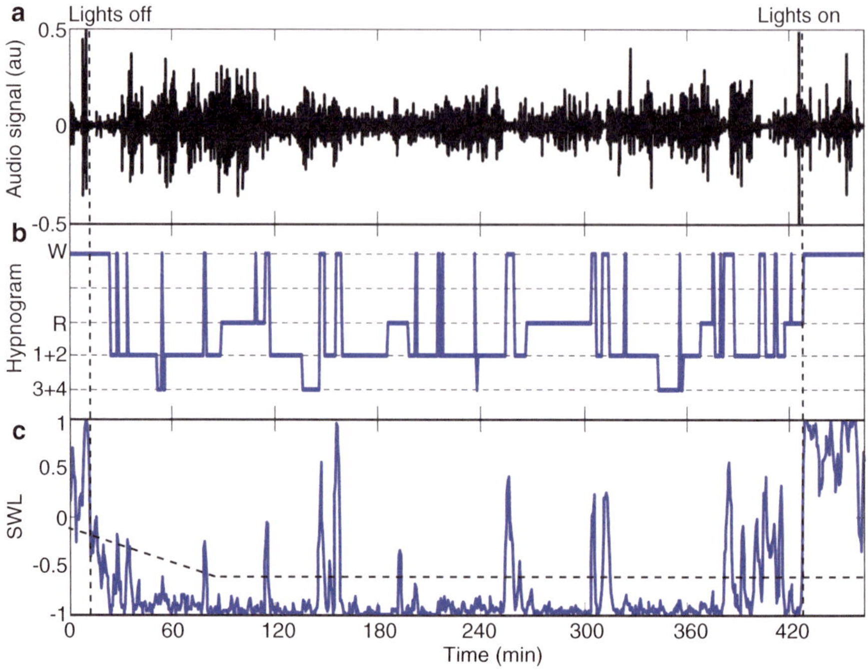

Fig. 14.4 Example of sleep-wake likelihood (SWL) score curve [22]. (**a**) Audio signal of whole-night recording. (**b**) Hypnogram. (**c**) The estimated whole-night SWL score curve. SWL was calculated using the eight acoustic features fed into the AdaBoost classifier. Higher values of SWL indicate increased likelihood toward wake state. When focusing on sleep and wake phases, note the similarity between the hypnogram (**b**) and the SWL (**c**). The horizontal dashed line represents the corresponding individual decision threshold over time; for more details, see main body. Data was collected from 52-year-old male, BMI 31

(Fig. 14.4b) and the proposed acoustic-based SWL curve (Fig. 14.4c). It should be emphasized that there is a considerable increase in SWL values as soon as wake initiates, and it declines immediately during sleep onset.

Once an estimation of the sleep-wake pattern across the entire sleep period is achieved, a clinical report can be generated. We decided to measure five common sleep parameters including TST, total sleep time; SL, sleep latency; SE, sleep efficiency; WASO, wake after sleep onset; and AwI, awakening index [22].

14.2.2.2 Experimental Setup and Results

In this study, 150 adult subjects were recorded in the Sleep-Wake Disorder Unit, Soroka University Medical Center, Israel. A condenser microphone (Rode, NTG-1) with a 20–20,000 Hz frequency response was placed about 1 m above the subject's head. The microphone was linked to an Edirol R-4 pro-audio recording device. The acquired signal was digitized at a sampling frequency of 44.1 kHz with 16 bit resolution. Since most of the breathing sound signal spectral information is below 8 kHz, the signal was down-sampled to 16 kHz to reduce computation time. The database contained the whole-night sound recordings of these subjects.

We found very good agreement of sleep parameters between the proposed audio-based method and the PSG [22]. The disagreement between PSG and our method (epoch-by-epoch comparison) was 3.9 ± 5.4% for SL, 11.4 ± 9.1% for TST, and 8.2 ± 8.3% for WASO. The total accuracy was 83.3% in detection of sleep-wake epochs.

We evaluated the audio-based sleep-wake classification according to anthropometric parameters of these subjects and the signal quality [22]. The classification performances were calculated using Cohen's kappa score [61], which is a more adequate measurement when inequality in class abundance is present (more sleep epochs than wake epochs). In this evaluation, we found insignificant correlation between system performance and anthropometric parameters (AHI, BMI, age, and gender); however, it seems that system performance is influenced by the signal quality (SNR), suggesting the importance of signal enhancement.

14.2.3 Macro-Sleep Stages (MSS) Classification

Recently, we introduced a novel concept to estimate macro-sleep stages [wake/rapid eye movement (REM)/non-REM (NREM)] from breathing sounds using non-contact microphone and audio analysis [35]. The basic physiological idea behind this concept is that transitions from sleep to wake and vice versa strongly affect control of ventilation and upper airway patency [20, 62, 63]. There are also changes in breathing patterns between REM and NREM sleep. REM sleep respiration is typically characterized by an increased frequency and reduced regularity. Tidal volume is reduced further in comparison with that of NREM sleep, resulting in the lowest level of normal ventilation [62].

14.2.3.1 Method

The main concept is to extract breathing and body movement sounds from the whole-night audio signal and then to estimate the macro-sleep stages due to breathing sound properties and movement. Therefore, the first step was signal enhancement based on a spectral subtraction approach [36]. This step is crucial since it reduces the background noise, which is subject-independent, and emphasizes the transient events that were recorded during sleep such as quiet breaths and body movements. The second step is breathing sound detection (see Sect. 14.2.1). The third step is feature extraction—the features were designed to discriminate between the three classes of MSS: Wake, REM, and NREM, and were categorized into two types: breathing characteristics and noise characteristics. The fourth step is MSS classification—this step involves estimation of the MSS using information from both acoustic features (regarding breathing and body movements) and information regarding the "natural" sleep pattern, i.e., taking into account the temporal relations between adjacent epochs. We constructed a classifier that is composed of time-variant hidden Markov model and an artificial neural network [35].

Once an estimation of the MSS across the entire sleep period is achieved, a handy clinical report can be generated. We decided to measure seven sleep parameters including TST, SL, SE, WASO, AwI (see Sect. 14.2.2), RL—REM latency, and RP—REM percentage [2]. These sleep parameters are commonly used in sleep medicine and are suitable for most sleep-disordered diagnosis [13].

14.2.3.2 Experimental Setup and Results

This study was performed on a database that consists of 213 patients who were referred to a routine polysomnography study. Thirty-five of these patients were simultaneously recorded with an ambient microphone that was attached to the ceiling and hung about 1 m above the patient's head. We used the hypnogram data from the PSG to train the time-dependent hidden Markov model (HMM) to better capture a natural sleep pattern and trained the ANN from the patients with both hypnogram and audio records. For each subject, we compared epoch-by-epoch MSS between the audio-based approach and the PSG annotated sleep stages. The comparison was measured using simple agreement (detection rate) and using Cohen's kappa, which also takes into account the inequality of states' proportions. We also tested the performance of the ANN alone and the contribution of the time-series model (HMM). For the ANN model, the agreement was 0.63 ± 0.10 and Cohen's kappa 0.32 ± 0.12. After applying the HMM, the performance was increased to 0.75 ± 0.09 and 0.42 ± 0.17, respectively [35].

For the clinical report, we compared the 7 sleep parameters mentioned above (TST, SL, SE, WASO, AwI, RL, and RP) between our approach and the PSG, using 20 patients who had audio recordings and were used in our validation dataset. Our comparison involved two-tailed paired *t*-test among each sleep parameter. TST, SL, SE, WASO, and RP comparison showed insignificant differences with p values of 0.26 for TST, 0.70 for SL, 0.62 for SE, 0.69 for WASO, and 0.09 for RP, showing that our approach is giving a similar result that cannot be ruled out. The sleep parameters AwI and RL showed a greater difference with p values of <0.01, 0.04, respectively. We hypothesized that the estimated AwI was lower in our approach due to the HMM states' "prolonging" properties. This might be addressed with a proper post-algorithm that searches awakening episodes among the sleep stages. In addition, REM latency (RL) can be significantly different once the first REM episode is undetected.

Figure 14.5 shows a typical example of MSS estimation on a 62-year-old male. The upper panel of Fig. 14.5 presents the estimated probabilities for each MSS across the night (the MSS of a given epoch is summed to (1). The middle panel of Fig. 14.5 presents the most probable MSS sequence across the night using the HMM, i.e., using the temporal relations between adjacent epochs. The lower panel of Fig. 14.5 shows the referenced hypnogram according to the gold standard PSG annotation. One can notice the similarities between the middle and lower panels of Fig. 14.5.

14.2.4 Obstructive Sleep Apnea Detection

In another endeavor, we developed a system that detects OSA and estimates OSA severity (AHI estimation) in subjects using whole-night audio signals (during sleep) and speech signals (during wakefulness).

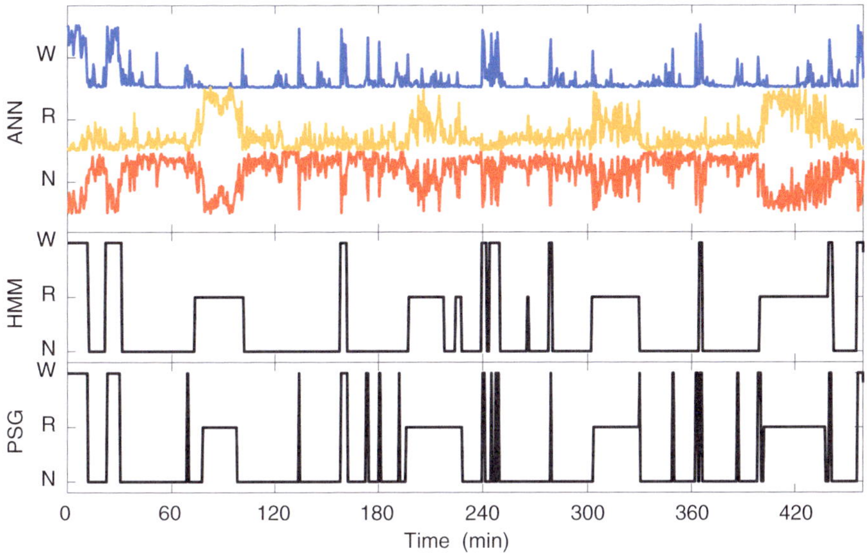

Fig. 14.5 Typical example of MSS estimation. Upper panel presents the three classes' MSS scores (probabilities) estimated by the ANN classifier (scores are summed to one). Center panel presents the HMM's most probable MSS sequence given the ANN scores, i.e., ANN + HMM. Lower panel presents the PSG annotation. W, Wake; R, REM; N, NREM. Subject: Male, age = 62, BMI = 26, AHI = 16. This example exhibits an accuracy rate of 89% and Cohen's kappa of 0.76

14.2.4.1 OSA Detection During Sleep

A strong association between upper airway patency and breathing sounds was demonstrated, enabling the detection of respiratory abnormalities during sleep [42, 44, 45, 64].

Method

The OSA detection and estimation system exploits the output of the breathing (and snoring) detection system in order to calculate breathing-related features; it also exploits the output of the sleep-wake state estimation system in order to calculate the relevant features only from sleep states and to estimate the AHI for each subject.

The system consists of two major phases—design phase for system training and validation phase for system evaluation. Once the snores are detected, an analysis of all snore events across the night is performed; various acoustic features are extracted. The OSA severity estimation (AHI_{EST}) is performed according to a fitting (regression) model.

In an early system [42], five features were developed and extracted per subject; these features express the acoustic properties of the snores and emphasize the differences between apneic snorers and simple snorers. The features were *mel-cepstability*, a measure of the entire night spectrum's stability; *running variance*, quantifies the inter-snore energy variability across the night; *apneic phase ratio*, represents the relative duration when the upper airways are collapsed; *inter-event silence*, counts the silence between two sound events; and *pitch density*, a measure of the stability of the tissue's vibration frequency.

In a later system [44], many different features were examined; these features were calculated using time or spectral domains. The *time domain features* can be further categorized into (a) periodicity features, (b) duration and sample scattering features, and (c) energy features. The *spectral domain features* can be further categorized into (a) spectral parameterization, (b) bio-characteristic frequencies, and (c) dynamic frequencies features. Based on these time-dependent (breathing event-based) features, a single (global) score was calculated for each feature using statistical measurements (probability distribution properties) such as min, max, variance, skewness, and kurtosis. To reduce features' dimensionality, a feature selection (genetic algorithm) was applied, and the chosen features were fed into a Gaussian mixture regression model in order to predict AHI.

Results

Figure 14.6 [44] shows the AHI estimation results of 155 subjects (women and men) referred to in-laboratory polysomnography (PSG) study. The performances of the proposed system were evaluated with Pearson correlation of $\rho = 0.89$ (for the testing set; 75 out of 155), AHI error of 7.35 events/h, and diagnostic agreement of 77.3%. These results show encouraging performances and a reliable non-contact alternative method for OSA severity estimation.

In a later study [45], we developed an algorithm to detect apnea and hypopnea events at their exact time locations during sleep. The algorithm enabled distinguishing between regular breathing sound events and A/H events using a binary random forest classifier. In this study, OSA severity was also estimated from 93 subjects (out

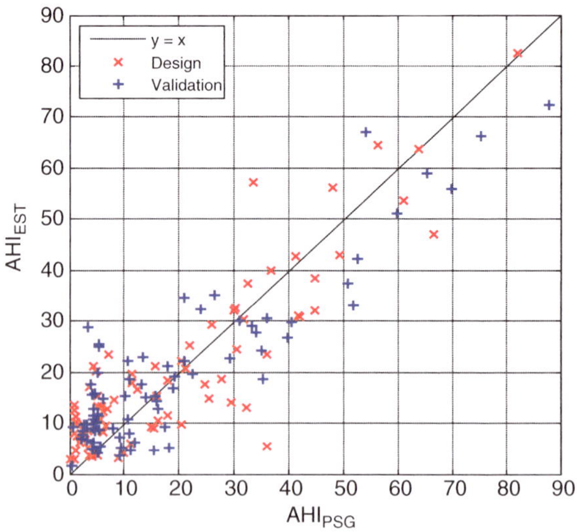

Fig. 14.6 AHI estimation using audio analysis vs. PSG-based AHI [44]. © 2013 IEEE. Reprinted, with permission, from Dafna E, Tarasiuk A, Zigel Y OSA severity assessment based on sleep breathing analysis using ambient microphone. In 2013 35th Annual International Conference of the IEEE Engineering in Medicine and Biology Society (EMBC), pp. 2044–2047

of 186) in at-home conditions. Total accuracy rate of 86.3% was achieved in A/H event detection. Correlation of $\rho = 0.87$ ($\rho = 0.74$), diagnostic agreement of 76% (81.7%), and average absolute difference AHI error of 7.4 (7.8) (events/hour) were achieved in in-laboratory (at-home) conditions, respectively.

14.2.4.2 OSA Detection During Wakefulness

OSA detection in awake subjects is very challenging. Recently, the ability to assess OSA during wakefulness was explored, using tracheal breath sounds analysis [65, 66] and speech signal processing [46–49, 67].

The idea behind OSA estimation using speech signals is that the acoustic parameters of speech are affected by the physiological and anatomical properties of the vocal tract and soft tissue characteristics [47, 48]. In the upper airway, there are changes in muscle properties and neural drive in patients with OSA. These changes lead to upper airway remodeling that affect its function during sleep [68] and speech during wakefulness. Several studies explored the association between speech and OSA [69]. In a series of studies, we developed several systems for the detection of OSA and estimation of AHI using speech signals acquired from subjects (men and women) reading a 1- to 2 min protocol (in Hebrew).

Methods

We developed a system that distinguishes between OSA and non-OSA (healthy) subjects using their speech signal [48]. One hundred acoustic features that were considered to be affected by the specific OSA physiology were extracted and analyzed. Two different feature sets were suggested, one represented mostly the short-time dynamics (short-term features) and the other represented the stationary configuration (long-term features). Feature selection was performed on each feature set to pinpoint the most discriminative features. The selected features indicated a difference in perception, structure, and nasalization between healthy and OSA speakers. Two GMM-based systems were evaluated—one for each feature set, and finally, the two systems were fused.

In a later study, the severity of OSA (AHI) was also estimated using speech signals [46, 47, 49].

Experimental Setup and Results

In the first study [48], we explored acoustic speech features of 93 subjects who were recorded using a text-dependent speech protocol and a digital audio recorder (ZOOM H4) immediately prior to polysomnography study. Following analysis of the study, subjects were divided into OSA ($n = 67$) and non-OSA ($n = 26$) groups. A classification error rate was estimated using the leave-one-out (LOO) method. Specificity and sensitivity of 83% and 79% were achieved for the male and 86% and 84% for the female OSA patients, respectively.

In the later studies, AHI was estimated using the speech signals of additional subjects. A diagnostic agreement of 67.3% between the speech-estimated AHI and the PSG-determined AHI and an absolute error rate of 10.8 events/h were achieved in a population of 198 subjects [46].

14.3 Discussion and Future Work

We reviewed several audio-based systems for sleep evaluation that were developed in the Biomedical Signal Processing Research Laboratory, Ben-Gurion University of the Negev, in collaboration with the Sleep-Wake Disorder Unit, Soroka University Medical Center. These systems evaluate snoring and breathing, sleep-wake stages and sleep quality parameters, macro-sleep stages, and obstructive sleep apnea using non-contact microphones.

These systems were validated on hundreds of subjects routinely referred to sleep evaluation including a wide range of age, BMI, and AHI distribution and both genders. Most of the subjects underwent PSG evaluation in the sleep laboratory, and some of the subjects underwent a reduced-channel sleep evaluation at home. Further studies are needed to confirm our findings in the general population.

The main idea beyond this audio-based approach is that central control of ventilation and upper airway patency are strongly affected by sleep and wake activity [20, 62]. During sleep, there is a considerable increase of upper airway resistance [20, 57, 58, 70] due to decreased activity of the pharyngeal dilator muscles [59, 60]. This elevated resistance is reflected by amplification of air-pressure oscillations in the upper airways during breathing. These air-pressure oscillations are perceived as typical breathing sounds during sleep. In contrast, during wakefulness, there is an increase in activity of the upper airway dilating muscles, hence decreased upper airway resistance [60] and airway oscillations [22].

We used a non-contact microphone to record breathing and snoring sounds since this approach enables more natural sleep that is not affected by equipment. Some other studies used a contact microphone that was taped to the nasion [38] or to the trachea [19, 71] or used a microphone embedded in a face mask [72].

Analyzing respiratory sounds across sleep time using a non-contact microphone is challenging since it was essential to improve SNR in order to also expose the relatively quiet breathing sounds that are of interest. To achieve this, we used an adaptive spectral subtraction technique that subtracted the estimated adjacent background noise. The spectral subtraction technique improved SNR with some effect on respiratory spectral content and with a minimal effect on sound intensity.

It is generally accepted that snoring and AHI are very dependent on the body position [73]. Further studies are needed to explore the effect of body position on breathing and snoring sound characteristics, as well as to explore the effect of bed partner sounds on the different sleep evaluation algorithms and to find ways to reduce these effects.

The recent increase in the use of smartphones with different onboard sensors has led to the proliferation of different sleep screening applications running on the phones [74] including audio-based applications. However, as far as we know, no existing sensor-based sleep-related application for smartphones has yet been scientifically validated. Since non-contact microphones are safe and convenient, and available in every smartphone, tablet, or personal computer, we assume that in the future, the accessibility to audio-based sleep evaluation applications will increase. The research on non-contact audio-based respiratory evaluation has the potential to advance new scientific-technological directions involving other types of respiratory sounds, such as the monitoring of inhaler use [75–77] and coughs [78].

Finally, many people have unrecognized and undiagnosed sleep disorders; early diagnosis and treatment improve health and quality of life. An audio-based method can be integrated with an existing technology (such as reduced channel PSG or accelerometer-based movement monitoring) for the evaluation of sleep, breathing, and follow-up after interventions (surgical or drugs). This concept will simplify data acquisition and will potentially increase accessibility to valid home-based diagnostic testing.

Acknowledgements We would like to thank Ms. Bruria Freidman from the Sleep-Wake Disorder Unit of Soroka University Medical Center, for her support and collaboration. This study was supported in part by the Israeli Ministry of Industry and Trade, The Kamin Program, award no. 46168 and by the Israel Science Foundation (ISF) grant no. 1403/15.

References

1. Bruni O, Fabrizi P, Ottaviano S, Cortesi F, Giannotti F, Guidetti V (1997) Prevalence of sleep disorders in childhood and adolescence with headache: a case-control study. Cephalalgia 17(4):492–498
2. Hillman DR, Murphy AS, Antic R, Pezzullo L (2006) The economic cost of sleep disorders. Sleep 29(3):299
3. Kales JD, Healey S (1979) Prevalence of sleep disorders in the Los Angeles metropolitan area. Am J Psychiatry 36(10):1257–1262
4. Mastronarde JG, Wise RA, Shade DM, Olopade CO, Scharf SM, Centers ALAACR (2008) Sleep quality in asthma: results of a large prospective clinical trial. J Asthma 45(3):183–189
5. Pillar G, Lavie P (2008) Upper airway in obstructive sleep apnea—controversies continue. J Sleep Res 17(2):123–124
6. Ronksley PE, Hemmelgarn BR, Heitman SJ, Flemons WW, Ghali WA, Manns B, Faris P, Tsai WH (2011) Excessive daytime sleepiness is associated with increased health care utilization among patients referred for assessment of OSA. Sleep 34(3):363
7. Sanna A (2013) Obstructive sleep apnoea, motor vehicle accidents, and work performance. Chron Respir Dis 10(1):29–33
8. Susan Redline M, Newman AB (2002) The relationship between chronically disrupted sleep and healthcare use. Sleep 25(3):289
9. Tarasiuk A, Reuveni H (2004) Obstructive sleep apnea syndrome: the diagnostic strategy dilemma. Israel Med Assoc J 6(11):686–690
10. Tarasiuk A, Reuveni H (2013) The economic impact of obstructive sleep apnea. Curr Opin Pulm Med 19(6):639–644
11. Tarasiuk A, Greenberg-Dotan S, Simon T, Tal A, Oksenberg A, Reuveni H (2006) Low socioeconomic status is a risk factor for cardiovascular disease among adult obstructive sleep apnea syndrome patients requiring treatment. Chest 130(3):766–773. https://doi.org/10.1378/chest.130.3.766
12. Flemons WW (2002) Clinical practice. Obstructive sleep apnea. N Engl J Med 347(7):498–504. https://doi.org/10.1056/NEJMcp012849
13. Iber C, Ancoli-Israel S, Chesson AL, Quan S (2007) The AASM manual for the scoring of sleep and associated events: rules, terminology, and technical specifications, 1st edn. The American Academy of Sleep Medicine, Westchester, IL
14. Collop N, Anderson WM, Boehlecke B, Claman D, Goldberg R, Gottlieb D, Hudgel D, Sateia M, Schwab R (2007) Clinical guidelines for the use of unattended portable monitors in the diagnosis of obstructive sleep apnea in adult patients. J Clin Sleep Med 3(7):737–747

15. Verginis N, Davey MJ, Horne RS (2010) Scoring respiratory events in paediatric patients: evaluation of nasal pressure and thermistor recordings separately and in combination. Sleep Med 11(4):400–405
16. Whyte K, Gugger M, Gould G, Molloy J, Wraith P, Douglas N (1991) Accuracy of respiratory inductive plethysmograph in measuring tidal volume during sleep. J Appl Physiol 71(5):1866–1871
17. Reuveni H, Schweitzer E, Tarasiuk A (2001) A cost-effectiveness analysis of alternative at-home or in-laboratory technologies for the diagnosis of obstructive sleep apnea syndrome. Med Decis Mak 21(6):451–458
18. Abeyratne UR, Karunajeewa AS Hukins C (2004) Higher-order spectra for the estimation of total-airway-response (TAR) in snore-based diagnosis of apnoea. In: Control, automation, robotics and vision conference. ICARCV. IEEE, pp 925–930
19. Azarbarzin A, Moussavi Z (2012) Snoring sounds variability as a signature of obstructive sleep apnea. Med Eng Phys. https://doi.org/10.1016/j.medengphy.2012.06.013
20. Colrain IM, Trinder J, Fraser G, Wilson G (1989) Ventilation during sleep onset. University of Tasmania, Tasmania
21. Dafna E, Tarasiuk A, Zigel Y (2012) Sleep-quality assessment from full night audio recordings of sleep apnea patients. In: Conference of the proceedings of the IEEE engineering in medicine and biology society. IEEE, pp 3660–3663
22. Dafna E, Tarasiuk A, Zigel Y (2015b) Sleep-wake evaluation from whole-night non-contact audio recordings of breathing sounds. PLoS One 10(2):e0117382
23. Hedner J, Pillar G, Pittman SD, Zou D, Grote L, White DP (2004) A novel adaptive wrist actigraphy algorithm for sleep-wake assessment in sleep apnea patients. Sleep 27(8): 1560–1566
24. Marino M, Li Y, Rueschman MN, Winkelman J, Ellenbogen J, Solet J, Dulin H, Berkman LF, Buxton OM (2012) Measuring sleep: accuracy, sensitivity, and specificity of wrist actigraphy compared to polysomnography. Sleep 36(11):1747–1755
25. Sadeh A, Acebo C (2002) The role of actigraphy in sleep medicine. Sleep Med Rev 6(2):113–124
26. Scharf SM, Garshick E, Brown R, Tishler PV (1990) Screening for subclinical sleep-disordered breathing. Sleep 13(4):344–353
27. Sola-Soler J, Fiz JA, Morera J, Jané R (2011) Bayes classification of snoring subjects with and without sleep apnea hypopnea syndrome, using a Kernel method. In: Engineering in Medicine and Biology Society, EMBC, 2011 annual international conference of the IEEE. IEEE, pp 6071–6074
28. Sola-Soler J, Jane R, Fiz JA, Morera J (2007) Automatic classification of subjects with and without sleep apnea through snoring analysis. In: Engineering in medicine and biology society, 2007. EMBS 2007. 29th Annual international conference of the IEEE. IEEE, pp 6093–6096
29. Berthomier C, Drouot X, Herman-Stoïca M, Berthomier P, Prado J, Bokar-Thire D, Benoit O, Mattout J, d'Ortho M-P (2007) Automatic analysis of single-channel sleep EEG: validation in healthy individuals. Sleep 30(11):1587
30. Choi JH, Kim EJ, Kim YS, Choi J, Kim TH, Kwon SY, Lee HM, Lee SH, Shin C, Lee SH (2010) Validation study of portable device for the diagnosis of obstructive sleep apnea according to the new AASM scoring criteria: Watch-PAT 100. Acta Otolaryngol 130(7):838–843
31. Hwang S, Chung G, Lee J, Shin J, Lee S-J, Jeong D-U, Park K (2012) Sleep/wake estimation using only anterior tibialis electromyography data. Biomed Eng Online 11:1–15
32. Sommermeyer D, Schwaibold M, Schöller B, Grote L, Hedner J Bolz A 2010 Detection of sleep disorders by a modified matching pursuit algorithm. In: World congress on medical physics and biomedical engineering, 7–12, 2009, Munich. Springer, pp 1271–1274
33. Akhter S, Abeyratne U, Swarnkar V (2013) Variations of snoring properties with macro sleep stages in a population of obstructive sleep apnea patients. In: Engineering in Medicine and Biology Society (EMBC), 2013 35th annual international conference of the IEEE. IEEE, pp 1318–1321
34. Ben-Israel N, Tarasiuk A, Zigel Y (2010) Nocturnal sound analysis for the diagnosis of obstructive sleep apnea. Conference proceedings: annual international conference of the IEEE

engineering in medicine and biology society IEEE engineering in medicine and biology society conference 2010:6146–6149. https://doi.org/10.1109/IEMBS.2010.5627784
35. Dafna E, Halevi M, Ben Or D, Tarasiuk A, Zigel Y (2016) Estimation of macro sleep stages from whole night audio analysis. In: Engineering in Medicine and Biology Society (EMBC), 2016 IEEE 38th annual international conference of the IEEE, pp 2847–2850
36. Dafna E, Tarasiuk A, Zigel Y (2013a) Automatic detection of whole night snoring events using non-contact microphone. PLoS One 8(12):e84139
37. De Chazal P, Fox N, O'HARE E, Heneghan C, Zaffaroni A, Boyle P, Smith S, O'CONNELL C, McNicholas WT (2011) Sleep/wake measurement using a non-contact biomotion sensor. J Sleep Res 20(2):356–366
38. Hoffstein V, Mateika S, Anderson D (1994) Snoring: is it in the ear of the beholder? Sleep 17(6):522–526
39. Maimon N, Hanly PJ (2010) Does snoring intensity correlate with the severity of obstructive sleep apnea. J Clin Sleep Med 6(5):475–478
40. Itamar Medical Ltd. http://www.itamar-medical.com/
41. Levartovsky A, Dafna E, Zigel Y, Tarasiuk A (2016) Breathing and snoring sound characteristics during sleep in adults. J Clin Sleep Med 12(3):375–384
42. Ben-Israel N, Tarasiuk A, Zigel Y (2012) Obstructive apnea hypopnea index estimation by analysis of nocturnal snoring signals in adults. Sleep 35(9):1299–1305C. https://doi.org/10.5665/sleep.2092
43. Dafna E, Rosenwein T, Tarasiuk A, Zigel Y (2015) Breathing rate estimation during sleep using audio signal analysis. In: 2015 37th annual international conference of the IEEE Engineering in Medicine and Biology Society (EMBC). IEEE, pp 5981–5984
44. Dafna E, Tarasiuk A, Zigel Y (2013) OSA severity assessment based on sleep breathing analysis using ambient microphone. In: 2013 35th annual international conference of the IEEE Engineering in Medicine and Biology Society (EMBC). IEEE, pp 2044–2047
45. Rosenwein T, Dafna E, Tarasiuk A, Zigel Y (2015) Breath-by-breath detection of apneic events for OSA severity estimation using non-contact audio recordings. In: 2015 37th annual international conference of the IEEE Engineering in Medicine and Biology Society (EMBC). IEEE, pp 7688–7691
46. Ben Or D, Dafna E, Tarasiuk A, Zigel Y (2016) Obstructive sleep apnea severity estimation: fusion of speech-based systems. In: Engineering in Medicine and Biology Society (EMBC), 2016 IEEE 38th annual international conference of the IEEE, pp 3207–3210
47. Elisha O, Zigel Y, Tarasiuk A (2012) Automatic detection of obstructive sleep apnea using speech signal analysis. In: Afeka-AVIOS speech processing conference
48. Goldshtein E, Tarasiuk A, Zigel Y (2011) Automatic detection of obstructive sleep apnea using speech signals. IEEE Trans Biomed Eng 58(5):1373–1382
49. Kriboy M, Tarasiuk A, Zigel Y (2014) Detection of Obstructive sleep apnea in awake subjects by exploiting body posture effects on the speech signal. In: 2014 36th annual international conference of the IEEE engineering in medicine and biology society, 2014, IEEE, pp 4224–4227
50. Rosenwein T, Dafna E, Tarasiuk A, Zigel Y (2014) Detection of breathing sounds during sleep using non-contact audio recordings. 35th Annual international IEEE EMBS conference, Chicago, IL
51. Sadeh A (2011) The role and validity of actigraphy in sleep medicine: an update. Sleep Med Rev 15(4):259–267
52. Johnson NL, Kirchner HL, Rosen CL, Storfer-Isser A, Cartar LN, Ancoli-Israel S, Emancipator JL, Kibler AM, Redline S (2007) Sleep estimation using wrist actigraphy in adolescents with and without sleep disordered breathing: a comparison of three data modes. Sleep 30(7):899
53. Blackwell T, Redline S, Ancoli-Israel S, Schneider JL, Surovec S, Johnson NL, Cauley JA, Stone KL, Group SoOFR (2008) Comparison of sleep parameters from actigraphy and polysomnography in older women: the SOF study. Sleep 31(2):283
54. Tilmanne J, Urbain J, Kothare MV, Wouwer AV, Kothare SV (2009) Algorithms for sleep–wake identification using actigraphy: a comparative study and new results. J Sleep Res 18(1):85–98
55. Malhotra A, Huang Y, Fogel R, Lazic S, Pillar G, Jakab M, Kikinis R, White DP (2006) Aging influences on pharyngeal anatomy and physiology: the predisposition to pharyngeal collapse. Am J Med 119(1):72.e79

56. Pillar G, Malhotra A, Fogel RB, Beauregard J, Slamowitz DI, Shea SA, White DP (2000) Upper airway muscle responsiveness to rising PCO 2 during NREM sleep. J Appl Physiol 89(4):1275–1282
57. Trinder J, Kay A, Kleiman J, Dunai J (1997) Gender differences in airway resistance during sleep. J Appl Physiol 83(6):1986–1997
58. Trinder J, Whitworth F, Kay A, Wilkin P (1992) Respiratory instability during sleep onset. J Appl Physiol 73:2462–2462
59. Edwards BA, White DP (2011) Control of the pharyngeal musculature during wakefulness and sleep: implications in normal controls and sleep apnea. Head Neck 33(S1):S37–S45
60. Worsnop C, Kay A, Kim Y, Trinder J, Pierce R (2000) Effect of age on sleep onset-related changes in respiratory pump and upper airway muscle function. J Appl Physiol 88(5):1831–1839
61. Cohen J (1960) A coefficient of agreement for nominal scales. Educ Psychol Meas 20(1):37–46
62. Malik V, Smith D (2012) Respiratory physiology during sleep. Sleep Med Clin 7(3):497–505
63. Phillipson EA (1978) Respiratory adaptations in sleep. Annu Rev Physiol 40(1):133–156
64. Halevi M, Dafna E, Tarasiuk A, Zigel Y (2016) Can we discriminate between apnea and hypopnea using audio signals? In: Engineering in Medicine and Biology Society (EMBC), 2016 IEEE 38th annual international conference of the IEEE, pp 3211–3214
65. Montazeri A, Giannouli E, Moussavi Z (2012) Assessment of obstructive sleep apnea and its severity during wakefulness. Ann Biomed Eng 40(4):916–924
66. Solà-Soler J, Fiz JA, Torres A, Jané R (2014) Identification of obstructive sleep apnea patients from tracheal breath sound analysis during wakefulness in polysomnographic studies. In: 2014 36th Annual international conference of the IEEE engineering in medicine and biology society. IEEE, pp 4232–4235
67. Espinoza-Cuadros F, Fernández-Pozo R, Toledano DT, Alcázar-Ramírez JD, López-Gonzalo E, Hernández-Gómez LA (2016) Reviewing the connection between speech and obstructive sleep apnea. Biomed Eng Online 15(1):1
68. Saboisky JP, Butler JE, Gandevia SC, Eckert DJ (2012) Functional role of neural injury in obstructive sleep apnea. Front Neurol 3:95
69. Fox AW, Monoson PK, Morgan CD (1989) Speech dysfunction of obstructive sleep apnea. A discriminant analysis of its descriptors. Chest J 96(3):589–595
70. Smith L, Schwartz AR (2012) Effect of end-expiratory lung volume on upper airway. J Appl Physiol 113(5):691–699
71. Yadollahi A, Moussavi Z (2007) Acoustical flow estimation: review and validation. IEEE Eng Med Biol Mag 26(1):56–61
72. Alshaer H, Levchenko A, Bradley TD, Pong S, Tseng W-H, Fernie GR (2013) A system for portable sleep apnea diagnosis using an embedded data capturing module. J Clin Monit Comput 27(3):303–311
73. Nakano H, Ikeda T, Hayashi M, Ohshima E, Onizuka A (2003) Effects of body position on snoring in apneic and nonapneic snorers. Sleep 26(2):169–176
74. Joachim B, Aoife R, João SD, Elnaz G, Gari DC (2013) A review of current sleep screening applications for smartphones. Physiol Meas 34(7):R29
75. Holmes MS, D'Arcy S, Costello RW, Reilly RB (2014) Acoustic analysis of inhaler sounds from community-dwelling asthmatic patients for automatic assessment of adherence. IEEE Trans Health Med 2:2700210
76. Taylor TE, De Looze C, MacHale P, Holmes MS, Sulaiman I, Costello RW, Reilly RB (2016a) Characterization of patient inhaler inhalation sounds using non-contact and tracheal microphones. Biomed Phys Eng Express 2(5):055021
77. Taylor TE, Holmes MS, Sulaiman I, Costello RW, Reilly RB (2016b) Monitoring inhaler inhalations using an acoustic sensor proximal to inhaler devices. J Aerosol Med Pulm Drug Deliv 29(5):439–446. https://doi.org/10.1089/jamp.2015.1276
78. Zigel Y, Goldbart A, Freud T, Erew A, Abu Leil M, Tocker Y, Levi I, Urkin J (2016) Diurnal and seasonal variation of cough episodes in healthy young adults. J Asthma 53(3):295–300

15 Cough Sounds

Saikiran Gopalakaje, Tony Sahama, and Anne B. Chang

15.1 Introduction

15.1.1 Cough: An Important Symptom

Cough is the most symptom of an airway disease. Thus, when chronic and/or associated with other respiratory symptoms, its presence often signifies an underlying lung disease. In a multicentre Australian study involving 346 children newly referred for chronic cough, only 13.9% of children did not have an underlying respiratory illness [1, 2]. Thus, understanding and careful evaluation of people with chronic cough are important. Delayed diagnosis (e.g. foreign body) may cause chronic respiratory morbidity [3]; early diagnosis of chronic diseases leading to appropriate management and subsequent resolution of cough and improved QoL [1] is important. Further, various aspects of the cough sound are as it is used in guidelines and research studies [4–6]. While clinical evaluation is important, it is outside the realms of this chapter, and readers are referred to exciting chronic cough guidelines.

S. Gopalakaje, M.B.B.S., M.D., M.R.C.P.C.H (✉)
Lady Cilento Children's Hospital, South Brisbane, QLD, Australia
e-mail: saikiran.gopalakaje@health.qld.gov.au

T. Sahama, B.Sc., M.Phil., Ph.D.
Queensland University of Technology, Brisbane, QLD, Australia
e-mail: t.sahama@qut.edu.au

A. B. Chang, M.P.H.T.M., Ph.D., F.R.A.C.P
Child Health Division, Menzies School of Health Research, Darwin, NT, Australia

Department of Respiratory and Sleep Medicine, Queensland Children's Medical Research Institute, Queensland Children's Health Service, Queensland University of Technology, South Brisbane, Australia
e-mail: anne.chang@menzies.edu.au

K. N. Priftis et al. (eds.), *Breath Sounds*, https://doi.org/10.1007/978-3-319-71824-8_15

15.1.2 Cough: The Burden

In countries where data is available, cough is the most common symptom that results in new medical consultations [7]. In the USA, approximately 29.5 million doctor visits per year are for cough [8], and $6.8 billion dollars are spent a year [7]. In Australia acute bronchitis/bronchiolitis is consistently the most common new problem encountered by general practitioners, ranging from annual rate of 2.2 to 3.2 per 100 encounters (1999–2009 data) [9]. The burden of cough is also reflected in the number of consultations (per child) sought for cough in children. A uni-centre Australian study described that the number of medical consultations for their coughing illness in the last 12 months was high: >80% of children had ≥5 doctor visits, and 53% had >10 [10]. This high consultation rate was later confirmed in a multicentre Australian study [1].

Although some medical practitioners consider chronic cough as a trivial symptom, cough is associated with significant morbidity in both children and their parents [1, 11]. In addition to the above, the burden of cough is also reflected in impaired quality of life (QoL). In a multicentre study on 346 children using a generic paediatric health-related QoL tool (PedsQL®), the mean normalized PedsQL® score of 74.7 was in the realm of children with other chronic illnesses (cardiac, 79.4; diabetes, 76.6; obesity, 75; gastrointestinal conditions, 72.4) but better than children with cancer (68.5) and end-stage renal disease (69.6) [1]. Further, the presence of cough (particularly when chronic) may be reflective of an underlying serious disorder [1, 12].

Thus, cough is important not only because of the commonality of the clinical problem of cough but also cough is an important symptom in clinical medicine. This chapter focuses on the sounds of cough as a symptom and some basic pathophysiological correlates, but not clinical management.

15.1.3 What Is a Cough

An overall review of the mechanisms of cough is beyond the scope of this article. However, to understand the sound of cough as a symptom, a basic understanding of the physiology of cough is required and briefly outlined below.

Physiologically cough has three phases: inspiratory, compressive and expiratory [13]. The inspiratory phase consists of inhaling a variable amount of air which serves to lengthen the expiratory muscles, optimizing the length-tension relationship. The compressive phase consists of a very brief (200 ms) closure of the glottis to maintain lung volume as intrathoracic pressure builds (up to 300 mmHg in adults) due to isometric contraction of the expiratory muscles against a closed glottis. The expiratory phase starts with opening of the glottis, releasing a brief (30–50 ms) supramaximal expiratory flow [14] (up to 12 L/s in adults, also termed the 'cough spike') followed by lower (3–4 L/s) expiratory flows lasting a further 200–500 ms [13]. Dynamic compression of the airways occurs during the expiratory phase, and the high-velocity expulsion of gas (air) sweeps airway debris along. Airway debris and secretions are also swept proximally by ciliary activity. Cough also enhances mucociliary clearance in both healthy individuals and those with lung disease [15].

Cough can be voluntarily initiated or suppressed except when it is part of the laryngeal expiratory reflex when the larynx is mechanically stimulated by foreign materials. Physiologists describe two basic types of cough: laryngeal cough (a true reflex, also known as 'expiratory reflex') and tracheobronchial cough. Laryngeal cough thus protects the airways from airway aspiration. Tracheobronchial cough is initiated distal to the larynx and can be volitional. It is primarily stimulated by chemoreceptors in the lower airways and can also be mechanically stimulated [16]. The primary function of tracheobronchial cough is airway clearance and maintenance of the mucociliary apparatus. It has been argued that differentiating the types of cough and what constitutes as a cough is important [17]. However clinicians remain certain what cough is in the clinical setting.

The knowledge of cough neurophysiology has significantly advanced in recent years although much of the work is based on animal models and may have limited applicability to humans as significant interspecies differences exist [18]. Readers are referred to recent reviews of cough mechanisms and cough receptors [19–21] for in-depth aspects of cough-related neurophysiology. As a gross oversimplification, the cough pathway can be compartmentalized to the afferent arm (from cough stimulus to the respiratory centre), and efferent arms (from the respiratory centre to the respiratory muscles, larynx and pelvic muscles) of the cough pathway are likely to be influenced by a bidirectional feedback loop, but this has not yet been clearly established. Receptors involved in cough are terminations of vagal afferents in airway mucosa and submucosa [18, 22]. These afferent receptors have different sensitivities to different stimuli and are unequally distributed in the airways; generally the larynx and proximal large airways are more mechanosensitive and less chemosensitive than peripheral large airways. The existence of distinct cough receptors, widely assumed to be present and first proposed by Widdicombe [23], is now proven [22, 24]. Generation of action potentials (depolarization of the terminal membrane) from these receptors are subclassified into two: ionotropic receptors (cause generator potentials by acting on ligand-gated ion channels) and metabotropic receptors (act indirectly on ligand-gated ion channels via G-protein-coupled receptors) [18, 25]. These include the transient receptor potential cation channel subfamily V member 1 (TRPV1), transient receptor potential cation channel subfamily A member 1 (TRPA1) and G-protein-coupled opioid-like receptor-1 (NOP1) receptors [26].

These cough and airway receptors mediated through the vagus nerve, jugular and nodose ganglions extend to the nucleus tractus solitarius (NTS), which is the first central nervous system (CNS) synaptic contact of these afferent fibres [27]. Second-order neurons from the NTS have polysynaptic connections with the central cough generator which is also the respiratory pattern generator [27, 28]. NTS is postulated to be the site of greatest modulatory influence and plasticity. The mechanisms underpinning chronic cough have been likened to that of chronic pain [16], and increased neurogenic markers have been described in children with increased cough receptor sensitivity (CRS) [29]. The intrathoracic pressure and effects of it generated by cough may also perpetuate the chronic cough cycle as suggested by a recent animal study that showed pressure effects enhance cough sensitivity [30].

A particularly important finding is the presence of small amounts of secretions in children with dry cough which may have implications in the management of suppurative lung disease; a dry cough may represent early disease process where only a small amount of mucus is present.

15.1.4 Normal Cough Sound

How are cough sounds generated? The sound of a cough is due to vibration of larger airways and laryngeal structures during turbulent flow in expiration [31, 32]. Thus physiologically, all components involved in the generation of the sound would affect the acoustic characteristics.

15.1.5 Physiological Influences

15.1.5.1 Age

There is direct and indirect evidence that age influences physiological domains that influence the clinical manifestation of conditions where cough is a dominant feature [33, 34]. These physiological domains can be simplified to (1) cough-specific physiology, (2) general respiratory physiology, (3) other direct systems such as the immune system that influence the respiratory system and (4) other general physiologies. Much of this data is available elsewhere [33]. Examples of cough-specific physiological differences include age- and sex-related variation in cough sensitivity [34]. In children, sex does not influence cough sensitivity, whereas in post-pubertal adolescents and adults, females have significantly increased sensitivity [34]. The cough reflex is weak in premature infants and develops with maturity. Exactly when the cough reflex is fully matured is unknown, but it is likely around 5 years of age, which is the cutoff age for risk of accidental nut inhalation, and thus parents are advised not to give nuts to their children prior to age of 5 years. Also, adults easily expectorate when airway secretions are present, whereas children do not even when secretions are abundant. Thus classical adult terms like productive cough cannot be applied to young children [35].

Examples of general respiratory physiology include differences in calibre of large and small airways and percentage of time spent in random eye movement (REM) sleep, which influences cough frequency [36]. Smaller airway calibre (which influences airflow exponentially as opposed to linearly) and lack of collateral ventilation in immature lungs influence likelihood of presence of wheeze and atelectasis in respiratory conditions where chronic cough is also common such as chronic suppurative lung disease and right middle lobe syndrome [35].

Specific for the sounds of cough, as the sound is dependent on flow, age-related issues that influence flow are volume (from where the cough starts), and the size of the airways also influences flow. The normal cough in children has different acoustic properties to adults as further described below, and this is not surprising as the same is clearly discernible from voices.

15.1.5.2 Sex

A person's sex influences their cough characteristics. While sex does not influence objective cough counts or subjective cough scores in children [37], adult data showed that sex significantly influenced objective cough scores [38]. In adults with chronic cough, objective cough counts and CRS were higher in females than males [38, 39]. In young or pre to early pubertal children, sex does not influence CRS [40, 41].

As sex also influences lung volumes and airway calibre, as reflected in spirometry reference ranges, [42] and cough characteristics are dependent on lung volume and airway calibre, invariably, sex influences the acoustics of cough in normal people.

15.1.6 Pathological Influences

The generation of cough sounds and some factors that influence cough sounds have been examined in the laboratory [31, 43]. Using cough sound analysis (spectrogram and time-expanded waveform), productive and nonproductive cough can be differentiated in the laboratory [43]. Unsurprisingly, the dimension of cough quality is used in management and diagnostic guidelines [4–6]. Thus, an understanding on the different constructs used to classify cough sounds is important.

15.1.7 Types of Cough Sounds

In addition to the construct based on cough duration (acute, subacute, chronic), the other constructs of cough include quality (wet/productive or dry, brassy, honking), timing (predominant nocturnal), character (paroxysmal, staccato) and strength or loudness (weak or strong/soft-feeble or loud). Here we focus on the sound characteristics rather than on the timing which relates to some clinical pathology.

Cough quality, specifically dry versus wet [44] or productive cough, is often used in epidemiological [45–47] and clinical research [40, 48]. Clinically, physicians also often differentiate between dry and wet cough [6, 49, 50]. In adults, productive cough is usually obvious, but children however often swallow their sputum, and hence a 'wet cough' is used interchangeably with 'productive cough' to describe cough quality in young children who are unable to expectorate [49, 51]. It is known that nocturnal cough is unreliably reported in both children [52] and adults [53].

15.1.7.1 Mucus

There is little doubt that the presence of secretions in the airways influences the cough quality. In addition to the volume of the secretions, the rheological properties of airway mucus also influence cough sound [32]. However, this has been studied mainly in relation to central airways, and it is not known how airway secretions in the more peripheral airways influence the sound of cough. It is not known which generation of the airways is involved when the human ear identifies a wet cough, and currently there are no validated human models that allow measurement of increased airway mucus. Mucus hypersecretory states in human diseases can occur from a variety of mechanisms which include hypersecretion of stored mucin, hypertrophy or hyperplasia of goblet cells and/or increased synthesis from overexpression of mucin genes [54]. In disease states, it is not known which mechanism or site of production is the most important, but in smokers with chronic bronchitis, a common cause of productive cough in adults, the larger bronchi (bronchi of diameter >4 mm, i.e. segmental bronchi and above) [55], are the site of greatest inflammation [54].

In humans, it is not known how much mucus is required and where it has to be located for the human ear to detect presence of a moist cough. It is likely that mucus in the large airways is required for detectable difference in cough quality as the sound of cough is generated from vibration of larger airways and laryngeal structures during turbulent flow in expiration [31, 32]. Laminar airflow, which occurs in smaller airways, is inaudible [56]. In an animal model, Korpas and colleagues showed that a certain amount of mucus is required to alter cough sound; 0.5 mL of mucus instilled into the trachea of cats altered cough sound; too little mucin had no effect on cough quality, while too much mucin impaired breathing [57].

15.1.7.2 Lower Airway Abnormalities

Tracheomalacia and bronchomalacia can be due to intrinsic (foreign body and other endobronchial obstructions) or extrinsic airway lesions [58]. In tracheomalacia, expiratory stridor may be present concurrently. If there is malacia of the extrathoracic trachea, inspiratory stridor may be present. The cough in children with tracheomalacia is often described as barking or brassy [59]. The quality of the cough related to tracheomalacia is thought to be related to the juxtaposition of the anterior and posterior walls of the trachea, resulting in recurrent vibrations and irritation of the airway [60].

One study involving 106 children (62 boys, 44 girls; median age = 2.6 years (IQR 5.7)) objectively evaluated cough quality in relation to airway abnormality [59]. When the clinicians detected the presence of a brassy cough, tracheomalacia was usually present at bronchoscopy performed several hours after the cough recording [59]. The intra- and interobserver clinician agreement for brassy cough was both good, kappa of 0.79 (95% CI 0.73–0.86), but the sensitivity of brassy cough (compared to tracheomalacia determined by the good standard, i.e. bronchoscopy) was poor at 0.57. The specificity of brassy cough for tracheomalacia was good at 0.81, respectively [59]. A second study [61] examined the predictive value of a clinically expected diagnosis of airway malacia prior to bronchoscopy. Of the 324 outpatients, airway malacia was found in 126 patients (115 cases of primary airway malacia) [61]. Prior to bronchoscopy, paediatric pulmonologists expected a malacia, based on history, physical examination and/or lung function in 82 patients of whom 61 actually had malacia (positive predictive value, 74%). In 65 of 126 patients, airway malacia was not suspected prior to bronchoscopy (false-negative rate of 52%). They recorded the clinical features in 96 children with primary airway malacia and without a concurrent medical condition. Cough was present in 80 out of 96 (83%) patients. The character and timing of the cough were described as night-time cough in 40 (42%), productive cough in 58 (60%), exercise-induced cough in 34 (35%) and barking, seal-like cough in 41 (43%).

A prospective study examined the relationship between malacia lesions and their respiratory illness profiles in 116 children (malacia $n = 81$ and control subjects $n = 35$) [62]. The median age of the group was 2.1 years (age range, 0.2–17.3 years). The adjusted relative risk of illness frequency was 2.1 (95% confidence interval [CI], 1.3–3.4) and of significant cough was 7.2 (95% CI, 1.01–27.22) for the malacia group. Significant coughing and cough disrupting daily activities were both more likely in the malacia group than in the control group. When compared to control subjects, the severity of illness was 66% higher at the initial presentation of illness, while a significant cough score was four times more likely, and a cough that disrupted or stopped daily activities during the first 2 weeks of illness was seven times more likely [62].

15.1.7.3 Muscle Strength

A cough is considered effective when it is able to displace and result in expulsion of secretions from the bronchial tree. This requires sufficient expiratory muscle strength to generate increased intrathoracic pressure leading to dynamic compression of the airways and reduction of their cross-sectional area [63]. Several studies have documented the correlation between expiratory muscle strength and cough [63, 64]. Adults with a MEP (maximal expiratory pressure) value of 60 cmH_2O or more are able to generate transients of peak flow during coughing and thus may be considered as having an effective cough [63].

Respiratory muscle strength correlates to cough capacity in patients with respiratory muscle weakness [65]. In a study, pulmonary function tests including forced vital capacity (FVC) and respiratory muscle strength (maximal expiratory pressure, MEP; maximal inspiratory pressure, MIP) were performed in 45 patients with amyotrophic lateral sclerosis (ALS), 43 with cervical spinal cord injury (SCI) and 42 with Duchenne muscular dystrophy (DMD) [65]. In the SCI group, MIP was more closely correlated with Peak Cough Flow (PCF), but MEP was more closely correlated with PCF in the ALS and DMD groups [65]. This is explained by the relative weakness of different respiratory muscle groups. In patients with Duchenne muscular dystrophy (DMD) and in high cervical spinal cord injury (SCI), diaphragmatic function is relatively well preserved despite generalized muscle dysfunction, and patients with amyotrophic lateral sclerosis (ALS) experience profound diaphragm weakness, early in the disease process.

If the lung volume attained before expiratory muscle contraction is insufficient, due to inspiratory muscle weakness, cough capacity decreases in spite of functional expiratory muscles. This can lead to atelectasis and loss of elasticity and compliance of the lung and chest wall. This may exacerbate cough weakness by restricting dynamic airway compression [65]. While there are no studies, the strength of cough alters the sound of cough when there is marked muscle weakness.

15.1.8 Cough Quality in Diseases

As described above, cough quality is used in clinical medicine. Here we focus on clinical correlates and the validity of the character, where data is available. In some conditions, cough is characteristic such as with pertussis, but in most, the cough reflects the pathophysiological process. As cough occurs in almost all airway diseases and other respiratory illnesses, it is beyond the scope of the chapter to describe all conditions. Here we limit this section to conditions were the quality of cough is altered.

15.1.9 Endobronchial Secretions: Wet/Dry Cough

Many airway diseases are associated with increased lower airway secretions such as protracted bacterial bronchitis, bronchiectasis and recurrent small volume aspiration lung disease [59]. When these children are clinically assessed and endobronchial secretions are present, their cough quality of wet/dry cough generally relates to the amount of bronchoscopic secretions determined using a standardized scoring system (BS grades) [59]. The study briefly mentioned above involving 106 children used digital recording of cough onto a high-quality recorder (for that era) using music compact disc quality format (44.1 kHz, 16 bit) on the morning of their bronchoscopy [59]. These stored cough sounds were later replayed (using headphones 30–10,000 Hz) and assessed by another clinician blinded to the bronchoscopy and what the first clinician scored [59]. The children without a known underlying respiratory diagnosis had a bronchoscopy undertaken 0.5–3 h after the digital recording [59]. Parents also independently reported what their child's cough was like (wet or dry; when it was mixed, the default was wet). Kappa (K) statistics was used for agreement, and inter-rater and intra-rater agreement examined on digitally recorded cough [59]. A receiver operating characteristic (ROC) curve was used to determine if cough quality related to the amount of airway secretions present at bronchoscopy [59]. The study found that when the cough was assessed as wet, secretions were always present, when the cough was dry secretions if present, were usually minimal or mild [59]. When compared to bronchoscopic findings, the study showed that a wet cough is always associated with BS grades of 3 or more [59]. Parent's assessment of cough quality (wet/dry) agreed with clinicians' ($K = 0.75$, 95% CI 0.58–0.93) [60]. When compared to bronchoscopy (bronchoscopic secretion grade 4), clinicians' cough assessment had the highest sensitivity (0.75) and specificity (0.79) and was marginally better than parent(s) [59]. The area under the ROC curve was 0.85 (95% CI 0.77–0.92). Intra-observer ($K = 1.0$) and inter-clinician agreement for wet/dry cough ($K = 0.88$, 95% CI 0.82–0.94) was very good [59]. Weighted K for inter-rater agreement for bronchoscopic secretion grades was 0.95 (95% CI 0.87–1) [59]. However, dry cough is less valid as the presence of dry cough does not necessarily indicate the absence of secretions. However, BS grades are less in dry cough as shown in the ROC curve [59].

Accuracy and reliability of symptoms are important in clinical and research settings. The above results are in contrast to other common respiratory sounds. For example, Cane and colleagues [66, 67] found that parental reports of wheeze and stridor are often not accurately reported in a clinic setting. Hay and colleagues showed that interobserver agreement for clinical signs of fever, tachypnoea and chest signs was poor to fair (kappa of 0.12–0.39) in the primary care setting, but these signs are known to have good agreement in secondary care settings [68]. This is not surprising as cough is common and a distinct sound for the untrained ear in contrast to sounds like stridor.

However, wet/dry cough has really only been validated in young children, and a study on older children is required given the possibility of the influence of airway size relative to the amount of secretions in the generation of a wet sounding cough (as mentioned in section above). Clinically and anecdotally, an adolescent with a productive cough may have a dry cough when requested to cough. Further, the quality of wet/dry or productive/nonproductive cough is non-diagnostic of a clinical entity as it only reflects the presence of excessive airway secretions. Nevertheless, in terms of children with chronic dry cough, a preliminary study reported that dry cough was significantly more likely to naturally resolve than wet cough [69]. Further follow-up cohort studies with strict clinical diagnostic categories would be useful.

15.1.9.1 Respiratory Infections

Viral Tracheobronchitis

Acute respiratory infection (ARI) caused by viruses is a transient and self-limited condition. Transient-enhanced cough sensitivity has been shown in children with influenza infection. The length of cough in ARI most likely depends on the patient and environment factors [58]. ARI is typically nonproductive at the beginning and quite annoying; later it becomes productive of mucus or mucopurulent sputum before it begins to subside. Often it is an isolated cough (otherwise well) with no other significant signs and symptoms. The most common cause for prolonged acute cough in children is postviral or postinfectious cough. This begins with symptoms related to the common cold and persists. This is seen in 10% of normal children who are still coughing with a simple head cold after 2–3 weeks. If the child is otherwise normal and the cough is resolving, no further investigations would be indicated. It has a high rate of spontaneous resolution without any therapeutic intervention [70].

Pneumonia

In pneumonia, there is increased stimulation of peripheral cough receptors and an increase in secretions. While there are reports that the cough sound relating to pneumonia is diagnostic, the biological plausibility is weak; clinicians are well aware that the cough quality of pneumonia is dependent on the time progression of the pneumonic illness. An initial dry cough is usually followed by varying sputum production causing wet cough dependent on the cause. There will be associated systemic symptoms of infection.

In lung abscess there can be sudden onset or increase in amount of purulent, often foul-smelling sputum. In chronic infections like tuberculosis, there is chronic, usually productive, cough, and there can be associated haemoptysis. However depending on the pulmonary pathology, tuberculosis can also present with chronic dry cough particularly if there are enlarged lymph nodes compressing airway or involving pleura [71].

Pertussis

Cough in pertussis is typically described as paroxysmal spasmodic cough with or without an inspiratory 'whoop' and vomiting [72]. In a study that examined the presence of common symptoms and signs of pertussis in identified cases, paroxysmal cough had a sensitivity of 86% and specificity of 26%, post-tussive whoop had a sensitivity of 50% and specificity of 73% and post-tussive vomit had a sensitivity of 70% and specificity of 61% [73]. The authors also reported that pertussis accounted for 32% of prolonged acute cough, and this was seen even when the classical pertussis symptoms are not present [73]. Another hospital-based study examined the characteristics of 57 infants suspected of having pertussis [74]. They described that [74] 'cough followed by inspiratory stridor and cough accompanied by cyanosis were significant predictors of pertussis (positive predictive values of 100% and 84%, respectively). Leukocyte count >20,000 cells/mm^3 and lymphocyte count >10,000 cells/mm^3 showed predictive values of 92% and 85%, respectively. However, these variables showed low negative predictive values for the diagnosis of pertussis (40%, 60%, 52% and 64%, respectively)'. A study on school-aged children with persistent cough for longer than 2 weeks (5–16 years of age) described that 37% of them had serological evidence of a recent pertussis infection with median of 112 days (range: 38–191 days) of coughing. All children had complete resolution of the cough [75].

Thus, while pertussis infection is associated with a characteristic cough, this is unsurprisingly not 100% precise and somewhat dependent on the age of the child and presence of immunity status [76]. For example, in adults with pertussis, a whoop is rarely present [76]. Further, a cough may be absent in babies with pertussis, and instead the illness is manifested as apnoea [77].

Chlamydia

The quality of cough in chlamydia infections is often described as staccato-like cough. This is seen in infancy. In a series of 115 cases, the authors noted chlamydia infection led to a gradual onset of respiratory tract symptoms [78]. The infant is often afebrile and a staccato cough is present [72, 78].

15.1.9.2 Asthma

While people with asthma often cough, not everyone with asthma coughs, and most children with a cough without other symptoms do not have asthma [16]. In children, clinicians sometimes describe a 'tight asthma cough' during acute asthma. However, this has not been validated. In general, cough associated with asthma without a coexistent respiratory infection is usually dry [4].

15.1.9.3 Non-respiratory Causes of Cough

Chronic cough has been reported as a side effect of ACE inhibitors (2–16.7%), inhaled ICS and as a complication of chronic vagus nerve stimulation. Chronic cough associated with ear canal stimulation from wax impaction and cholesteatoma due to the presence of auricular branch of the vagus nerve has been reported [79]. The cough in these circumstances is usually dry.

15.1.9.4 Habitual and Psychogenic Cough

Habitual cough can be a symptom of a 'vocal tic'. This is a dry repetitive cough and disappears with sleep. Habit cough is seen in younger children with the mean age range from 4 to 15 years. This can be transient or chronic [58, 72]. Psychogenic cough is usually seen in an older child/adolescent. The quality of cough is bizarre disruptive honking cough with child exhibiting 'la belle indifference'. Cough goes away with concentration or sleep. Bizarre honking coughs usually serve a purpose with some secondary gain [72].

In a recent review [80] of the use of habit cough and psychogenic cough for these disorders, an expert panel suggested that:

1. In adults or children with chronic cough, the presence or absence of night-time cough or cough with a barking or honking character should not be used to diagnose or exclude psychogenic or habit cough.
2. In adults and children with chronic cough that has remained medically unexplained after a comprehensive evaluation based upon the most current evidence-based management guideline, the diagnosis of tic cough should be made when the patient manifests the core clinical features of tics that include suppressibility, distractibility, suggestibility, variability and the presence of a premonitory sensation whether the cough is single or one of many tics.
3. In adults and children with chronic cough, substituting the diagnostic term tic cough for habit cough should be made consistent with the DSM-5 classification of diseases and because the definition and features of a tic capture the habitual nature of cough.
4. In adults and children, substituting the diagnostic term somatic cough disorder for psychogenic cough should be made consistent with the DSM-5 classification of diseases.

15.1.10 Measuring Cough Sounds

The cough sounds can be measured by its *intensity* (the respiratory muscle strength), *frequency* (number of coughs per hour—the cough patterns) of cough occurrence and *quality* (dry, moist, productive, brassy, hoarse, wheezy and barking). Cough can also be classified by the *severity* (e.g. associated urge that impacts quality of life). While the intensity and frequency of the cough are subjected to quantitative but subjective analysis, the severity of the cough is objective, qualitative and specific to the episode. The practical complexity of measuring the severity of the cough ranges from patient to patient and varies among the diagnosis.

A number of validated tools have been developed to measure the severity of cough. Various aspects of cough including symptom severity, frequency, intensity and impact on quality of life can be measured using these tools (Table 15.1). For this chapter we focus on cough sounds and will not discuss the other methods of assessing cough as an outcome (e.g. QoL, cough sensitivity, etc.). Cough sound analysis has also been used in veterinary medicine {ref.}.

15.1.11 Cough Recorders

Currently, cough frequency assessment is considered the gold standard for the objective assessment of cough frequency [81]. However, the analysis of cough frequency has proven problematic. Because cough is episodic, data collection over many hours is required, along with real-time aural analysis [82]. Various methods have been used to capture cough (Table 15.2).

The earliest systems consisted of tape recorders, and the recorded cough sounds were counted manually. The manual cough counting was time-consuming and the patients were restricted to a single room [82]. To optimally classify a sound event as cough or non-cough, the feature vectors of coughs from different subjects should

Table 15.1 Cough measurement tools (adapted from [81])

Assessment focus		Assessment tool	Limitations
Symptom based		Visual analogue scale (VAS)	Less comprehensive compared to HRQOL tools in assessing different components of health status
		Cough severity score (CSS)	
		Cough severity diary (CSD)	
Questionnaire-based health-related quality of life (HRQOL)		Leicester Cough Questionnaire (LCQ)	Largely subjective measures
		Chronic Cough Impact Questionnaire (CCIQ)	
		Cough-Specific Quality of Life Questionnaire (CQLQ)	
		Paediatric Cough Quality of Life Questionnaire (PC-QLQ)	
Objective measures	Cough reflex sensitivity	Capsaicin, citric acid, fog, tartaric acid	Techniques not standardized, hence difficult to compare between centres
	Cough monitors	*Older devices* Hull Automated Cough Monitor LifeShirt PulmoTrack	Poor discrimination between cough sound and sound from environment Not suitable for field trials
		Newer devices Leicester cough monitor (LCM) VitaloJAK	Some manual input still needed to complete cough frequency counting

Table 15.2 Signals and sensor types for monitoring cough (adapted from [83, 84])

Signal	Sensor
Sound detection based	Free-field microphone
	Air-coupled microphone
	Contact microphone
Movement detection based	Electromyography
	Accelerometer
	Induction plethysmography Optoelectronic plethysmography Impedance plethysmography Piezo transducer based

have similar values, whereas non-cough events should give dissimilar feature vectors. The measuring system should not depend on the sound amplitude because the cough loudness is not the same for different people, and it makes the relative distance of the microphone less important [85]. These principles are similar to those used in speech recognition [85].

Initial products developed include Hull Automated Cough Monitor, LifeShirt and PulmoTrack [85–87]. The discrimination of cough sounds from speech and other noise was suboptimal with these earlier devices. Two newer cough monitoring systems are more widely in use in clinical research [88, 89]: the Leicester cough monitor (LCM) and the VitaloJAK [81]. A group from the UK published [85] their study on 33 smoking subjects, 20 male and 13 female aged between 20 and 54 with a chronic troublesome cough studied in the hour after rising using a programme for the analysis of digital audio recordings. The Hull Automatic Cough Counter (HACC) uses digital signal processing (DSP) to calculate characteristic spectral coefficients of sound events, which are then classified into cough and non-cough events by the use of a probabilistic neural network (PNN). Parameters such as the total number of coughs and cough frequency as a function of time can be calculated from the results of the audio processing. In their study with this automated system HACC, the average sensitivity was calculated to be 0.80 with a range of 0.55–1.00, while the specificity was 0.96 with a range of 0.92–0.98. Using HACC it was possible to identify coughs in an hour long recording in an average time of 1 min 35 s, a reduction of 97.5% in counting time [85]. Reproducibility of repeated HACC analysis was 100%. The average percentage of false positives compared to true positives was calculated to be 20%. False positives were caused by similar sounds such as laughter, loud bangs and other subjects coughing [85].

The VitaloJAK consists of two microphones (contact and free-field) and an MP3 recorder [90]. The counting has to be done manually but on a condensed version of 24-h recording into 1.5-h-long version [90]. Thus human factor plays a role in its accuracy which increases with experience of the user and makes this system more time-consuming compared to fully automated system like Leicester cough monitor (LCM) [90]. In contrast, the LCM comprises of a free-field microphone and an MP3 recorder [91]. It has automated specifically designed software for cough detection.

This system also requires minor refinement by an operator (5 min per 24-h recording). The sensitivity and specificity for cough detection are very good [91, 92].

One study examined the accuracy of a sound-based cough monitor for detecting and discriminating patient cough from environmental cough [93]. In a hospital ward, they obtained sound recordings from five patients; each has 15-min recordings using the Leicester Cough Monitor (LCM), a sound-based cough monitor ('semi-automated counts'). There were 65 patient coughs and 78 environmental coughs (manual counts). Absolute agreement for patient cough count between all three measurement methods (LCM automated, live and manual sound counts) was high, with intra-class correlation coefficient of 0.94 [95% confidence intervals (CI): 0.74, 0.99]. The proportion of exact agreements for patient cough between LCM and manual count was 0.92, and kappa was 0.84 (95% CI: 0.75, 0.93). The LCM showed sensitivity of 0.94 (95% CI: 0.84, 0.98), specificity of 0.91 (95% CI: 0.82, 0.96), positive predictive value of 0.90 (95% CI: 0.79, 0.95) and negative predictive value of 0.95 (95% CI: 0.86, 0.98) for detecting patient coughs [93].

15.2 Future Directions for Cough Recorders

Cough recorders assessing multidimensional data such as cough intensity, frequency, coughing patterns over time and sound quality would help in holistically assessing the impact of cough as a symptom for the patient [83]. There is no gold standard to compare in currently available cough recorders. Simple, portable and ambulatory monitors would help monitor cough in real-life situations [83].

15.2.1 Other Methods of Cough Sound Analyses

In addition to cough frequency, cough sounds can be analysed using a variety of methods. Most cough sound recorders are based on the acoustic sound analysis principles and aim to capture quasi-periodic waveforms and harmonic frequencies. These can produce signatures in higher-order spectrums (e.g. bispectral or trispectral). In some instances when using conventional techniques, these higher-order spectral signatures can be segregated. Depending on the cough sound quality recorded, conventional analytical techniques would not be appropriate and largely inefficient.

The validity and practicability of several cough sound analysis protocols in scientific literature are worth exploring. To start with, modern voice recognition software has been used to distinguish pertussis cough from other coughs [94], contributing to the robust classifier that assists in tracing possible pertussis cases. When the chronic condition of the cough is reported, it is a different challenge to assess the cough for asthma and/or pneumonia. It is rather complex when this condition is among adults and children and is not conservative. Assessing chronic cough in children is not straightforward and requires different protocols to assessing adult coughs [95].

While cough sound analysis research is advancing, it is apparent that different computer science and engineering techniques are required to analyse cough sound qualities to distinguish the types of cough. For instance, finite element analyses and higher-order spectral (bispectral or trispectral) analyses are promising endeavours to tackle the cough sound quality analysis challenge.

15.2.1.1 Apps for Cough

In recent years, the clinical uses of app-based identification of cough sounds and identifying the likely diagnosis have emerged [96–99]. A study [100] on an automated objective classification model to categorize cough sounds into wet and dry class used first-, second- and third-order statistical features (e.g. formant frequencies, mel-cepstrum, non-Gaussianity, bispectrum, etc.) of the cough sounds. Model was trained and tested on a comprehensive database of 536 coughs from 78 subjects (41 male, 37 female) with age range of 1 month to 15 years. The subjects included in the study had a range of respiratory illnesses such as asthma, pneumonia, bronchitis and rhinopharyngitis. The data was collected in Indonesia. The inclusion criteria were patients with symptoms of chest infection: at least two of cough, sputum, increased breathlessness and temperature >37.5. In those with advanced disease where recovery was not expected, droplet precautions and NIV requirement were excluded. According to the authors [100], their model had a high negative predictive value (NPV = 93%), when scorer consensus data is used as the ground truth. This means that if the model classifies a cough as non-wet (dry), it is most likely that the two expert scorers would independently reach the same conclusion. However, the positive predictive value of the method compared to human scorers was lower (PPV = 55%). Thus, a sizable fraction of coughs classified by the model as wet ends up being consensus-classified as dry by human scorers. As no clinical correlation was undertaken, the significance of the above results is unknown.

In a study published in 2015 [99], the authors detailed a novel technique of cough recording system. Their cough recording system consisted of a low-noise microphone having a cardioid beam pattern (Model NT3, RODE®, Sydney, Australia), followed by a preamplifier and an A/D converter (model: Mobile Pre-USB, M-Audio®, CA, USA) [99]. The output of the MobilePre USB was connected to the USB port of a laptop computer [99]. The nominal distance from the microphones to the mouth of subjects was 50 cm [99]. The actual distance could vary from 40 to 100 cm due to the subject movement [99]. The sampling rate was Fs = 44.1 ksamples/s and 16-bit resolution to obtain the best sound quality [99]. The inclusion criteria used in the recruitment were patients with at least two of the following symptoms: cough, sputum, breathlessness and temperature higher than 37.5 °C [99]. The duration of recording for each subject was between 4 and 6 h in 24 paediatric subjects aged 3–71 months having respiratory diseases such as pneumonia, bronchiolitis and nasopharyngitis [99]. The study showed sensitivity and specificity of >90% [99]. They concluded that the cough segmentation method proposed in their paper achieved accuracy, sensitivity and specificity of 97.3%, 92.8% and 97.5%, respectively [99]. They also recorded Kappa agreement between the automated method and the human observer which was 0.65 [99].

There is current ongoing research on 'Analysis of cough and breathing sounds obtained from clinical sites using iPhones and other recording devices' and 'ResApp Research Project: Phase 2'. ResApp Company explains their approach to development of cough apps. They have a machine learning approach to develop highly accurate algorithms which diagnose disease from cough and respiratory sounds. Machine learning is an artificial intelligence technique that constructs algorithms with the ability to learn from data. Signatures that characterize the respiratory tract are extracted from cough and breathing sounds. Then matching of signatures in a large database of sound recordings with known clinical diagnoses is performed. The machine learning tools then find the optimum combination of these signatures to create an accurate diagnostic test or severity measure (called classification). The company developing these apps also described the ability to diagnose pneumonia from cough sounds as mentioned above.

Further, the complexities of having overlapping or unclear diagnosis have not been considered in the above. For instance, the cough sounds associated with asthma and pneumonia are confounded with the disease conditions in children. Several research publications that involve distinguishing asthmatic cough sounds have been reported [97, 101–105]. Most cough sounds are described as having two phases—expulsive (or burst) and steady-state phases. Asthmatic cough sounds have a quasi-periodic expulsive phase (resulting in a wheezing sound), and the dominant frequency is in the range of 300—600 Hz [101]. Such quasi-periodic waveforms have phase relationships between fundamental and other harmonic frequencies, which can produce signatures in higher-order spectral (bispectral or trispectral) domains [106–117]. The estimation and analysis of higher-order spectral features are challenging. The waveform envelopes and frequency content differ between asthmatic and non-asthmatic coughs in subtle ways that we expect to robustly capture sounds with bispectral features. Features can be extracted in many ways; however there is currently a lack of international experts who can extract time-varying bispectral features [116, 117]. The potential of these features in the analysis of cough sounds has not yet been fully investigated although [105] the use of two other bispectrum features has been reported along with wavelet and time-frequency features for cough sound analysis.

For cough apps, it is vital that the smartphone apps in this juncture are designed with a comprehensive understanding of users and the outcomes anticipated. Thorough consideration of the design (the user interface), the screen that will be used to interact with the users, the amount of information the user should input and the amount of information the user will notice and acquire are required. These approaches are developed to meet the user expectations and decision-makers' efficient attention and, finally, reach an effective and accurate outcome where possible with minimal risk. The sixth generation of computer applications is close to human cognitive capabilities, hence collecting data from apps must be conducted sensitively, with a faster reaction time than fifth- and fourth-generation computer applications.

15.3 Summary

Cough being an important symptom in terms of health-care utilization yields itself to investigation in multiple facets. This ranges from defining various aspects of cough such as duration, quality and type to high-tech fields of studying biomechanical properties of sounds generated in airways during the act of coughing enabling automated disease identification.

Irrespective of technological advances, children with cough require a systematic evaluation and approach. A complete review of cough is beyond the scope of this chapter, and readers are referred elsewhere for an evidenced-based approach and guidelines [72, 118, 119].

References

1. Chang AB, Robertson CF, Van Asperen PP (2012) A multicenter study on chronic cough in children: burden and etiologies based on a standardized management pathway. Chest 142:943–950
2. Schmit KM et al (2013) Evaluating cough assessment tools: a systematic review. Chest 144(6):1819–1826
3. Karakoc F et al (2002) Foreign body aspiration: what is the outcome? Pediatr Pulmonol 34(1):30–36
4. British Thoracic Society; Scottish Intercollegiate Guidelines Network (2003) British guideline on the management of asthma. Thorax 58(Suppl 1):i1
5. Morice AH, C Members (2004) The diagnosis and management of chronic cough. Eur Respir J 24(3):481–492
6. Chang AB, Asher MI (2001) A review of cough in children. J Asthma 38(4):299–309
7. Irwin RS et al (2014) Overview of the management of cough: CHEST guideline and expert panel report. Chest 146(4):885–889
8. Irwin RS (2006) Introduction to the diagnosis and management of cough: ACCP evidence-based clinical practice guidelines. Chest 129(1_Suppl):25S–227
9. Britt H et al (2009) General practice activity in Australia 1999–00 to 2008–09: 10 year data tables. General practice series no. 26. Cat. no. GEP 26. AIHW, Canberra, ACT
10. Marchant JM et al (2008) What is the burden of chronic cough for families? Chest 134(2):303–309
11. Faniran AO, Peat JK, Woolcock AJ (1998) Persistent cough: is it asthma? Arch Dis Child 79(5):411–414
12. Bush A (2002) Paediatric problems of cough. Pulm Pharmacol Ther 15(3):309–315
13. McCool FD (2006) Global physiology and pathophysiology of cough: ACCP evidence-based clinical practice guidelines. Chest 129(1_suppl):48S–53S
14. Bennett WD, Zeman KL (1994) Effect of enhanced supramaximal flows on cough clearance. J Appl Physiol 77(4):1577–1583
15. Oldenburg FA et al (1979) Effects of postural drainage, exercise and cough on mucus clearance in chronic bronchitis. Am Rev Respir Dis 120:739–745
16. Chang A.B (1999) State of the Art: Cough, cough receptors, and asthma in children. Pediatr Pulmonol 28(1):59–70
17. Widdicombe J, Fontana G (2006) Cough: what's in a name? Eur Respir J 28(1):10–15
18. Canning BJ (2006) Anatomy and neurophysiology of the cough reflex. Chest 129(1 Suppl):33S–47S
19. Haji A, Kimura S, Ohi Y (2013) A model of the central regulatory system for cough reflex. Biol Pharm Bull 36(4):501–508
20. De LF et al (2016) TRP functions in the broncho-pulmonary system. Semin Immunopathol 38(3):321–329
21. Canning BJ et al (2014) Anatomy and neurophysiology of cough: CHEST guideline and expert panel report. Chest 146(6):1633–1648
22. Mazzone SB (2004) Sensory regulation of the cough reflex. Pulm Pharmacol Ther 17(6): 361–368

23. Widdicombe J (2001) The race to explore the pathway to cough: who won the silver medal? Am J Respir Crit Care Med 164(5):729–730
24. Canning BJ et al (2004) Identification of the tracheal and laryngeal afferent neurones mediating cough in anaesthetized guinea-pigs. J Physiol 557(Pt 2):543–558
25. Lee MG et al (2004) Ionotropic and metabotropic receptor mediated airway sensory nerve activation. Pulm Pharmacol Ther 17(6):355–360
26. Spina D, Page CP (2013) Regulating cough through modulation of sensory nerve function in the airways. Pulm Pharmacol Ther 26:486–490
27. Bonham AC, Sekizawa S, Joad JP (2004) Plasticity of central mechanisms for cough. Pulm Pharmacol Ther 17:453–457
28. Shannon R et al (2004) Production of reflex cough by brainstem respiratory networks. Pulm Pharmacol Ther 17(6):369–376
29. Chang AB et al (2007) Calcitonin gene-related peptide relates to cough sensitivity in children with chronic cough. Eur Respir J 30(1):66–72
30. Hara J et al (2008) Effect of pressure stress applied to the airway on cough reflex sensitivity in guinea pigs. Am J Respir Crit Care Med 177:585–592
31. Korpas J et al (1987) The origin of cough sounds. Bull Eur Physiopathol Respir 23(Suppl 10):47s–50s
32. Hashimoto Y et al (2003) Influence of the rheological properties of airway mucus on cough sound generation. Respirology 8(1):45–51
33. Chang AB, Widdicombe JG (2006) Cough throughout life: children, adults and the senile. Pulm Pharmacol Ther 20(4):371–382
34. Chang AB et al (2011) Do gender and atopy influence cough outcome measurements in children? Chest 140:324–330
35. Chang AB, Redding GJ, Everard ML (2008) Chronic wet cough: protracted bronchitis, chronic suppurative lung disease and bronchiectasis. Pediatr Pulmonol 43:519–531
36. Widdicombe J, Eccles R, Fontana G (2006) Supramedullary influences on cough. Respir Physiol Neurobiol 152(3):320–328
37. El-Hennawi DM, Bou-Halawa AS, Zaher SR (2006) Management of clinically diagnosed subacute rhinosinusitis in children under the age of two years: a randomized, controlled study. J Laryngol Otol 120(10):845–848
38. Kelsall A et al (2009) Sex differences and predictors of objective cough frequency in chronic cough. Thorax 64(5):393–398
39. Fujimura M et al (1996) Female gender as a determinant of cough threshold to inhaled capsaicin. Eur Respir J 9:1624–1626
40. Chang AB et al (1997) Airway hyperresponsiveness and cough-receptor sensitivity in children with recurrent cough. Am J Respir Crit Care Med 155(6):1935–1939
41. Varechova S et al (2008) Role of gender and pubertal stage on cough sensitivity in childhood and adolescence. J Physiol Pharmacol 59(Suppl 6):719–726
42. Miller MR et al (2005) ATS/ERS Taskforce series: standardisation of spirometry. Eur Respir J 26(2):319–338
43. Murata A et al (1998) Discrimination of productive and non-productive cough by sound analysis. Intern Med 37(9):732–735
44. Jalaludin BB, O'Toole BI, Leeder SR (2004) Acute effects of urban ambient air pollution on respiratory symptoms, asthma medication use, and doctor visits for asthma in a cohort of Australian children. Environ Res 95(1):32–42
45. Spengler JD et al (2004) Housing characteristics and children's respiratory health in the Russian Federation. Am J Public Health 94(4):657–662
46. Robertson CF et al (1991) Prevalence of asthma in Melbourne schoolchildren: changes over 26 years. BMJ 302:1116–1118
47. Soto-Quiros ME, Soto-Martinez M, Hanson LA (2002) Epidemiological studies of the very high prevalence of asthma and related symptoms among school children in Costa Rica from 1989 to 1998. Pediatr Allergy Immunol 13(5):342–349

48. Coren ME et al (1998) The value of ultrafast computed tomography in the investigation of pediatric chest disease. Pediatr Pulmonol 26(6):389–395
49. De Jongste JC, Shields MD (2003) Chronic cough in children. Thorax 58(11):998–1003
50. Wubbel C, Faro A (2003) Chronic cough in children. Pediatr Case Rev 3(2):95–104
51. Chang AB et al (2003) Non-CF bronchiectasis-clinical and HRCT evaluation. Pediatr Pulmonol 35(6):477–483
52. Chang AB et al (1998) Subjective scoring of cough in children: parent-completed vs child-completed diary cards vs an objective method. Eur Respir J 11(2):462–466
53. Hsu JY et al (1994) Coughing frequency in patients with persistent cough: assessment using a 24 hour ambulatory recorder. Eur Respir J 7:1246–1253
54. Foster WM (2003) Mucus secretion and cough. In: Chung KF, Widdicombe JG, Boushey HA (eds) Cough: causes, mechanisms and therapy. Blackwell Science, London, pp 207–216
55. Nunn JF (1993) Functional anatomy of the respiratory tract. In: Applied respiratory physiology. Butterworths, London, pp 18–21
56. Nunn JF (1993) Non-elastic resistance to gas flow. In: Applied respiratory physiology. Butterworths, London, pp 61–89
57. Korpas J, Widdicombe JG, Vrabec M (1993) Influence of simulated mucus on cough sounds in cats. Respir Med 87(1):49–54
58. Chang AB (2003) Causes, assessment and measurement of cough in children. In: Widdicombe GJ, Chung KF, Boushey HA (eds) Cough: causes, mechanisms and therapy. Blackwell Publishing, Oxford, pp 58–73
59. Chang AB et al (2005) Cough quality in children: a comparison of subjective vs. bronchoscopic findings. Respir Res 6:3
60. Carden KA et al (2005) Tracheomalacia and tracheobronchomalacia in children and adults*: an in-depth review. Chest 127(3):984–1005
61. Boogaard R et al (2005) Tracheomalacia and bronchomalacia in children*: incidence and patient characteristics. Chest 128(5):3391–3397
62. Masters IB et al (2008) QUantified tracheobronchomalacia disorders and their clinical profiles in children. Chest 133(2):461–467
63. Szeinberg A et al (1988) Cough capacity in patients with muscular dystrophy. Chest 94(6):1232–1235
64. Schramm CM (2000) Current concepts of respiratory complications of neuromuscular disease in children. Curr Opin Pediatr 12(3):203–207
65. Park JH et al (2010) How respiratory muscle strength correlates with cough capacity in patients with respiratory muscle weakness. Yonsei Med J 51(3):392–397
66. Cane RS, McKenzie SA (2001) Parents' interpretations of children's respiratory symptoms on video. Arch Dis Child 84(1):31–34
67. Cane RS, Ranganathan SC, McKenzie SA (2000) What do parents of wheezy children understand by "wheeze"? Arch Dis Child 82(4):327–332
68. Hay AD et al (2004) The inter-observer agreement of examining pre-school children with acute cough: a nested study. BMC Fam Pract 5(1):4
69. Marchant JM, Masters IB, Chang AB (2004) Defining paediatric chronic bronchitis. Respirology 9(Suppl):A61
70. Shields MD, Thavagnanam S (2013) The difficult coughing child: prolonged acute cough in children. Cough 9(1):11
71. Farzan S (1990) Clinical methods: the history, physical, and laboratory examinations, 3rd edn. Butterworths, Boston, MA
72. Shields MD et al (2008) British Thoracic Society guidelines recommendations for the assessment and management of cough in children. Thorax 63(Suppl 3):iii1–iii15
73. Cornia PB et al (2010) Does this coughing adolescent or adult patient have pertussis? JAMA 304(8):890–896
74. Ferronato AE (2013) Respiratory viral infections in infants with clinically suspected pertussis. J Pediatr 89(6):549–553

75. Harnden A, Grant C, Harrison T (2006) Whooping cough in school aged children with persistent cough: a prospective cohort study in primary care. BMJ 333:174
76. Barlow RS et al (2014) Vaccinated children and adolescents with pertussis infections experience reduced illness severity and duration, Oregon, 2010–2012. Clin Infect Dis 58(11):1523–1529
77. Tozzi AE et al (2003) Clinical presentation of pertussis in unvaccinated and vaccinated children in the first six years of life. Pediatrics 112(5):1069–1075
78. Schaad UB, Rossi E (1982) Infantile chlamydial pneumonia—a review based on 115 cases. Eur J Pediatr 138(2):105–109
79. Chang AB (2005) Cough: are children really different to adults? Cough 1(1):7
80. Vertigan AE et al (2015) Somatic cough syndrome (previously referred to as psychogenic cough) and tic cough (previously referred to as habit cough) in adults and children: chest guideline and expert panel report. Chest 148(1):24–31
81. Spinou A, Birring SS (2014) An update on measurement and monitoring of cough: what are the important study endpoints? J Thorac Dis 6:S728–S734
82. Martinek J et al (2013) Cough sound analysis. Acta Med Martiniana 13:15–20
83. Morice AH et al (2007) ERS guidelines on the assessment of cough. Eur Respir J 29(6):1256–1276
84. Amoh J, Odame K (2013) Technologies for developing ambulatory cough monitoring devices. Crit Rev Biomed Eng 41(6):457–468
85. Barry SJ et al (2006) The automatic recognition and counting of cough. Cough (London, England) 2:8–8
86. Vizel E et al (2010) Validation of an ambulatory cough detection and counting application using voluntary cough under different conditions. Cough (London, England) 6:3
87. Coyle MA et al (2005) Evaluation of an ambulatory system for the quantification of cough frequency in patients with chronic obstructive pulmonary disease. Cough (London, England) 1:3
88. Ryan NM, Birring SS, Gibson PG (2012) Gabapentin for refractory chronic cough: a randomised, double-blind, placebo-controlled trial. Lancet 380(9853):1583–1589
89. Yousaf N et al (2010) Long-term low-dose erythromycin in patients with unexplained chronic cough: a double-blind placebo controlled trial. Thorax 65(12):1107–1110
90. Barton A et al (2012) Data reduction for cough studies using distribution of audio frequency content. Cough (London, England) 8:12
91. Birring SS et al (2008) The Leicester cough monitor: preliminary validation of an automated cough detection system in chronic cough. Eur Respir J 31(5):1013–1018
92. Yousaf N et al (2013) Cough frequency in health and disease. Eur Respir J 41(1):241–243
93. Kulnik ST et al (2016) Cough frequency monitors: can they discriminate patient from environmental coughs? J Thorac Dis 8(11):3152–3159
94. Parker D et al (2013) Detecting paroxysmal coughing from pertussis cases using voice recognition technology. PLoS One 8(12):e82971
95. Gilchrist FJ, Carroll WD (2016) Assessing chronic cough in children. Paediatr Child Health 26(6):273–275
96. Pramono RXA, Imtiaz SA, Rodriguez-Villegas E (2016) A cough-based algorithm for automatic diagnosis of pertussis. PLoS One 11(9):e0162128
97. Amrulloh Y et al (2015) Cough sound analysis for pneumonia and asthma classification in pediatric population. In: Proceedings of the 2015 6th international conference on intelligent systems, modelling and simulation. IEEE Computer Society, pp 127–131
98. Abeyratne UR et al (2013) Cough sound analysis can rapidly diagnose childhood pneumonia. Ann Biomed Eng 41(11):2448–2462
99. Amrulloh YA, Abeyratne UR, Swarnkar V, Triasih R, Setyati A (2015) Automatic cough segmentation from non-contact sound recordings in pediatric wards. Biomed Signal Process Control 21:126–136
100. Swarnkar V et al (2013) Automatic identification of wet and dry cough in pediatric patients with respiratory diseases. Ann Biomed Eng 41(5):1016–1028

101. Hiew YH et al (2002) DSP algorithm for cough identification and counting. In: IEEE international conference on acoustics speech and signal processing. Institute of Electrical and Electronics Engineers (IEEE), Piscataway, NJ
102. Al-khassaweneh M, Mustafa SB, Abu-Ekteish F (2012) Asthma attack monitoring and diagnosis: a proposed system. In: 2012 IEEE-EMBS conference on biomedical engineering and sciences. Institute of Electrical and Electronics Engineers (IEEE), Piscataway, NJ
103. Kosasih K, Abeyratne UR, Swarnkar V (2012) High frequency analysis of cough sounds in pediatric patients with respiratory diseases. In: 2012 annual international conference of the IEEE engineering in medicine and biology society. Institute of Electrical and Electronics Engineers (IEEE), Piscataway, NJ
104. Ranjani S, Santhiya V, Jayapreetha A (2012) A real time cough monitor for classification of various pulmonary diseases. In: 2012 third international conference on emerging applications of information technology. Institute of Electrical and Electronics Engineers (IEEE), Piscataway, NJ
105. Liu M, Huang M-C (2015) Asthma Pattern Identification via Continuous Diaphragm Motion Monitoring. IEEE Tran Multi-Scale Comput Syst 1(2):76–84
106. Kosasih K et al (2015) Wavelet augmented cough analysis for rapid childhood pneumonia diagnosis. IEEE Trans Biomed Eng 62(4):1185–1194
107. Chandran V, Ning D, Sridharan S (2004) Speaker identification using higher order spectral phase features and their effectiveness vis–a–vis Mel-Cepstral features. In: Biometric authentication. Springer Nature, New York, NY, pp 614–622
108. Kuang Chua C (2009) Cardiac health diagnosis using higher order spectra and support vector machine. Open Med Inform J 3(1):1–8
109. Chua KC et al (2009) Higher order spectra based support vector machine for arrhythmia classification. In: IFMBE proceedings. Springer Nature, New York, NY, pp 231–234
110. Mookiah MRK et al (2015) Application of higher-order spectra for automated grading of diabetic maculopathy. Med Biol Eng Comput 53(12):1319–1331
111. EtehadTavakol M et al (2013) Breast cancer detection from thermal images using bispectral invariant features. Int J Therm Sci 69:21–36
112. Chandran V, Elgar S (1991) Shape discrimination using invariants defined from higher-order spectra. In [Proceedings] ICASSP 91: 1991 international conference on acoustics, speech, and signal processing. Institute of Electrical and Electronics Engineers (IEEE), Piscataway, NJ
113. Chandran V, Elgar S (1994) A general procedure for the derivation of principal domains of higher-order spectra. IEEE Trans Signal Process 42(1):229–233
114. Chandran V, Elgar S, Pezeshki C (1993) Bispectral and trispectral characterization of transition to chaos in the duffing oscillator. Int J Bifurcat Chaos 03(03):551–557
115. Chua KC et al (2009) Analysis of epileptic EEG signals using higher order spectra. J Med Eng Technol 33(1):42–50
116. Chandran V (2012) Time-varying bispectral analysis of visually evoked multi-channel EEG. EURASIP J Adv Signal Process 2012(1):140
117. Chandran V (2012) Time-varying bispectral analysis of auditory evoked multi-channel scalp EEG. In: 2012 11th international conference on information science, signal processing and their applications (ISSPA). Institute of Electrical and Electronics Engineers (IEEE), Piscataway, NJ
118. Chang AB (2006) Guidelines for evaluating chronic cough in pediatrics: ACCP evidence-based clinical practice guidelines. Chest 129:260S–283S
119. Chang AB et al (2017) Management of children with chronic wet cough and protracted bacterial bronchitis: CHEST guideline and expert panel report. Chest 151(4):884–890

Part IV

Where Are We Going?

16 Future Prospects for Respiratory Sound Research

Alda Marques and Cristina Jácome

16.1 Introduction

Respiratory sounds, first presented by René Laennec in his book in 1819, following his invention of the stethoscope in 1816 [1], are still valuable indicators of respiratory health. Although other measures have become available to diagnose and monitor respiratory diseases (e.g., spirometry and medical imaging techniques), the information derived from respiratory sounds is both different and complementary to these measures. Respiratory sounds acquired through auscultation are nearly universally available [2, 3], inexpensive, noninvasive, comfortable (no need to tolerate a face mask or seal around a mouthpiece), and cost-effective, can be repeated as often as necessary, and require minimal patient cooperation [4] and health professionals' training. Nevertheless, the subjectivity of auscultation is widely recognized, which has led to a new era of developments in computerized techniques for the acquisition and analysis of respiratory sounds. These techniques consist of recording patients' respiratory sounds with an electronic device and classifying/analyzing them based on specific signal characteristics [5–7]. Respiratory sounds are promising, simple measures that are sensitive to changes in the respiratory system of healthy people [8–10], in the presence of a respiratory condition [11–14], in different phases of the same respiratory condition [15], or in response to respiratory therapy [16].

A. Marques (✉)
Lab 3R—Respiratory Research and Rehabilitation Laboratory, School of Health Sciences, University of Aveiro (ESSUA), Aveiro, Portugal

Institute for Research in Biomedicine (iBiMED), University of Aveiro, Aveiro, Portugal
e-mail: amarques@ua.pt

C. Jácome
Lab 3R—Respiratory Research and Rehabilitation Laboratory, School of Health Sciences, University of Aveiro (ESSUA), Aveiro, Portugal

Centro de Investigação em Tecnologias e Serviços de Saúde (CINTESIS), University of Porto, Porto, Portugal
e-mail: cristinajacome@ua.pt

K. N. Priftis et al. (eds.), *Breath Sounds*, https://doi.org/10.1007/978-3-319-71824-8_16

16.2 What Has Been Hindering Its Wide Application?

In the year 2000, the European Community funded a Biomed 1 Concerted Action project entitled Computerized Respiratory Sound Analysis—CORSA—where the investigations on respiratory sounds were summarized [17]. This action published recommendations for standardized data acquisition, procedures, and signal processing techniques. However, these recommendations were not successfully transferred into clinical and research practice, as the different scientific areas (i.e., medicine, physics, informatics, and engineering) and industries continued to work independently. To date, high-quality scientific research on respiratory sounds has been conducted in three main areas: (1) development of equipment to acquire respiratory sounds data [18, 19], (2) development of algorithms to analyze respiratory sounds [20–24], and (3) understanding the mechanisms behind the generation of respiratory sounds and their clinical meaning in healthy people and in people with a respiratory condition [16, 25–29]. Nevertheless, experts within these areas have historically not communicated effectively, and therefore, despite decades of research, the scattered nature of the research produced has meant that there is still no accepted standard on the acquisition, analysis, and clinical interpretation of respiratory sounds. This lack of effective communication led to a significant amount of research being produced, even after the release of CORSA, with different methodologies and nomenclatures, making comparisons among studies very difficult and hindering knowledge advance on respiratory sounds.

More specifically, the wide application of respiratory sounds has been limited by the:

1. Uncertainties on respiratory sounds origin, mechanisms, acoustic characteristics, and clinical meaning
2. Difficulties acquiring high-quality data at the bedside with minimal setup
3. Paucity of algorithms providing real-time analysis and simple reports
4. Lack of consensus on the terminology used worldwide to describe respiratory sounds
5. Challenges with integrating respiratory sounds into electronic health records systems
6. Lack of consensus on respiratory sounds acquisition, analysis, and interpretation considering the new advances of research
7. Scarce investment in training students and health professionals on respiratory sounds

16.3 Future Prospects for Respiratory Sound Research

The future prospects for respiratory sound research should focus on overcoming these identified barriers, which we here proposed to be organized in three main areas: (1) basic and clinical research, (2) equipment, and (3) knowledge translation (Fig. 15.1).

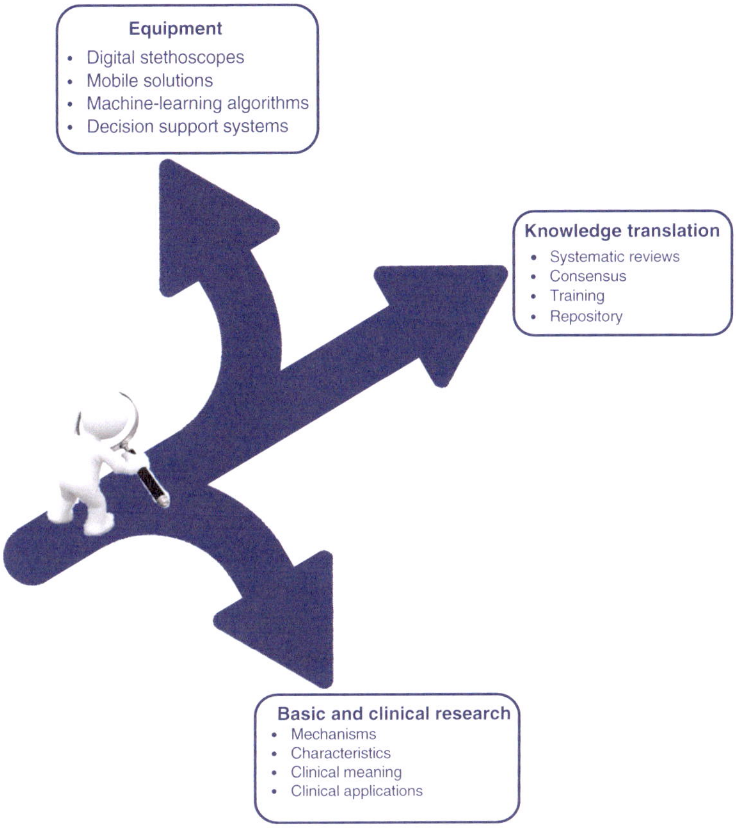

Fig. 15.1 Areas identified for respiratory sounds future research

The future prospects for each of these three areas are discussed next, aiming at encouraging research within this field and enhancing the routine use of respiratory sounds.

16.3.1 Basic and Clinical Research

Although many advances on respiratory sound research, namely, their origin, mechanics, acoustic characteristic, and clinical meaning, have been achieved [9, 27, 30–38], much remains unknown and needs validation or further expansion. For example, there is still debate regarding the sounds of contentious classification: (1) rhonchus and low-pitched wheezes; (2) origin and mechanisms of squawk [4, 34] and wheezes, beyond the "fluttering" mechanism [27]; (3) normal respiratory sounds at different ages; and (4) sounds of extra-thoracic origin (e.g., stridor and grunting).

It is clear that the present era, which is based on technology, offers immense potential for acquiring, storing, analyzing, and transferring respiratory sounds, but the basic acoustic characteristics of many respiratory conditions remain to be established: What are the differences among them (obstructive, restrictive, infectious respiratory conditions)? How do they vary considering age, gender, body position, airflow, and environmental noise? How do they respond to different therapies among others? It is therefore inconclusive how the new technology and respiratory sounds can contribute for the routine diagnosis and management of respiratory conditions in different populations and settings. Thus, basic science, as well as the application of basic research in clinical settings, needs to be conducted to further enhance our understanding on respiratory sounds, their clinical meaning, and potential applications.

It is known that frequencies and intensities of respiratory sounds, even in healthy people, vary between different chest locations [39] and strongly correlate with airflow [40] and that low frequencies are mainly due to sound wave propagation through the parenchyma, while higher frequency sounds are mainly propagated through airways [41]. Additionally, frequency and intensity of respiratory sounds have been found to be sensitive even to small changes (changes as little as 10% in forced expiratory volume in 1 s—FEV_1) [42–44]. An equipment capable of detecting and displaying this information quickly and in a user-friendly manner would provide noninvasive valuable information about the regional ventilation and airflow obstruction within the lung and trachea. Such information is currently not possible to obtain with any other simple measures and would be much informative to monitor sleep apnea [45]. However, further clinical research is needed.

Adventitious respiratory sounds have also shown to be promising to contribute for the diagnosis [11] and monitoring [16] of several respiratory conditions, but the old-dated studies based on relatively low-quality data reported have limited conclusions. Nevertheless, it seems established that wheezes (i.e., percentage of the respiratory cycle occupied by wheezes) provide crucial information on the degree of airflow obstruction in adults [43, 46] and children [47–51], being particularly important in children as pulmonary function tests are difficult or impossible to perform. The presence of crackles has also been considered an early sign and associated with several respiratory conditions. Characteristics of crackles, such as type (i.e., coarse or fine), frequency, duration, and number per respiratory phase and cycle, have been also considered as differentiator parameters across conditions and in (non)response to therapy [13, 52–58]. Therefore, given the promise value of adventitious respiratory sounds for the assessment of respiratory health status, further research should also focus on the analysis of the main parameters of crackles and wheezes, in healthy people [10] and in people with respiratory conditions [11, 16].

Another area that needs to be further explored is the potential of respiratory sounds as outcome measures in respiratory conditions. This may include investigating the effect of therapeutic interventions (e.g., invasive and noninvasive ventilation, bronchodilator, bronchoprovocation challenge test, exercise training, respiratory physiotherapy, and pulmonary rehabilitation) on respiratory sounds. In addition, it is important to define the parameters of respiratory sounds with higher sensitivity to change.

16.3.2 Equipment

Much equipment for respiratory sounds acquisition exists [7, 19, 59–64]. However, none has ever fully meet health professionals' standards for clinical implementation. Developing, testing, and using new, highly portable, user-friendly, with minimal setup, and low-cost equipment (hardware and software) for respiratory sounds acquisition and analysis are essential to have a simple and quick way to obtain rich information about a person's respiratory health. Such equipment would be easily used in diverse populations (even in noncooperative patients, such as infants, those with impaired cognitive function, or ventilated patients), and in diverse environments (e.g., bedside or tele-monitoring patients). This is currently available for other biomedical signals, such as blood pressure or peripheral oxygen saturation.

16.3.2.1 Acquisition of Respiratory Sounds

The challenge is to have a sensor and/or several sensors with minimal mass, wide bandwidth as possible, be relatively insensitive to environmental noise, and combine processing power, storage, analysis programs [38], and audiovisual displays in real time in a hand-held user-friendly device. To answer these needs, technological developments and research in two target areas are crucial: digital stethoscopes and mobile solutions.

Advances in digital stethoscopes have been the main focus of universities and companies in the last decade, which currently allows acquiring high-quality respiratory sounds. However, the relatively high cost of these devices has limited its use both in developing and developed countries [65]. In the next years, more efforts should be made to produce smaller, lighter, and low-cost digital stethoscopes, maintaining the achieved quality of the recordings. This would facilitate the widespread use of respiratory sounds.

Mobile solutions, such as mobile apps, also have the potential to increase the use of respiratory sounds by delivering ubiquitous, dynamic, and user-centered solutions. Smartphones are now common in most parts of the world [66] and have the advantages of being personal, portable, connected, increasingly low cost, and computationally powerful. It is believed that the development of mobile solutions would facilitate the use of respiratory sounds by students and health professionals. In addition, it would be an important step to increase the use of respiratory sounds for self-monitoring purposes by patients and caregivers. Some encouraging first steps have already happened, as is the example of the Lung Sound Recorder app (https://play.google.com/store/apps/details?id=com.mobiletechnologylab.lungsoundrecorder&hl=en) or the CliniCloud app (https://clinicloud.com/en/app), however, much more is needed.

In addition, equipment and systems to acquire and analyze respiratory sounds in real time should connect respiratory sounds information to other clinical data, namely, with electronic health records systems. Even though we live in the era of telecommunications and mobile solutions, such products are not yet available. It is therefore clear that much has to be done before we can have a system "off-the-shelf" to be used in routine clinical practice.

16.3.2.2 Analysis of Respiratory Sounds

The automated recognition and rejection of artefacts, as well as identification of normal and adventitious respiratory sounds and noise cancellation, need to be refined. Significant work has been developed [67], and several algorithms have been proposed to detect normal respiratory sounds [68, 69], crackles [24, 70–73], wheezes [20, 74–78], and respiratory cycles [5, 79–82], to perform active noise cancellation in high-noise environments [83, 84], and to separate adventitious respiratory sounds [73, 85, 86] and/or heart sounds [87, 88] from normal respiratory sounds. However, none has been widely accepted. Moreover, there is also a need to have algorithms adjusted to the parameters that influence respiratory sounds, such as gender, age, body size, body position, place where the sound is being auscultated, airflow, and presence or absence of a respiratory condition. Machine-learning algorithm, which possesses artificial intelligence that learns from past experiences, allowing the tools to function more accurately, is believed to be one of the best strategies to deal with respiratory sounds' characteristics, and it is where research has been currently focusing. A recent systematic review showed that the use of machine-learning techniques for respiratory sounds analysis is still preliminary, with the artificial neural networks and k-nearest neighbor algorithms being the most used [89]. This work also recommended that future research should focus on more advanced machine-learning algorithms and also hybrid machine-learning techniques for respiratory sounds analysis [89]. Therefore, accelerating the development of machine-learning algorithms is another area where much research is needed to commercialize respiratory sounds for use in a clinical environment.

16.3.2.3 Integration of Respiratory Sounds in Decision Support Systems

Respiratory sounds have diagnostic and monitoring potential not only for health professionals but also for community health workers, first-line care providers, and patients themselves.

If user-friendly and low-cost equipment become available, what is then essential is to integrate respiratory sounds information, using audiovisual techniques, in electronic health records, where other clinical information should be already compiled. This would allow the development of robust clinical decision support systems and would have potential to positively impact on healthcare delivery. The centralization of the information will also reshape the healthcare provided by allowing bedside or remote assessment in different populations and settings, transmission to specialists for second opinions, and activation of decision support algorithms.

Recordings could be performed by any person, and reports could be automatically generated, providing clinical guidance, even in lay language. This would empower not just health professionals but also patients and the whole community to manage their own health and disease. The vision is that every citizen, irrespective of professional background or literacy (e.g., health professionals, community health workers, patients, caregivers, citizens), would benefit from the integration of respiratory sounds with other clinical data in real time to help in the estimation of respiratory health status in the short and intermediate term. In the long term, predictive computer models integrated in decision-making systems could process clinical data (including respiratory sounds) in real time to predict how the patient's health would evolve in the near future. Such predictions could then be used in wearables to empower patients, carers, and citizens for self-management of health and well-being.

It is known that self-management and prompt treatment of respiratory exacerbations in patients with asthma, COPD, and other respiratory conditions reduce the use of health resources (e.g., hospitalizations, pharmacologic therapies), saving healthcare costs [90, 91]. By enabling access to this comprehensive information in telecommunications and mobile apps, empowerment to manage health and disease will be given not only to health professionals but also to community health workers, first-line providers, caregivers, and patients themselves. This may result in more cost-effective healthcare systems by enabling the management of respiratory diseases outside healthcare services and improving outcomes, and/or by encouraging healthy citizens to remain healthy.

Approaches that provide patients with active information suppliers have already demonstrated their viability in preventing and following up heart diseases. These systems integrate displays in personal health records and electronic health records, resulting in higher adherence to clinical guidelines [92]. A good example of these systems is the *MobiGuide*, which is a telemedicine system based on computerized clinical guidelines and adapted to a mobile environment. *MobiGuide* provides personalized medical decision support for patients with chronic illnesses, such as cardiac arrhythmias, diabetes, and high blood pressure (http://www.mobiguide-project.eu/). There are also promising results in respiratory sounds: tele-monitoring respiratory sounds for predicting acute exacerbations of COPD [93], tracheal sounds for distinguishing people with and without asthma [94], and phonopneumogram for the analysis of respiratory sounds based on smartphones [95]. Therefore, much research is needed to ultimately empower people and decrease the burden of respiratory diseases worldwide.

16.3.3 Knowledge Translation

The value of respiratory sounds does not depend only on evidence-based research and technological advances but also on making different stakeholders (i.e., health professionals, researchers, patients, and caregivers) communicate using the same terms and follow the same methodologies and principles of interpretation that new advances of science propose. This falls into the concept of knowledge translation.

Knowledge translation is a relatively new concept that has been highly recommended to facilitate the transfer of high-quality research evidence into clinical practice and community [96, 97]. Different terms have been found in the literature to define knowledge translation, e.g., knowledge transfer, knowledge exchange, research utilization, implementation, dissemination, and diffusion [98, 99]. According to Rubio et al., knowledge translation is when research findings are moved from the researcher's bench to the patient's bedside and community [100]. It develops in two stages: stage 1, transfers knowledge from basic research to clinical research, and stage 2, transfers findings from clinical studies or clinical trials to practice settings and communities, where the findings improve health [100]. The primary aim of knowledge translation is to address the gap between evidence-based research and its implementation by stakeholders (i.e., researchers and knowledge users—health professionals, decision-makers, and patients) with the intention of efficiently improving healthcare system and health outcomes [101].

Knowledge translation has been successfully applied in several areas of health research, such as mental health [102, 103] and cancer [104], with short- and long-term benefits. The benefits observed in different healthcare areas have been receiving increasing interest from national and international respiratory societies [105], mainly due to recognition that the traditional approaches used to move research into practice (i.e., approaches based on education, such as continuing professional development, did not lead to optimal care [97]).

Respiratory sounds need an urgent basic unit of knowledge translation. This unit may develop up-to-date systematic reviews or other syntheses of research findings to identify the key messages for different target audiences. Then, these messages have to be fashioned in language, and knowledge translation products that are easily assimilated by different audiences [97].

In the light of the new scientific advances, the terminology, acquisition, analysis, and interpretation of respiratory sounds need consensus and knowledge transfer to different audiences. A recent European Respiratory Society Task Force was conducted, and several recommendations to standardize respiratory sounds nomenclature at international and national levels have been published [106]. This initiative started to address a need identified a long time ago [107]. However, it is known that historically the adoption of new terminology has been slow and not uniform [106]. Thus, it is imperative to conduct research on strategies to disseminate these recommendations, based, for example, on the knowledge transfer strategies previously proposed [97], and to assess the impact of their use in clinical practice. Some examples could include:

- Using audio-visual recordings of respiratory sounds, with the recommended terminology, for training auscultation skills and examining students and for advance training of health professionals
- Using audio-visual recordings of respiratory sounds in educational materials, meetings, and outreach activities
- Adding audio-visual recordings of respiratory sounds as a measure in studies that collect other respiratory measures, namely, pulmonary function and structural and functional medical imaging studies, which may lead to better appreciation of the strengths and limitations of respiratory sounds

Significant advances since the last standardization of computerized respiratory sound analysis [36] have been achieved. Almost two decades have passed, and it is now the time to develop new standards for acquiring, analyzing, and interpreting respiratory sounds by critically evaluating the current knowledge on respiratory sounds profile, acquisition, and analysis procedures. A Delphi survey with different stakeholders (e.g., researchers, health professionals, engineers, patients, industry) followed by a consensus meeting could also be conducted in the near future. This new consensus would be fundamental to boost respiratory sounds used in different contexts and populations and would start the knowledge transfer on respiratory sounds to different audiences, reducing the evidence-practice and policy gaps.

It would also be of great value to have a publicly available repository of large datasets of respiratory sounds, based on high-quality recordings and annotated by several experts (e.g., respiratory phases and adventitious respiratory sounds). This repository could then be used as gold standard to train students and health professionals on respiratory sounds and to develop, train, and validate algorithms. Additionally, it would also be a simple and standardized way to share information and could then be used by different stakeholders to develop and consolidate knowledge and disseminate respiratory sounds. A good starting point that could be further expanded is the "Reference Database of Respiratory Sounds" in the e-learning resources of the European Respiratory Society (http://www.ers-education.org/e-learning/reference-database-of-respiratory-sounds.aspx).

Conclusion

Future prospects for respiratory sound research holds some exciting challenges that can be summed into:

- Developing basic and clinical research on respiratory sounds
- Developing a hand-held, user-friendly, and low-cost equipment to collect and automatically analyze respiratory sounds frequency, intensity, and presence and characteristic of adventitious respiratory sounds
- Integrating the information acquired with equipment developed into electronic health information databases to be used as part of decision support systems
- Establishing a knowledge translation package composed by several strategies, namely, systematic reviews and consensus for the terminology; acquisition, analysis, and interpretation of respiratory sounds based on new research; and integrating several stakeholders

Together all these advances will take respiratory sounds from bench to routine clinical practice and ultimately contribute for decreasing the burden with respiratory diseases.

Acknowledgments We would like to thank Ms. Bruria Freidman from the Sleep-Wake Disorder Unit of Soroka University Medical Center for her support and collaboration. This study was supported in part by the Israeli Ministry of Industry and Trade, the Kamin Program, award no. 46168, and by the Israel Science Foundation (ISF) grant no. 1403/15.

References

1. Bishop PJ (1981) Reception of the stethoscope and Laënnec's book. Thorax 36(7):487–492
2. Bauserman M, Hailey C, Gado J, Lokangaka A, Williams J, Richards-Kortum R, Tshefu A, Bose C (2015) Determining the utility and durability of medical equipment donated to a rural clinic in a low-income country. Int Health 7(4):262–265
3. Ellington LE, Gilman RH, Tielsch JM, Steinhoff M, Figueroa D, Rodriguez S, Caffo B, Tracey B, Elhilali M, West J, Checkley W (2012) Computerised lung sound analysis to improve the specificity of paediatric pneumonia diagnosis in resource-poor settings: protocol and methods for an observational study. BMJ Open 2(1):e000506
4. Bohadana A, Izbicki G, Kraman SS (2014) Fundamentals of lung auscultation. N Engl J Med 370(8):744–751
5. Moussavi ZK, Leopando MT, Pasterkamp H, Rempel G (2000) Computerized acoustical respiratory phase detection without airflow measurement. Med Biol Eng Comput 38(2):198–203
6. Kandaswamy A, Kumar CS, Ramanathan RP, Jayaraman S, Malmurugan N (2004) Neural classification of lung sounds using wavelet coefficients. Comput Biol Med 34(6):523–537
7. Polat H, Guler I (2004) A simple computer-based measurement and analysis system of pulmonary auscultation sounds. J Med Syst 28(6):665–672
8. Gavriely N, Nissan M, Cugell D, Rubin A (1994) Respiratory health screening using pulmonary function tests and lung sound analysis. Eur Respir J 7(1):35–42
9. Pasterkamp H, Powell RE, Sanchez I (1996) Lung sound spectra at standardized air flow in normal infants, children, and adults. Am J Resp Crit Care 154(2):424–430
10. Oliveira A, Marques A (2014) Respiratory sounds in healthy people: a systematic review. Respir Med 108(4):550–570
11. Gurung A, Scrafford CG, Tielsch JM, Levine OS, Check W (2011) Computerized lung sound analysis as diagnostic aid for the detection of abnormal lung sounds: a systematic review and meta-analysis. Respir Med 105(9):1396–1403
12. Jácome C, Marques A (2015) Computerized respiratory sounds in patients with COPD: a systematic review. COPD 12(1):104–112
13. Murphy RLH (2008) In defense of the stethoscope. Respir Care 53(3):355–369
14. Bettencourt PE, Del Bono EA, Spiegelman D, Hertzmark E, Murphy RL Jr (1994) Clinical utility of chest auscultation in common pulmonary diseases. Am J Respir Crit Care Med 150(5 Pt 1):1291–1297
15. Jácome C, Oliveira A, Marques A (2015) Computerized respiratory sounds: a comparison between patients with stable and exacerbated COPD. Clin Respir J 11(5):612–620
16. Marques A, Oliveira A, Jácome C (2014) Computerized adventitious respiratory sounds as outcome measures for respiratory therapy: a systematic review. Respir Care 59(5): 765–776
17. Sovijärvi A, Dalmasso F, Vanderschoot J, Malmberg L, Righini G, Stoneman S (2000) Definition of terms for applications of respiratory sounds. Eur Respir Rev 10(77):597–610
18. Sánchez Morillo D, Astorga Moreno S, Fernández Granero MÁ, León Jiménez A (2013) Computerized analysis of respiratory sounds during COPD exacerbations. Comput Biol Med 43(7):914–921
19. Pinho C, Oliveira A, Oliveira D, Dinis J, Marques A (2014) RIBS@UA: interface to collect and store respiratory data, a preliminary study. Comput Biol Med 47:44–57
20. Taplidou SA, Hadjileontiadis LJ (2007) Wheeze detection based on time-frequency analysis of breath sounds. Comput Biol Med 37(8):1073–1083
21. Serbes G, Sakar CO, Kahya YP, Aydin N (2013) Pulmonary crackle detection using time–frequency and time–scale analysis. Digital Signal Process 23(3):1012–1021
22. Benedetto G, Dalmasso F, Guarene MM (1983) A method for the acoustical analysis of respiratory crackles in cryptogenic fibrosing alveolitis. IEEE T Bio-Med Eng 30(9):620–623
23. Ono M, Arakawa K, Mori M, Sugimoto T, Harashima H (1989) Separation of fine crackles from vesicular sounds by a nonlinear digital-filter. IEEE T Bio-Med Eng 36(2):286–291

24. Cátia P, Oliveira A, Jácome C, Rodrigues JM, Marques A (2016) Integrated approach for automatic crackle detection based on fractal dimension and box filtering. IJRQEH 5(4):34–50
25. Fredberg JJ, Holford SK (1983) Discrete lung sounds: crackles (rales) as stress-relaxation quadrupoles. J Acoust Soc Am 73(3):1036–1046
26. Gavriely N, Kelly KB, Grotberg JB, Loring SH (1985) Forced expiratory wheezes are a manifestation of airway flow limitation. J Appl Physiol 62(6):2398–2403
27. Gavriely N, Shee TR, Cugell DW, Grotberg JB (1985) Flutter in flow-limited collapsible tubes: a mechanism for generation of wheezes. J Appl Physiol 66(5):2251–2261
28. Grotberg JB, Gavriely N (1989) Flutter in collapsible tubes: a theoretical model of wheezes. J Appl Physiol 66(5):2262–2273
29. Vyshedskiy A, Alhashem RM, Paciej R, Ebril M, Rudman I, Fredberg JJ, Murphy R (2009) Mechanism of inspiratory and expiratory crackles. Chest 135(1):156–164
30. Forgacs P (1967) Crackles and wheezes. Lancet 290(7508):203–205
31. Nath AR, Capel LH (1974) Inspiratory crackles – early and late. Thorax 29(2):223–227
32. Nath AR, Capel LH (1974) Inspiratory crackles and mechanical events of breathing. Thorax 29(6):695–698
33. Forgacs P (1978) Lung sounds. Bailliere Tindall, London
34. Forgacs P (1978) The functional basis of pulmonary sounds. Chest 73(3):399–405
35. Grotberg JB, Davis SH (1980) Fluid-dynamic flapping of a collapsible channel: Sound generation and flow limitation. J Biomech 13(3):219–230
36. Sovijärvi A, Vanderschoot J, Earis J (2000) Standardization of computerized respiratory sound analysis. Eur Respir Rev 10(77):585
37. Pasterkamp H, Kraman SS, Wodicka GR (1997) Respiratory sounds: advances beyond the stethoscope. Am J Respir Crit Care 156:974–987
38. Earis JE, BMG C (2000) Future perspectives for respiratory sound research. Eur Respir Rev 10(77):641–646
39. Gavriely N, Nissan M, Rubin A-H, Cugell DW (1995) Spectral characteristics of chest wall breath sounds in normal subjects. Thorax 50:1292–1300
40. Charbonneau G, Sudraud M, Soufflet G (1987) Method for the evaluation of flow rate from pulmonary sounds. Bull Eur Physiopathol Respir 23(3):265–270
41. Patel S, Lu S, Doerschuk PC, Wodicka GR (1995) Sonic phase delay from trachea to chest wall: spatial and inhaled gas dependency. Med Biol Eng Comput 33(4):571–574
42. Anderson K, Aitken S, Carter R, MacLeod JE, Moran F (1990) Variation of breath sound and airway caliber induced by histamine challenge. Am Rev Respir Dis 141(5 Pt 1):1147–1150
43. Malmberg LP, Sovijarvi ARA, Paajanen E, Piirila P, Haahtela T, Katila T (1994) Changes in frequency spectra of breath sounds during histaminic challenge test in adult asthmatics and healthy control subjects. Chest 105(1):122–132
44. Pasterkamp H, Consunji-Araneta R, Oh Y, Holbrow J (1997) Chest surface mapping of lung sounds during methacholine challenge. Pediatr Pulmonol 23(1):21–30
45. Alshaer H, Fernie GR, Maki E, Bradley TD (2013) Validation of an automated algorithm for detecting apneas and hypopneas by acoustic analysis of breath sounds. Sleep Med 14(6):562–571
46. Cortes S, Jane R, Fiz JA, Morera J (2005) Monitoring of wheeze duration during spontaneous respiration in asthmatic patients. Conference proceedings: annual international conference of the IEEE engineering in medicine and biology society IEEE engineering in medicine and biology society conference 6:6141–6144
47. Eising JB, Uiterwaal CS, van der Ent CK (2014) Nocturnal wheeze measurement in preschool children. Pediatr Pulmonol 49(3):257–262
48. Bentur L, Beck R, Berkowitz D, Hasanin J, Berger I, Elias N, Gavriely N (2004) Adenosine bronchial provocation with computerized wheeze detection in young infants with prolonged cough: correlation with long-term follow-up. Chest 126(4):1060–1065
49. Faber TE, Kamps AW, Sjoerdsma MH, Vermeulen S, Veeger NJ, Bont LJ (2015) Computerized assessment of wheezing in children with respiratory syncytial virus bronchiolitis before and after hypertonic saline nebulization. Respir Care 60(9):1252–1256

50. Beck R, Elias N, Shoval S, Tov N, Talmon G, Godfrey S, Bentur L (2007) Computerized acoustic assessment of treatment efficacy of nebulized epinephrine and albuterol in RSV bronchiolitis. BMC Pediatr 7(22):1–6
51. Sanchez I, Powell RE, Pasterkamp H (1993) Wheezing and airflow obstruction during methacholine challenge in children with cystic fibrosis and in normal children. Am Rev Respir Dis 147(3):705–709
52. Epler GR, Carrington CB, Gaensler EA (1978) Crackles (rales) in the interstitial pulmonary diseases. Chest 73(3):333–339
53. Piirila P, Sovijarvi ARA, Kaisla T, Rajala H-M, Katila T (1991) Crackles in patients with fibrosing alveolitis, bronchiectasis, COPD, and heart failure. Chest 99(5):1076–1083
54. Piirila P (1992) Changes in crackle characteristics during the clinical course of pneumonia. Chest 102(1):176–183
55. Bohadana AB (2000) Lung sounds in asthma and chronic obstructive pulmonary disease. Monaldi Arch Chest Dis 55(6):484–487
56. Piirila P, Lehtola H, Zitting A, Kivisaari L, Koskinen H, Luukkonen R, Salo SP, Vehmas T, Nordman H, Sovijarvi ARA (2000) Lung sounds in asbestos induced pulmonary disorders. Eur Respir J 16:901–908
57. Cottin V, Cordier JF (2012) Velcro crackles: the key for early diagnosis of idiopathic pulmonary fibrosis? Eur Respir J 40(3):519–521
58. Sellares J, Hernandez-Gonzalez F, Lucena CM, Paradela M, Brito-Zeron P, Prieto-Gonzalez S, Benegas M, Cuerpo S, Espinosa G, Ramirez J, Sanchez M, Xaubet A (2016) Auscultation of Velcro crackles is associated with usual interstitial pneumonia. Medicine 95(5):2573
59. Sun X, Cheetham BM, Earis JE (1998) Real time analysis of lung sounds. Technol Health Care 6(1):3–10
60. Jiang H, Chen J, Cao J, Mu L, Hu Z, He J (2015) Evaluation of vibration response imaging (VRI) technique and difference in VRI indices among non-smokers, active smokers and passive smokers. Med Sci Monit 21:2170–2177
61. Abbas A, Fahim A (2010) An automated computerized auscultation and diagnostic system for pulmonary diseases. J Med Syst 34(6):1149–1155
62. Foche-Perez I, Ramirez-Payba R, Hirigoyen-Emparanza G, Balducci-Gonzalez F, Simo-Reigadas FJ, Seoane-Pascual J, Corral-Penafiel J, Martinez-Fernandez A (2012) An open real-time tele-stethoscopy system. Biomed Eng Online 11(57):11–57
63. Palaniappan R, Sundaraj K, Sundaraj S, Huliraj N, Revadi SS (2015) A telemedicine tool to detect pulmonary pathology using computerized pulmonary acoustic signal analysis. Appl Soft Comput 37:952–959
64. Yu C, Tsai TH, Huang SI, Lin CW (2013) Soft stethoscope for detecting asthma wheeze in young children. Sensors 13(6):7399–7413
65. Chamberlain D, Mofor J, Fletcher R, Kodgule R (2015) Mobile stethoscope and signal processing algorithms for pulmonary screening and diagnostics. In: Global humanitarian technology conference (GHTC), 2015 IEEE, 8–11 Oct 2015. pp 385–392. doi:10.1109/GHTC.2015.7344001
66. Africa & Middle East Telecom-Week (2014) Africa & Middle East mobile factbook 2Q 2014. http://www.mikekujawski.ca/2009/03/16/latest-mobile-phone-statistics-from-africa-and-what-this-means/
67. Palaniappan R, Sundaraj K, Sundaraj S (2014) Artificial intelligence techniques used in respiratory sound analysis—a systematic review. Biomed Tech 59(1):7–18
68. Guler EC, Sankur B, Kahya YP, Raudys S (2003) Two-stage classification of respiratory sound patterns. Comput Biol Med 35(1):67–83
69. Mayorga P, Druzgalski C, Gonzalez OH, Lopez HS (2012) Modified classification of normal lung sounds applying quantile vectors. Conference proceedings: annual international conference of the IEEE engineering in medicine and biology society IEEE engineering in medicine and biology society conference 5(10):6346908
70. Vannuccini L, Rossi M, Pasquali G (1998) A new method to detect crackles in respiratory sounds. Technol Health Care 6(1):75–79

71. Lu X, Bahoura M (2008) An integrated automated system for crackles extraction and classification. Biomed Signal Process Control 3(3):244–254
72. Charleston-Villalobos S, Dorantes-Mendez G, Gonzalez-Camarena R, Chi-Lem G, Carrillo JG, Aljama-Corrales T (2011) Acoustic thoracic image of crackle sounds using linear and nonlinear processing techniques. Med Biol Eng Comput 49(1):15–24
73. Hadjileontiadis LJ, Panas SM (1997) Separation of discontinuous adventitious sounds from vesicular sounds using a wavelet-based filter. IEEE Trans Biomed Eng 44(12):1269–1281
74. Waris M, Helisto P, Haltsonen S, Saarinen A, Sovijärvi A (1998) A new method for automatic wheeze detection. Technol Health Care 6(1):33–40
75. Homs-Corbera A, Jane R, Fiz JA, Morera J (2000) Algorithm for time-frequency detection and analysis of wheezes. Proceedings of the 22nd annual international conference of the IEEE engineering in medicine and biology society, Vols 1–4 22:2977–2980
76. Hsueh M-L, Chien J-C, Chang F-C, Wu H-D, Chong F-C (2005) Respiratory wheeze detection system. Proceedings of the 2005 IEEE engineering in medicine and biology 27th annual conference, 1–4
77. Guntupalli KK, Alapat PM, Bandi VD, Kushnir I (2008) Validation of automatic wheeze detection in patients with obstructed airways and in healthy subjects. J Asthma 45(10):903–907
78. Lin BS, Yen TS (2014) An FPGA-based rapid wheezing detection system. Int J Environ Res Public Health 11(2):1573–1593
79. Huq S, Moussavi Z (2010) Automatic breath phase detection using only tracheal sounds. Conference proceedings: annual International conference of the IEEE engineering in medicine and biology society IEEE engineering in medicine and biology society conference 2010:272–275
80. Moussavi ZK, Leopando MT, Rempel GR (1998) Automated respiratory phase detection by acoustical means. Proceedings of the 20th annual international conference of the IEEE engineering in medicine and biology society 20(1):21–24
81. Yap YL, Moussavi Z (2001) Respiratory onset detection using variance fractal dimension. IEEE Eng Med Bio Soc 2:1554–1556
82. Yildirim I, Ansari R, Moussavi Z (2008) Automated respiratory phase and onset detection using only chest sound signal. 30th annual international conference of the IEEE engineering in medicine and biology society 1–8:2578–2581
83. Suzuki A, Sumi C, Nakayama K, Mori M (1995) Real-time adaptive cancelling of ambient noise in lung sound measurement. Med Biol Eng Comput 33(5):704–708
84. Chang GC, Lai YF (2010) Performance evaluation and enhancement of lung sound recognition system in two real noisy environments. Comput Methods Prog Biomed 97(2): 141–150
85. Hadjileontiadis LJ, Panas SM (1996) Nonlinear separation of crackles and squawks from vesicular sounds using third-order statistics. In: Engineering in medicine and biology society, 1996. Bridging disciplines for biomedicine. Proceedings of the 18th annual international conference of the IEEE, vol. 2215, 31 Oct to 3 Nov 1996, pp 2217–2219. doi:10.1109/IEMBS.1996.646504
86. Mastorocostas PA, Theocharis JB (2007) A dynamic fuzzy neural filter for separation of discontinuous adventitious sounds from vesicular sounds. Comput Biol Med 37(1):60–69
87. Cortes S, Jane R, Torres A, Fiz JA, Morera J (2006) Detection and adaptive cancellation of heart sound interference in tracheal sounds. Conference proceedings: annual international conference of the IEEE engineering in medicine and biology society IEEE engineering in medicine and biology society conference 1:2860–2863
88. Pourazad MT, Moussavi Z, Thomas G (2006) Heart sound cancellation from lung sound recordings using time-frequency filtering. Med Biol Eng Comput 44(3):216–225
89. Palaniappan R, Sundaraj K, Ahamed NU (2013) Machine learning in lung sound analysis: a systematic review. Biocybern Biomed Eng 33(3):129–135
90. Effing T, Kerstjens H, van der Valk P, Zielhuis G, van der Palen J (2009) (Cost)-effectiveness of self-treatment of exacerbations on the severity of exacerbations in patients with COPD: the COPE II study. Thorax 64(11):956–962

91. Casas A, Troosters T, Garcia-Aymerich J, Roca J, Hernández C, Alonso A, del Pozo F, de Toledo P, Antó JM, Rodríguez-Roisín R, Decramer M (2006) Integrated care prevents hospitalisations for exacerbations in COPD patients. Eur Respir J 28(1):123–130
92. Garcia-Saez G, Rigla M, Martinez-Sarriegui I, Shalom E, Peleg M, Broens T, Pons B, Caballero-Ruiz E, Gomez EJ, Hernando ME (2014) Patient-oriented computerized clinical guidelines for mobile decision support in gestational diabetes. J Diabetes Sci Technol 8(2):238–246
93. Fernandez-Granero MA, Sanchez-Morillo D, Leon-Jimenez A (2015) Computerised analysis of telemonitored respiratory sounds for predicting acute exacerbations of COPD. Sensors 15(10):26978–26996
94. Anderson K, Qiu Y, Whittaker AR, Lucas M (2001) Breath sounds, asthma, and the mobile phone. Lancet 358(9290):1343–1344
95. Reyes BA, Reljin N, Kong Y, Nam Y, Ha S, Chon KH (2016) Towards the development of a mobile phonopneumogram: automatic breath-phase classification using smartphones. Ann Biomed Eng 44(9):2746–2759
96. Wallace J (2008) Lost in translation: transferring knowledge from research to clinical practice. Adv Psychiatr Treat 19(4):250–258
97. Grimshaw JM, Eccles MP, Lavis JN, Hill SJ, Squires JE (2012) Knowledge translation of research findings. Implement Sci 7(50):1748–5908
98. Tetroe JM, Graham ID, Foy R, Robinson N, Eccles MP, Wensing M, Durieux P, Legare F, Nielson CP, Adily A, Ward JE, Porter C, Shea B, Grimshaw JM (2008) Health research funding agencies' support and promotion of knowledge translation: an international study. Milbank Q 86(1):125–155
99. McKibbon KA, Lokker C, Wilczynski NL, Ciliska D, Dobbins M, Davis DA, Haynes RB, Straus SE (2010) A cross-sectional study of the number and frequency of terms used to refer to knowledge translation in a body of health literature in 2006: a tower of babel? Implement Sci 5(16):1748–5908
100. Rubio DM, Schoenbaum EE, Lee LS, Schteingart DE, Marantz PR, Anderson KE, Platt LD, Baez A, Esposito K (2010) Defining translational research: implications for training. Acad Med 85(3):470–475
101. Graham ID, Logan J, Harrison MB, Straus SE, Tetroe J, Caswell W, Robinson N (2006) Lost in knowledge translation: time for a map? J Contin Educ Heal Prof 26(1):13–24
102. McGrath PJ, Lingley-Pottie P, Emberly DJ, Thurston C, McLean C (2009) Integrated knowledge translation in mental health: family help as an example. J Can Acad Child Adolesc Psychiatry 18(1):30–37
103. Bullock H, Watson A, Goering P (2010) Building for success: mental health research with an integrated knowledge translation approach. Can J Commun Ment Health 29(Special issue supplement 2010):9–21
104. O'Brien K, Brooks D (2006) Two episodic illnesses: lessons learned in rehabilitation. Physiother Can 58(4):251–254
105. Palange P, Noel JL, Simonds AK (2011) The European Respiratory Society: future directions in medical education. Eur Respir J 38(3):498–499
106. Pasterkamp H, Brand PL, Everard M, Garcia-Marcos L, Melbye H, Priftis KN (2016) Towards the standardisation of lung sound nomenclature. Eur Respir J 47(3):724–732
107. Postiaux G, Lens E (1999) Pulmonary stethacoustic nomenclature: why not a worldwide consensus? Rev Mal Respir 16(6):1075–1090

Check for updates

In Pursuit of a Unified Nomenclature of Respiratory Sounds

17

Kostas N. Priftis, Maria Antoniadi, and Hans Pasterkamp

17.1 Introduction

Audible noises associated with breathing are a common clinical sign. They may be of particular usefulness in clinical diagnosis. However, patients as well as caregivers use a variety of rather descriptive terms to report respiratory sounds, and this can often be misleading [1–3]. Physicians may also use confusing terminology when they try to convey various respiratory noises to colleagues [1, 2, 4–7]. Consequently, doctors' documentation and interpretation of their patients' respiratory sounds may differ, relying largely upon the wording they or their discussants use.

Correct interpretation of respiratory sounds that are reported by parents and caregivers, or even by health care professionals, depends on common medical and lay language terminology in various countries and regions [3, 5, 8, 9]. In each language, medical terminology has its own evolutionary dynamics according to the verbal richness, the depth, and the degree of dependence on other dominant languages. Even within the same language, regional dialects may create special difficulties in the understanding of certain terms [10–12].

This chapter will provide an overview of the survey undertaken in the context of the European Respiratory Society (ERS) Task Force on Respiratory Sounds (2012–2014) [13], investigating the current nomenclature in the languages of European countries.

K. N. Priftis (✉)
Children's Respiratory and Allergy Unit, Third Department of Paediatrics, "Attikon" Hospital, National and Kapodistrian University of Athens, Athens, Greece
e-mail: kpriftis@otenet.gr

M. Antoniadi
Community Health Service, Rhodos, Greece

H. Pasterkamp
Department of Pediatrics and Child Health, University of Manitoba, Winnipeg, MB, Canada
e-mail: hans.pasterkamp@umr.umanitoba.ca

K. N. Priftis et al. (eds.), *Breath Sounds*, https://doi.org/10.1007/978-3-319-71824-8_17

17.2 Terms Confusion

Laennec recognized early on that breath sounds were easier to distinguish than describe [14, 15]. The difficulty in description resulted in a variety of terms used for the same sound by different doctors and to different sounds described by the same term. This confusion may be even more pronounced when the same sound is described in different languages, e.g., in Sir John Forbes' famous translation of Laennec's terms "rale" and "rhonchus" as having different meanings rather than the same meaning as was originally intended [15, 16].

This situation is captured in the imaginary dialogue between Dr. Laennec and Dr. Forbes 140 years later, published in *The Lancet* in 1957 [17].

> You mean *adventitious sounds*, said Forbes. I was very pleased with my translation of *bruits étrangers* by *adventitious sounds*. But what about the word *râles*? It really is very desirable that some name might be found for the phenomenon which would prove generally acceptable to English physicians. In my first edition, I translated *râle* by the nearest synonym of *rattle* but hardly anyone would adopt it. In my next edition I put, *rattle* or *rhonchus*. In my fourth edition I put just *rhonchus* as a translation, and really prefer this, as did C. J. B. Williams. As a matter of fact, most people use the original French term *râle* in this country, but there are several objections to its use.

In 1985, at the tenth meeting of the International Lung Sounds Association, an ad hoc committee recognized that written or oral descriptions of what is heard with a stethoscope on auscultation of the lungs continued to be an "acoustic Tower of Babel" [18]. This was considered to be due primarily to the difficulty of physical qualification of auscultatory findings and consequently to the difficulties arising when terms of uncertain meaning are translated from one language to another. At this meeting the committee agreed on a classification that included fine and coarse crackles, wheezes, and rhonchi. This terminology was described in terms of acoustic properties without assuming any generating mechanism or location and has since been widely cited. In addition, matching terms were presented in French, German, Japanese, Portuguese, and Spanish [18, 19].

Although other classification attempts are well known in the literature, they did not aim at matching terms in other languages [17–22]. The European Respiratory Society (ERS) Task Force on Breath Sounds (2012–2014), in an effort to unify the nomenclature for respiratory sounds at national and international levels, investigated the current terminology in the languages of most European countries.

17.3 The European Survey

17.3.1 Methodology

17.3.1.1 National Collaborators and Languages

Collaborators in the survey of lung sound nomenclature in European countries had either volunteered at ERS Assembly meetings to participate in this project or were identified from the ERS directory as national representatives and/or ERS members.

In the recruitment of collaborators, priority was given to those who had author-related publications or otherwise expressed an interest in the area of lung sounds. The aim was to achieve national representation in both pediatric and adult respiratory medicine from each European country. The number of participants from each country at the original design was decided considering the size of the country and the number of official languages spoken.

The criterion for a European country to be included in the survey was the total population and the collaborators availability [22]. For practical reasons, only those with more than 1,000,000 inhabitants were considered [23]. The goal was to obtain at least two replies from each country.

17.3.1.2 Questionnaire

An invitation to participate in the survey was sent by email. National collaborators then received a link to an online questionnaire. To improve the response rate of completing, a total of three reminders were sent over the course of 2 months.

Collaborators were asked general questions regarding the difficulties in translating terms from the English breath sound nomenclature to their national language, terms in their language, which are different than the exact translations of the English equivalent, and their opinion in any need for an international nomenclature unification (Table 17.1).

In addition to these, there were questions about the translation of specific terms. The English nomenclature in the questionnaire was based on a recent review by Bohadana et al. [24] (Chap. 5).

The national collaborators were not asked for suggestions regarding terms to be used in their language but rather about the current use "in your language."

All the officially recognized European languages spoken in these countries were included [23], as European were considered not only current members of the European Union but the geographically determined countries. Dialects, as a particular form of language which is peculiar to a specific region or social group, were not considered.

17.3.2 Results

A total of 66 completed surveys (64 from countries other than the UK) were received from a total of 99 invitees. The response rate was 76% to the first mailing and 53%, 31% and 27% to the next iterations. The completed questionnaires represented 34 countries and 29 languages (Table 17.2).

In five languages responses were in non-Latin alphabets (Bulgarian, Greek, Macedonian, Russian, and Ukrainian). Google Translate and ushuaia.pl, as online transliteration tools for both of Latin- and non-Latin-alphabet languages were used.

The term "normal lung sounds" was used in 24 out of 29 languages, while the term "vesicular sounds" was used in 19 out of 29. "Murmur" was mentioned in 6 out of 29 languages to describe normal (basic) sounds.

Impressively, the term "stridor" was used literally the same in all but one language (Greek), while the term "wheeze" was listed in six.

Table 17.1 International nomenclature unification

Country	Language	Normal lung sounds	Bronchial breathing	Stridor	Wheeze	Rhonchus	Fine crackle	Coarse crackle	Pleural friction rub	Squawk
Albania	Albanian	Respiracion vesikular	Respiracion bronkial	Stridor	Wheezing	Rale	Krepitacione fine	Krepitacione te ashpra	Ferkime pleurale	
Austria	German	Vesikuläres Atemgeräusch	Bronchialatmen	Stridor	Giemen	Brummen	Feinblasige RG	mittel bis grobblasige RG	Pleurareiben	
Belgium	Dutch	Normaal vesiculair ademgeruis; normale longgeluiden	Bronchiaal ademgeruis, bronchiaal ademen	Stridor	Wheezing; piepende ronchi	Rhonchus	Fijne crepitaties; velcro crepitaties	Brommende ronchi; grofblazige (grove) crepitaties	Pleurale kraakgeluiden; pleuraal wrijfgeruis	
	French	Bruits respiratoires normaux; bruit respiratoire normal	Bruit respiratoire bronchique	Stridor	Sibilances	Ronchi	Crépitements fins; craquement de haute fréquence	Crépitements graves; craquement de basse fréquence	Frottement pleural	
Bulgaria	Bulgarian	везикуларно дишане; чисто везикуларно дишане	бронхиално дишане	стридор	сухи свиркащи хрипове; свиркане	ронхи; хъркащи сухи хрипове	крепитации; дребни влажни хрипове	влажни хрипове; едри влажни хрипове	плеврално триене	шумно дишане, крепитации
Croatia	Croatian	Normalan plućni zvuk; normalni šum disanja	Bronhalno disanje, bronhalni šum disanja	Stridor	Zvižduci; fijuk; fićuk	Hropac; krupni hropci	Fina krepitacija	Gruba krepitacija; hropci	Pleuralno trenje	
Cyprus	Greek	Αναπνευστικό ψιθύρισμα; φυσιολογικό αναπνευστικό ψιθύρισμα	Σωληνώδες φύσημα; βρογχικού τύπου αναπνοή	Σιγμός, εισπνευστικός συριγμός	Συριγμός	Ρόγχοι	Λεπτοί τρίζοντες	Παχείς τρίζοντες	Ήχος τριβής υπεζωκότα	

Czech Rep	Czech	Sklípkové dýchání	Trubicové dýchání	Stridor	Pískoty; piskot	Vrzoty	Chrůpky	Chropy	Pleurální třecí šelest	
Denmark	Danish	Normal lunge lyd	Bronchial vejrtrækning	Stridor	Hvæsen	Ronchi	Fin knitren	Grov knitren	Pleural gnidningslyd	
Estonia	Estonian	Vesikulaarne hingamiskahin	Bronhiaalne (kare) hingamiskahin	Stridor	Vilistav (vilinatega) hingamine	Kuivad räginad, jurinad	Peenemullilised räginad; krepitatsioonid	Suuremullilised räginad	Pleura hõõrdumiskahin	
Finland	Finnish	Normaali hengitysääni	Bronkiaalinen hengitysääni	Sisäänhengityksen vinkuna, stridor	Uloshengityksen vinkuna	Limarahina; rohina	Hienojakoinen rahina	Karkeajakoinen rahina	Pleuran hankausääni	
France	French	Murmure vésiculaire; bruits auscultatoires normaux	Bruits bronciques, souffle tubaire	Stridor	Sibilants; wheeze; sifflement	Rhonchus; râle bronchique	Crépitants fins	Gros crépitants; râles sous-crépitants	Frottement pleural; pleural friction	Squeak
FYROM	Macedonian	нормални белодробни звуци; Нормален белодробен наод	Бронхијално дишење	Стридор	Пискава хркулка; визинг	Стругава хркулка; кркори	Нежен пукот; фини пукања; влажни шушњеви	Нежен пукот; фини пукања; влажни шушњеви	Плеврално триење; плеврална линија	Писок
Germany	German	Normale Atemgeräusche; pueriles atemgeräusch	Bronchialatmung, bronchiales Atemgeräusch	Stridor	Juchzen; giemen; pfeifen	Brummen	Feinblasige rasselgeräusche; feinblasige atemgeräusche	Grobblasige rasselgeäusche; grobblasige atemgeräusche	Pleurales reiben; pleurareiben	
Greece	Greek	Φυσιολογικοί αναπνευστικοί ήχοι; φυσιολογικοί πνευμονικοί ήχοι	Βρογχική αναπνοή	Στγμός, εισπνευστικός συριγμός	Συριγμός; συρίττοντες	Ρόγχοι	Λεπτοί τρίζοντες	Παχείς τρίζοντες	Ήχος πλευριτικής τριβής; πλευριτική τριβή	

(continued)

Table 17.1 (continued)

Country	Language	Normal lung sounds	Bronchial breathing	Stridor	Wheeze	Rhonchus	Fine crackle	Coarse crackle	Pleural friction rub	Squawk
Hungary	Hungarian	Normál légzési hangok; puha sejtes alaplégzés	Hörgi légzés	Stridor, sípolás	Zihálál; nehézlégzés	Szörtyzörej; sípolás, búgás	Finom ropogás; apró hólyagú szörtyzörej	Durva ropogás; vegyes (közepes és nagy) hólyagú szörtyzörej	Pleurális dörzszörej	Durva zörej
Ireland	English	Normal breath sounds	Bronchial breathing	Stridor	Wheeze	Rhonchus	Fine crackles	Coarse crackles	Pleural friction rub	
Italy	Italian	Murmure vescicolare normale	Respiro bronchiale	Stridor	Fischio; sibili; broncospasmo	Ronco; ronchi	Rangoni fini; fini crepitii	Rantoli grossolani; rantoli crepitanti	Sfregamento pleurico	Squawk, gemiti
Latvia	Latvian	Vezikulāra elpošana; normāla plaušu skaņa	Bronhiāla elpošana	Stridor	Sēkšana; čīkstoša elpošana; svilpjoša elpošana	Rupjš sauss troksnis; patoloģiski elpošanas trokšņi	Sīks mitrs troksnis; smalka krepitācija	Rupjš mitrs troksnis; rupja krepitācija	Pleiras berzes troksnis	
Lithuania	Lithuanian	Normalus plaučių garsas; vezikulinis alsavimas	Bronchinis alsavimas	Stridoras	Sausi švilpiantys karkalai; švokštimas	Sausi birzgiantys karkalai	Smulkūs drėgni karkalai	Stambūs drėgni karkalai	Pleuros trynimosi užesys	
Netherlands	Dutch	Vesiculair ademgeruis; normaal ademgeruis	Bronchiaal ademgeruis	Stridor	Piepende rhonchi; hoogfrequente rhonchi; fluitende rhonchi	Ronchi; laagfrequente rhonchi; brommende rhonchi	Fijne crepetaties	Grove crepetaties	Pleurawrijven	Squawk; squeek; squeak
Norway	Norwegian	Normale lungelyder; vesikulær respirasjonslyd	Bronkial respirasjonslyd, bronkial blåst	Stridor	Piping	Rhoncus; pipelyder; lavfrekvent knatrelyd	Krepitasjoner	Grove knatrelyder; blærer	Pleural gnidningslyd; gnidningslyd	Bronkial blåst
Poland	Polish	Szmer pęcherzykowy prawidłowy	Szmer oskrzelowy	Stridor	Świsty	Rzężenia	trzeszczenia drobne	Trzeszczenia grube	Tarcie opłucnej	

Portugal	Portuguese	Murmúrio vesicular; sons respiratórios	Ruído brônquico, sons respiratórios	Estridor	Sibilos	Roncos	Fervores finos; crepitações finas; fervores subcrepitantes	Fervores grosseiros; crepitações grossas	Atrito pleural	
Romania	Romanian	Auscultatie normala; sunete pulmonare normale	Suflu tubar, bronhofonie	Stridor	Wheezing	Ronflante; ronhusuri	Crepitante fine; raluri crepitante	Crepitante; raluri subcrepitante	Frecatura pleurala	
Russia	Russian	Нормальное везикулярное дыхание; нормальный легочный звук	Бронхиальное дыхание	стридор	Свистящие хрипы	Хрипы	мелкопузырчатые влажные хрипы; сухие хрипы	грубые (групнопузырчатые) влажгын хрипы	Шум трения плевры	
Serbia	Serbian	Normalan disajni šum; normalan disajni zvuk	Bronhijalno disanje; bronhalno disanje	Stridor	Zviždanje	Krkori	Kasni inspirijumski pukoti	Rani inspirijumski pukoti	Pleuralno trenje	
Slovakia	Slovakian	Fyziologický posluchový nález; vezikulárne dýchanie; normálny auskultačný nález	Bronchálne dýchanie	Stridor; stridorózne dýchanie	Hvízdanie; pískanie	Chrôpky	Jemné praskanie; jemný krepitus	Drsné praskanie; drsný krepitus	Pleurálny trecí šelest	
Slovenia	Slovenian	Normalen dihalni šum	Bronhialno dihanje	Stridor	Piski; piskanje	Hropenje; grobi piski	Fino pokanje; drobni poki	Grobo pokanje; grobi poki	Plevralno trenje	

(continued)

Table 17.1 (continued)

Country	Language	Normal lung sounds	Bronchial breathing	Stridor	Wheeze	Rhonchus	Fine crackle	Coarse crackle	Pleural friction rub	Squawk
Spain	Spanish	Sonidos pulmonares normales; murmullo vesicular; ruidos o sonidos respiratorios normales	Soplo tubárico; respiración bronquial	Estridor	Sibilancias	Roncus	Crepitantes finos; crepitantes de fina burbuja o pequeña burbuja	Crepitantes gruesos	Roce pleural	
Sweden	Swedish	Normala andningsljud; vesikulärt andningsljud	Bronkiella andningsljud; bronkialandning	Stridor	Pipig och väsande andning; pipande eller väsande andning	Ronki	Fina krepitationer	Grova rassel; grova krepitationer; knastrande andningsljud	Gnidningsljud; pleurala gnidiningsljud	
Switzerland	German	Vesikuläres atemgeräusch; normales atemgeräusch	Bronchialatmung; bronchialatmen	Stridor	Giemen; pfeifendes atemgeräusch	Ronchi; rasselgeräusch	Feinblasiges rasselgeräusch; feinblasiges Knisterrasseln	Feuchtes rasselgeräusch; grobblasiges rasselgeräusch	Pleurareiben; pleurales reiben	Quäken kreischen
Turkey	Turkish	Normal (doğal) akciğer sesleri; veziküler ses	Bronşiyal solunum; tuberl sufl; bronsiyal ses	Stridor; hırıltı	Wheeze; sibilan ral, hışıltı, hırıltı, vizing	Ronkus	Ince ral; krepitasyon	Kaba ral	Frotman; plevral sürtünme sesi	
UK, Wales	English	Normal breath sounds; vesicular breath sounds	Bronchial breathing	Stridor	Wheeze	crackles; I do not use this word	Fine crackle	Coarse crackle	Pleural rub	Squeak
Ukraine	Ukrainian	Нормальний легеневий подих (Везикулярне дихання); vezicularne	Бронхіальне дихання; bronhialne	Свистяче дихання (стридорозне дихання); stridor	Свистяче дихання, ядуха; svistiaschee	Хрип	Дрібнопузирчастий хрип; vologi milkopuhirchati	Крупнопузирчастий хрип	Шум тертя плеври; shum tertia plevry	Клекотіння

Table 17.2 Countries and national collaborators from each participated in the survey

Country	Language	National collaborator(s)
Albania	Albanian	Hasan Hafisi
Austria	German	Horst Olschewski
Belgium	Dutch, French	Glenn Leemans, Christiane DeBoeck, Giuseppe Liistro, Guy Postiaux
Bulgaria	Bulgarian	Daniela Petrova, Stoyanova Guergana Petrova
Croatia	Croatian	Marko Jakopovic, Banac Srdan
Cyprus	Greek, Turkish	Tonia Adamide, Panayiotis Yiallouros
Czech Rep	Czech	Frantisek Salajka, Petr Pohunek
Denmark	Danish	Anders Lokke
Estonia	Estonian	Mall-Anne Riikjarv
Finland	Finnish	Matti Korppi
France	French	Emmanuel Andres, Bruno Crestani, Michael Fayon, Sylvain Blanchon
FYROM	Macedonian	Kamelija Busljetic, Emilija Vlashkie
Germany	German	Christophe Lange, Monika Gappa
Greece	Greek	Micheal Anthracopoulos, Petros Bakakos
Hungary	Hungarian	Ildiko Horvath, Bánfi Andrea
Ireland	English	Desmond Cox
Italy	Italian	Stefano Aliberti, Antonio Foresi, Diego Peroni, Fabio Midulla
Latvia	Latvian	Renate Snipe, Dace Gardovska
Lithuania	Lithuanian	Arunas Valiulis
Netherlands	Dutch	Peter Merkus, Luuk Willems
Norway	Norwegian	Espen Carslen, Kai-Håkon Carlsen
Poland	Polish	Joanna Domagala-Kulawik
Portugal	Portuguese	Antonio Bugalho, Ines Azevedo
Romania	Romanian	Diana Ionita, Mihai Craiu
Russia	Russian	Rustem Fassakhov, Elena Kondratyeva
Serbia	Serbian	Miodrag Vukcevic, Predrag Minic
Slovakia	Slovakian	Brezina Martin
Slovenia	Slovenian	Rozman Ales, Uros Krivec
Spain	Spanish	Julio Ancochea, Cesar Picado, Manuel Sánchez-Solís, Antonio Martinez-Gimeno
Sweden	Swedish	Gunilla Hedlin, Göran Wennergren
Switzerland	German	Juerg Barben, Daiana Stolz
Turkey	Turkish	Füsun Yildiz, Bülent Karadag
UK, Wales	English	Ian Ketchell, Iolo Doull
Ukraine	Ukrainian	Alexander Mazulov, Tetyana Pertseva

"Rhonchus" was used in the same or very similar form in 17 languages, while 4 used "rales" and 2 out of 29 used "crackles."

The term "crepitations" were reported in 16 out of 29 languages to describe fine crackles. One report from France mentioned the interchangeable use of "rale" and "rhonchus."

For the term "pleural friction rub," about all of the language either adopted the roots of the words or use the corresponding ones in the given language.

For only 10 out of 34 languages collaborators mentioned a term corresponding to "squawk," while 49 out of 64 responses stated that no such term exists in their language.

In general, 25 of collaborators considered that they were facing problems in translating the breath sounds terms in their own language. Sixty out of 64 (94%) agreed that there is a need for a unified international nomenclature on respiratory sounds.

There was no country with a complete agreement on all terms by the respective collaborators. In six there was agreement in at least one term. Interestingly, the difference was wider between adult and pediatric respondents, although the cases were too few to analyze.

17.4 Discussion

The initiative to unify the most common respiratory sounds nomenclature in the languages of European countries in the context of the ERS Task Force was presented. It was ascertained that many languages have their own terminology, while other have adopted the English terms verbatim or the corresponding translations. Furthermore, differing descriptions between collaborators from the same countries were frequently observed. The clarity of the meaning of terms varies. There are some that are used almost uniformly in the same sense, while some others used distinctly differently in different languages.

The most clear observation regarding the studied terms was for the term "stridor," since all of the collaborators indicated as the corresponding one in their own language the very same word, properly adopted, apart from Greeks. Nevertheless, even in Greek, the proposed terms were either exclusively used for stridor ("sigmos") or the one used for wheeze ("sirigmos") with the descriptive adjective "inspiratory" ("ispnefstikos"). By contrast, the term with the most confusing and contradictory usage in about all languages was the term "rhonchus." This finding has already extensively discussed in the recent literature [7, 11]. In half of the counties, collaborators reported the same (adapted) word as a translation of "rhonchus," whereas in a few, it was apparently used for other sounds as well. Interestingly, both of the abovementioned terms come from Latin. The word "stridor" originates from the Latin *stridere*, *stridēre* (shrill or harsh sound) of imitative origin [25]. The word "rhonchus" comes through Latin from the Greek *ῥόγχος* (*rhónkhos*), variant of *rhenkos*, *rhenkhos*, from *ῥέγχειν*, *ῥέγκειν* (*rhenkein*, to snore, snort) of imitative origin again [26, 27]. Nevertheless, the former term has been adopted unequivocally and almost uniformly (Norway and Finland may use "inspiratory wheezing" in their respective languages), whereas use of the latter remains confused. Obviously, it is not the term per se, but its use over the last two centuries.

Terms referred to noncontinuous respiratory sounds mostly used the word "crepitations" adapted to the corresponding language. No one outside of native English speakers used "crackles"; a few used the word "rales" and interestingly two the descriptive "Velcro rale" which has occasionally been reported for fine crackles as the sound heard when separating the joined strips of Velcro closures [28].

The main strength of this survey is the coverage of close to 1.5 billion first-language speakers. This is the largest sample of lung sound terms currently in use in Western languages through a structured approach with reference to English terminology.

However, there are also some limitations. Only a small number of specialists reported for each country. The aim of two responders and equal pediatric/adult representation from each country was not achieved in all cases. Also, there were some unresolved discrepancies, no ranking of multiple options, and no independent reverse translation.

In short, the nonuniform use of terms describing adventitious lung sounds, especially the noncontinuous and low-pitched continuous ones, is common and widespread in European languages. It appears that more formal research and educational initiatives are needed.

References

1. Elphick HE, Ritson S, Rodgers H, Everard ML (2000) When a "wheeze" is not a wheeze: acoustic analysis of breath sounds in infants. Eur Respir J 16:593–597
2. Saglani S, McKenzie SA, Bush A, Payne DNR (2005) A video questionnaire identifies upper airway abnormalities in preschool children with reported wheeze. Arch Dis Child 90:961–964
3. Michel G, Silverman M, Strippoli M-PF, Zwahlen M, Brooke AM, Grigg J, Kuehni CE (2006) Parental understanding of wheeze and its impact on asthma prevalence estimates. Eur Respir J 28:1124–1130
4. Van Sickle D (2005) Perceptions of asthma among physicians: an exploratory study with the ISAAC video. Eur Respir J 26:829–834
5. Pasterkamp H, Montgomery M, Wiebicke W (1987) Nomenclature used by health care professionals to describe breath sounds in asthma. Chest 92:346–352
6. Staszko KF, Lincho C, Engelke Vda C, Fiori NS, Silva KC, Nunes EI, Zhang L (2006) Pulmonary auscultation terminology employed in Brazilian medical journals between January of 1980 and December of 2003. J Bras Pneumol 32:400–404
7. Melbye H, Garcia-Marcos L, Brand P, Everard M, Priftis K, Pasterkamp H (2016) Wheezes, crackles and rhonchi: simplifying description of lung sounds increases the agreement on their classification: a study of 12 physicians' classification of lung sounds from video recordings. BMJ Open Respir Res 3(1):e000136
8. Wilkins RL, Dexter JR (1990) Comparing RCPs to physicians for the description of lung sounds: are we accurate and can we communicate? Respir Care 35:969–976
9. Wilkins RL, Dexter JR, Murphy RL, DelBono EA (1990) Lung sound nomenclature survey. Chest 98:886–889
10. Elphick HE, Sherlock P, Foxall G, Simpson EJ, Shiell NA, Primhak RA, Everard ML (2001) Survey of respiratory sounds in infants. Arch Dis Child 84:35–39
11. Phankingthongkum S, Daengsuwan T, Visitsunthorn N, Thamlikitkul V, Udompunthuruk S, Vichyanond P (2002) How do Thai children and adolescents describe asthma symptoms? Pediatr Allergy Immunol 13:119–124
12. Wilkins RL, Dexter JR, Smith JR (1984) Survey of adventitious lung sound terminology in case. Chest 85:523–525
13. Pasterkamp H, Brand PL, Everard M, Garcia-Marcos L, Melbye H, Priftis KN (2016) Towards the standardisation of lung sound nomenclature. Eur Respir J 47:724–732
14. Laënnec RTH (1819) De l'ausculatation médiate, un Traité du diagnostic des maladies des poumons et du coeur, fonde, principalement sur ce naveau moyen d'exploration. (A treatise on the diseases of the chest and on mediate auscultation) Paris, Brosson et Chande

15. Lethbridge R, Everard ML (2018) The stethoscope: historical considerations. In: Priftis KN, Hadjileontiadis L, Everard ML (eds) Breath sounds: from basic science to clinical practice. Springer, New York
16. Laënnec RTH (1821) A treatise on the diseases of the chest, in which they are described according to their anatomical characters, and their diagnosis established on a new principle by means of acoustic instruments (Translator Forbes J). Underwood, London
17. Robertson AJ (1957) Rales, Rhonchi, and Laennec. After an evening with Robert Coope. Lancet 2:417–423
18. Mikami R, Murao M, Cugell DW, Chretien J, Cole P, Meier-Sydow J, Murphy RL, Loudon RG (1987) International symposium on lung sounds. Synopsis of proceedings. Chest 92:342–345
19. Cugell DW (1987) Lung sound nomenclature. Am Rev Respir Dis 136:1016
20. ACCP-ATS Joint Committee on Pulmonary Nomenclature (1975) Pulmonary terms and symbols. Chest 67:583–593
21. Sovijärvi ARA, Malmberg LP, Charbonneau G, Vanderschoot J, Dalmasso F, Sacco C, Rossi M, Earis JE (2000) Characteristics of breath sounds and adventitious respiratory sounds. Eur Respir Rev 10(77):591–596
22. https://en.wikipedia.org/wiki/Demographics_of_Europe. Accessed 22 May 5 2017
23. https://en.wikipedia.org/wiki/Languages_of_Europe. Accessed 28 May 5 2017
24. Bohadana A, Izbicki G, Kraman SS (2014) Fundamentals of lung auscultation. N Engl J Med 370:744–751
25. The American Heritage Dictionary. https://www.ahdictionary.com/word/search.html?q=stridor. Accessed 28 May 5 2017
26. https://www.ahdictionary.com/word/search.html?q=rhonchus. Accessed 28 May 5 2017
27. Liddell HJ, Scott R (1889) Liddell & Scott: an intermediate Greek-English Lexicon, vol 4. Harper & Brothers, New York, NY, p 10, 21
28. Cottin V, Cordier JF (2012) Velcro crackles: the key for early diagnosis of idiopathic pulmonary fibrosis? Eur Respir J 40:519–521

18 Epilogue

Mark L. Everard, Kostas N. Priftis, and Leontios J. Hadjileontiadis

It is argued that the coming two decades will see a fundamental revolution in 'medicine' and health that will completely transform the field and how health care is viewed [1, 2]. In a world in which many predict that health care and 'wellness' will be transformed by the power of the smartphones, computerisation and the ever more rapid advances in sequencing technologies, what is the future of the humble, low-tech conventional stethoscope? In considering this question, it should be remembered that the revolution in European health care that was taking place around the late eighteenth and early nineteenth centuries was just as dramatic as that that is apparently underway in the first half of the twenty-first century. Laennec was a key player in this revolution in which the physician evolved from a professional operating largely on beliefs based on pseudo-'philosophical' ideas with no scientific basis to one that has a belief in trying to apply sound scientific insights (the sensible physician knowing that much of what he believes is scientifically sound may prove to be false as knowledge progress over time). Laennec's insights, largely derived from his expertise in morbid anatomy, generated new knowledge and help embed the notion that, in order to develop effective therapy, we needed to try and understand the disease process based on scientific rigor rather than abstract speculation.

M. L. Everard
Division of Child Health, University of Western Australia,
Perth Children's Hospital, Perth, Australia
e-mail: mark.everard@uwa.edu.au

K. N. Priftis (✉)
Children's Respiratory and Allergy Unit, Third Department of Paediatrics, "Attikon" Hospital, National and Kapodistrian University of Athens, Athens, Greece
e-mail: kpriftis@otenet.gr

L. J. Hadjileontiadis
Department of Electrical and Computer Engineering, Aristotle University of Thessaloniki, Thessaloniki, Greece
e-mail: leontios@auth.gr

K. N. Priftis et al. (eds.), *Breath Sounds*, https://doi.org/10.1007/978-3-319-71824-8_18

He was one of the pioneers of that era who developed the concept that all contemporary 'knowledge' needs to be challenged and revised where it is found wanting.

In developing the stethoscope, he launched the concept that information regarding the nature of an individual's ill health may be inferred from interpretation of data generated with tools that augmented the clinicians' five senses. In the respiratory field, it was the first of a number of technologies that have been developed in the intervening two centuries that includes X-rays, bronchoscopy, spirometry, CT scanning and PET scanning. With effort, the radiation exposure from a CT scan can be reduced to less than that of an AP+ lateral chest X-ray (Murray C, personal communication) providing infinitely greater information with no additional radiation, yet there is no expectation of the immediate demise of the CXR. It remains by far the most widely used adjunct to clinical assessment, and despite predictions of its imminent demise that have been repeated over the decades, sales of stethoscopes continue to rise [3]. Much of the rise in sales of conventional stethoscopes is occurring in developing countries, while sales of electronic stethoscopes for bedside and telehealth use continue to grow in developed countries [3, 4]. In the veterinary world, a very large pharmaceutical company has recently made a considerable invested in a 'stethoscope' and automated analysis system that would directly inform farmers when to consider treating cattle being monitored, indicating that such systems will continue given the economic impact they may have [5].

The symbolic power of the stethoscope should not be underestimated even in this high-tech era. In a recent study in which members of the public were shown photographs of a man in which one or more items associated with doctors, such as the stethoscopes, otoscope, theatre scrubs and tendon hammer, the individual in the photographs containing a stethoscope scored consistently higher as appearing to manifest each of the following attributes—honest, trustworthy, genuine, ethical and moral [6]. This boost in the effectiveness of consultations in itself would justify the small investment in a stethoscope.

However, it is as a practical, valuable, adjunct to the clinical assessment that will see the stethoscope remaining the first medical device a medical student will invest in (other than their smartphone). The problem with any piece of technology is that when used effectively and appropriately, it can enhance our lives and effectiveness but if misused, because of lack of effective training and a failure to appreciate its strengths and weaknesses, its application may be deleterious. Most doctors, hopefully, understand that a 'silent chest' is of great concern in someone with a significant exacerbation of asthma; yet, few seem to appreciate that the lack of 'added' or adventitial sounds does not exclude significant pathology, as, for example, in those with a persistent bacterial bronchitis who typically have a clear chest but a wet cough when asked to cough. Similarly, most medical students appear to be taught that additional respiratory sounds are either crackles or wheeze. Hence, if an added sound is not clearly a crackle, then it must be a wheeze or a 'transmitted sound' (a curious term given that all sounds are transmitted from somewhere, but, in this context, the clinician is assuming, often erroneously, that it is apparently transmitted from the upper airways).

The preceding chapters highlight the ongoing challenges in trying to describe the sound reaching our ears via this apparently simple device and communicate this in a meaningful manner to another. The suggestion that automated analysis will help clear this confusion is yet to be confirmed despite decades of work.

Two hundred years ago, Laennec described five sounds that he repeatedly heard when listening to patients with pulmonary disease and through his obsessional attention to details developed an in-depth understanding of the likely implication. While not perfect, his work still stands as probably the most logical and least confusing approach to nomenclature being developed at a time when there were no other tools available. Since then, the development of a variety of imaging modalities and techniques for assessing 'lung function' has greatly enhanced our ability to characterise the nature of pulmonary disease, but none to date has replaced the need for a good history and careful examination. It remains to be seen whether the latest 'medical revolution' utilising the power of systems biology approaches to integrate data including that generated by the new 'omnics' technologies, such as phenomics, epigenetics and microbiome sequencing, will, eventually, replace the need for the central role of the doctor-patient discussion and examination, thus, eventually seeing the stethoscope relegated to the museum. In fact, medicine is moving back to the patient's narration of his/her disease, a narration given by various types of gadgets and new communication means, even via "medical selfies"! Not only will these gadgets mean medical staff will need to touch patients less, they will also put a mass of data about a person's body into his/her own hands. This clearly raises the question: "What does this do to the professional - does the doctor become a coach, a servant or an adviser - what will the new role be?" Doctor, eventually, must go back to the bedside; to be an interpreter of symptoms—so she/he can learn every possible aspect of what the patient is feeling and experiencing. From this perspective, there is no immediate prospect that the stethoscope will disappear during our professional lifetime!

References

1. Topol E (2015) The patient will see you now. Basic Books, New York
2. Price ND, Magis AT, Hood L et al (2017) A wellness study of 108 individuals using personal, dense, dynamic data clouds. Nat Biotechnol. https://doi.org/10.1038/nbt.3870
3. http://www.grandviewresearch.com/industry-analysis/stethoscopes-market
4. http://telehealthtechnology.org/toolkits/electronic-stethoscopes/about-electronic-stethoscopes/technology-overview
5. http://investors.merck.com/news/press-release-details/2016/Merck-Animal-Health-to-Acquire-Worldwide-Rights-to-Whisper-Veterinary-Stethoscope-System/default.aspx
6. Jiwa M, Millett S, Meng X, Hewitt VM (2012) Impact of the presence of medical equipment in images on viewers' perceptions of the trustworthiness of an individual on-screen. J Med Internet Res 14(4):e100. https://doi.org/10.2196/jmir.1986

MIX
Papier aus verantwortungsvollen Quellen
Paper from responsible sources
FSC® C105338

If you have any concerns about our products,
you can contact us on
ProductSafety@springernature.com

In case Publisher is established outside the EU,
the EU authorized representative is:
Springer Nature Customer Service Center GmbH
Europaplatz 3, 69115 Heidelberg, Germany

Printed by Libri Plureos GmbH
in Hamburg, Germany